JUNE 2016

TO MARISA & BRANDON

THIS BOOK IS WRITTEN IN CONSULTATION WITH
PROFESSORS OBSTETRICS,
MIDWIVES HAVE EXCELLENT RESOURCES AVAILABLE WHICH
THEY WOULD HAVE PROVIDED IN U.K
ATTENDING CHILDBIRTH/PARENTING EDUCATION GROUPS MOST
COUPLES FIND VERY HELPFUL WITH THEIR FIRST CHILD.

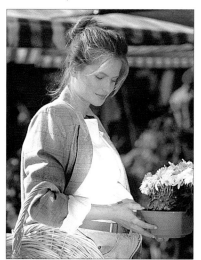

GW00707613

Pregnancy

the complete
Australian guide
to planning and birth

I ALSO LIKED THIS BOOK BECAUSE DAD'S AND
SUPPORT PEOPLE ARE INCLUDED, WORKING IN LABOUR
SUITES & BEING A CHILDBIRTH/PARENTING EDUCATOR FOR
MANY YEARS HAS BEEN SUCH AN HONOUR/PRIVILEDGE
FOR ME.   LOVE LAUREL XX   (LEONARD)

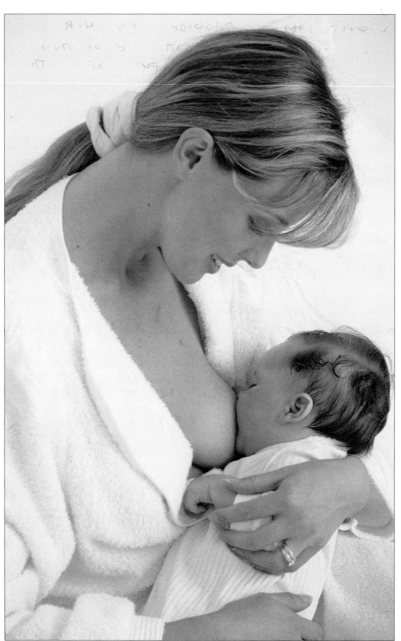

Pregnancy

the complete Australian guide to planning and birth

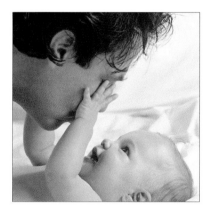

A practical and reassuring guide to
the changes in your body,
your baby and your life

Heather Welford

Consultant

Professor M.G.Elder

A Marshall Edition
Conceived, edited and designed by
Marshall Editions
The Old Brewery, 6 Blundell Street
London N7 9BH

This edition published in 2010 by
Cameron House
an imprint of The Scribo Group
Equinox Centre
18 Rodborough Rd
Frenchs Forest, NSW, 2086

Reprinted 2004, 2006, 2007, 2008, 2009

ISBN 10: 1-877082-29-5
ISBN 13: 978-1-8770-8229-0

Project editor Anne Yelland
Editor Caroline Taggart
Art editor Hugh Schermuly
Picture editor Zilda Tandy
DTP editors Mary Pickles, Lesley Gilbert
Copy editors Isabella McIntire, Maggi McCormick
Proof reader Clare Stewart
Managing editor Lindsay McTeague
Editorial co-ordinator Rebecca Clunes
Editorial director Sophie Collins
Art director Sean Keogh
Production Nikki Ingram

The pronouns he and she, used on alternate spreads, refer to both
sexes, unless a topic applies only to a boy or a girl.

Printed in China by 1010 Printing International Ltd

CONTENTS

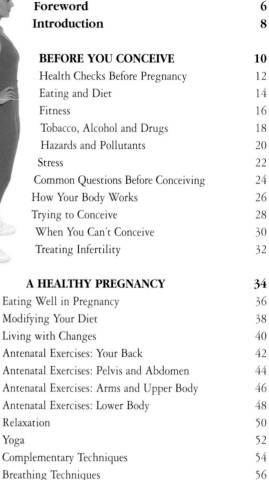

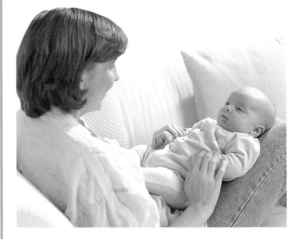

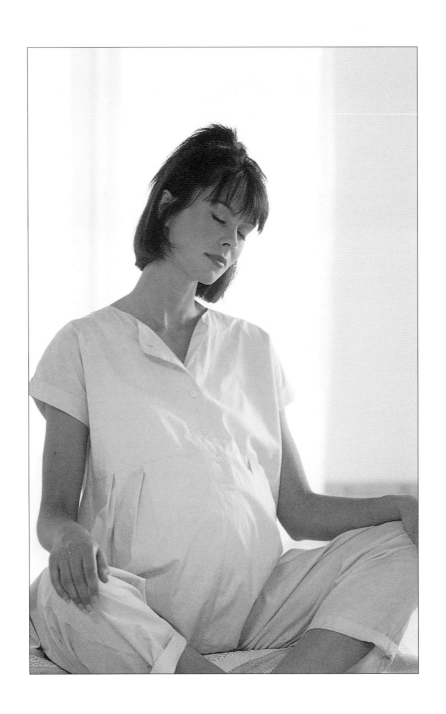

FOREWORD

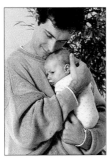

Being a gynaecologist and obstetrician today is an exciting challenge. Our patients have become our partners in their care, eager to learn all they can about pregnancy and childbirth. They want to be well informed, so that they are able to participate fully in every aspect of pregnancy, labour and delivery. They want detailed information, in layperson's language, to enable them to plan ahead, think through options and make decisions.

This book is a wonderful resource. It answers the questions most commonly posed by patients in an accurate, sympathetic manner. It contains up-to-date medical information, but acknowledges the full spectrum of prospective parents' concerns, emotional as well as physical. Our goal as parents is to give ourselves every chance of raising healthy, happy children. This book gives parents-to-be the best possible start.

PROFESSOR M. G. ELDER
PROFESSOR MICHAEL J. BENNETT

INTRODUCTION

Pregnancy is a time of great physical and emotional change, of tremendous anticipation and occasional doubts, as you nurture a new life growing inside you.

There has never been a better time to have a baby. Advances in obstetrics have made birth safer than ever for mothers, even for those who have underlying health problems as they enter their pregnancies. Greater knowledge of what can harm babies in the uterus – and heightened awareness of what parents-to-be can do to minimize risks – has resulted in more babies being born healthy and at a good weight. Breakthroughs in identifying and treating fertility problems have meant that many more couples who want a baby will succeed in having one. And work with small or sick babies has given even the tiniest and most vulnerable infants a better-than-ever chance of surviving with no lasting problems.

For many parents, however, plentiful information about how doctors are successfully treating problems actually heightens couples' fears about the problems themselves. Because expectant parents are so well informed about the risk factors and physical demands of pregnancy and childbirth, they let exaggerated worries rob them of their joy. Remember that worrying without acting does no good. If your love for each other has resulted in a new life growing inside you, enjoy it fully as one of life's greatest gifts.

Attitudes towards pregnancy have also changed. At the same time that the medical profession has been making pregnancy and birth safer for mother and baby, parents-to-be have become more discerning consumers of healthcare and more knowledgeable about pregnancy. Antenatal care and childbirth are now recognized as partnerships, in which parents and medical staff together identify options, discuss treatments and

A baby is the ultimate bond between a couple, a testament to all of the strength of their love and partnership. Planning a pregnancy can provide strong motivation for both of you to start taking care of youselves, to be fit and healthy for the challenging – but infinitely rewarding – years of family life that lie ahead.

work towards a common goal – the safe and happy birth of a healthy baby.

USING THIS BOOK

In an ideal world, a man and a woman decide to have a baby, and both spend a few months getting in shape before trying to conceive. They assess, then modify, their lifestyle. They identify and work at reducing causes of stress, take up some exercise, and pay attention to eating healthily. They eliminate alcohol, tobacco and other drugs, and evaluate whether their workplace may have an effect on either conception or the progress of their pregnancy.

For many couples, pregnancy arrives without such thorough preparation, but don't let that become a source of worry for you if you are among the surprised. If you are pregnant already, read the advice in Chapter 1, then start following the guidelines detailed in Chapter 2: A Healthy Pregnancy. Many problems in pregnancy result from cumulative action – the more you do, the worse the effect. So rather than dwelling on what you have or have not done in the past, concentrate on what you should be doing now.

Chapters 3, 4 and 5 describe the trimesters of pregnancy. As the months pass, read the information describing how your body will change, how you might feel physically and emotionally, and what to expect of antenatal check-ups. Note the answers to the most common questions parents-to-be pose, and keep a record yourself of questions to ask your practitioners – and the

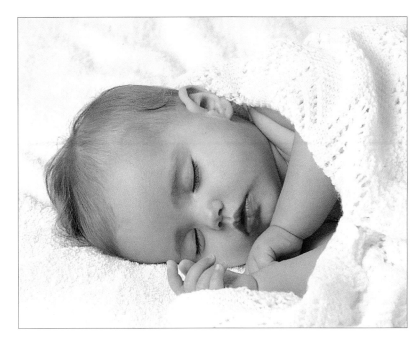

answers you receive – throughout your pregnancy.

Chapter 6 details what happens when you go into labour, how labour is likely to progress, and what you can expect during childbirth. Finally, Chapter 7 gives a general overview of your first few days at home with your baby.

YOUR PREGNANCY

No two people are alike, nor are any two pregnancies or birth experiences identical. For most women, the second or third time around still offers some surprises. But many experiences are similar.

Most women have times during their pregnancies when they do not feel or look their best, and most also experience periods of great vitality and blooming good looks. Some women never have a second thought about their decision to become pregnant, but most admit to one or two misgivings (Will I manage? What will the baby do to our relationship?). Most births are

Taking the best possible care of yourself both before you conceive and while you are pregnant is one of the best ways to ensure that your pregnancy reaches a happy conclusion, with the birth of a beautiful healthy baby.

problem-free, but if circumstances become less than ideal, parents will want to be prepared to cope with a birth that does not go as planned. This book explains a typical birth and offers reassurance and information about unusual situations.

Pregnancy is not about waiting for your baby to be born. It is a time to savour moods and feelings that you have never experienced before and may never experience again. It's a period of loving preparation for a whole new phase of a couple's life. It's a time to enjoy what you have, as well as looking forward to what this new life will bring to you, and to other members of your family – the baby's grandparents, aunts and uncles will share your joy at his or her arrival.

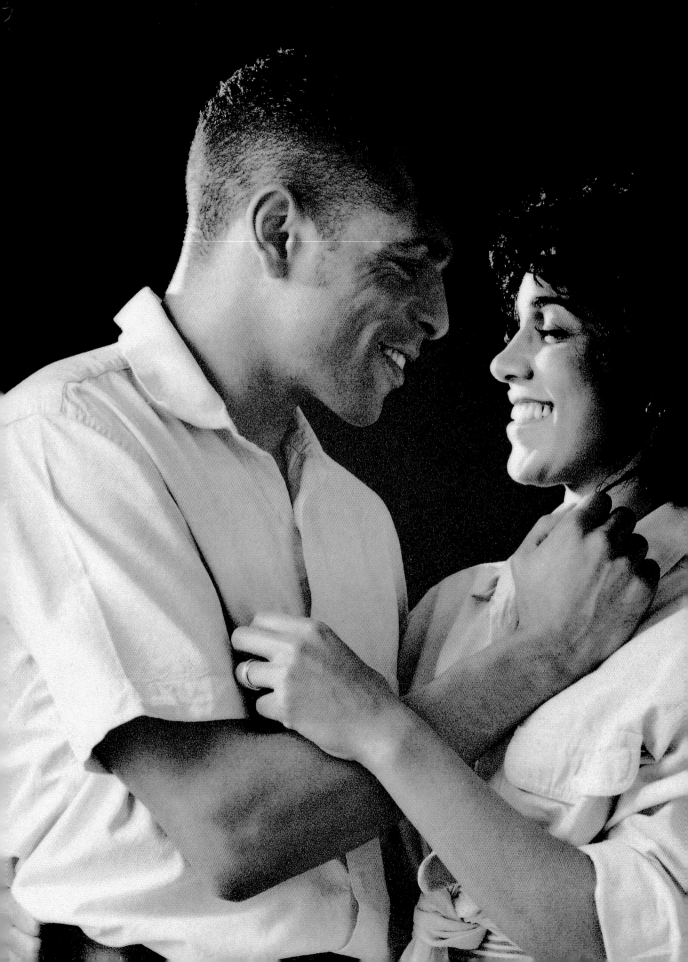

Before you conceive

BY MAKING SURE that you and your partner are in good health before you try to conceive a baby, you will:

- Speed conception
- Reduce the chances of miscarriage
- Have an easier pregnancy, with fewer potential problems
- Give your baby the best opportunity to develop and grow in your womb
- Promote the health and strength of your baby at birth and beyond
- Cope more successfully with labour and delivery
- Recover more quickly and thoroughly from pregnancy and childbirth
- Feel fit and energetic for the demanding early weeks and months of parenthood.

HEALTH CHECKS BEFORE PREGNANCY

Give your baby the best possible start in life by making sure that you and your partner are fit and healthy before trying to conceive.

You can start to prepare for a healthy pregnancy now by improving your diet, regularly exercising, and working with your doctor on any existing health issues. The more medical matters you deal with before you are pregnant, the better for both you and your baby.

It's important to check with your doctor if you have previously suffered a miscarriage, fertility problem or other gynaecological difficulties. The doctor may recommend special treatment or precautions. Make sure as well that your doctor knows you are trying to conceive if you have an ongoing health problem, such as asthma, diabetes, hypertension or a circulatory disorder. Regular medication sometimes needs to be changed or adjusted during the early weeks of pregnancy.

If you have an acute illness or injury, give yourself plenty of time to make a full recovery. Have any minor operations, dental X-rays or other treatments done now.

SCREENING FOR IMMUNITIES
Diseases such as rubella, measles and chickenpox are rare, but becoming more common as parents choose not to have their children immunized. While not all of these diseases endanger the foetus, many doctors recommend updating vaccinations for these conditions and such others as mumps, hepatitis B and tetanus.

Immunity can be tested by a simple blood test. In the case of rubella (German measles) – which can create risks for your baby if you contract it in early pregnancy – you will be advised to wait for three months after vaccination before conceiving. There are, however, no known cases of damage to a foetus from rubella vaccine, so don't worry if you accidentally become pregnant.

GENETIC COUNSELLING
Obstetricians recommend that men and women with a family history of inheritable diseases, the most common of which are cystic fibrosis and muscular dystrophy, seek genetic counselling before conceiving a child. Counselling helps to establish any risk to the health of a future baby.

Counselling may also be advisable if you are at risk from genetic illnesses linked to your ethnic background, most commonly sickle-cell trait for people of African origin; thalassemia for those of Mediterranean (chiefly Italian or Greek), Southeast Asian or Philippino descent; and Tay–Sachs or Gauchers disease for people of Ashkenazi Jewish origin.

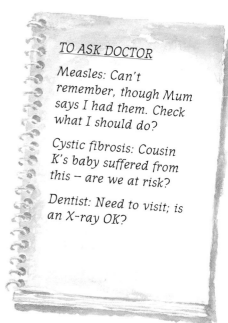

Measles: Can't remember, though Mum says I had them. Check what I should do?

Cystic fibrosis: Cousin K's baby suffered from this – are we at risk?

Dentist: Need to visit; is an X-ray OK?

Keep a notebook handy to jot down questions to ask your doctor as you think of them. It's sometimes hard to remember everything in the midst of an examination. Note the answers and your doctor's recommendations so that you have no doubts later about what was said.

PARTNERS: YOUR HEALTH
Two healthy people have the best chances of making a healthy baby. A man's health affects the quantity and quality of his sperm and hence his fertility.

Sperm require 100 days to mature fully (see pp. 26–27), and this delicate process can be affected by a number of factors: stress; smoking; alcohol and drug intake; poor nutrition; and environmental pollution, including exposure to chemicals and toxins in the workplace.

Contraception

If you are planning a baby, you will obviously stop using any contraceptive devices. If you have been taking birth control pills, allow your body at least two normal menstrual cycles before trying to conceive. Both the combined oral contraceptive pill (which uses oestrogen and progesterone) and the progesterone-only pill, or mini-pill (which thickens cervical mucus and alters the lining of the womb to make pregnancy less likely), usually prevent conception. It may take a few months for "natural" periods to resume. If you had hormonal injections, your cycle may take up to 18 months to return to normal.

There is also some evidence that the pill can reduce the body's ability to absorb certain vitamins and minerals. Coming off the pill in advance allows you time to recover from this effect as well.

In the meantime, use a barrier method such as condoms or a diaphragm (cap) with spermicide.

Either of these methods should provide adequate birth control during this time.

Since an IUD does not disrupt your menstrual cycle, in theory you can become pregnant as soon as you have it removed. Such symptoms as an urge to urinate frequently, a burning sensation on doing so, or abnormal periods (heavier or more painful than usual) could be a sign of pelvic inflammatory disease (PID), which an IUD can trigger. If you display any of the symptoms, ask your doctor to check for this before you try to conceive. PID can be treated with antibiotics.

If you become pregnant while taking the pill, don't be alarmed. There is no evidence that the pill increases the risk of foetal abnormality. It is also possible to become pregnant with an IUD in place. Your doctor will be able to advise you on whether it should be removed or not. If your doctor thinks it safer to leave it, be alert for pain or bleeding (see p. 91).

If you are routinely exposed to any of these factors, taking action to eliminate or minimize them at least three months before conception could make a significant difference. You will almost certainly produce healthier sperm and increase your sperm count (the number of healthy, or viable, sperm). By following the advice on pages 14 to 23, you may also speed conception and help to give your baby a strong start.

If you seek a genetic counsellor's advice, you will need information on both families. In rare cases the counsellor may want you both to have a blood test. Some diseases can be passed on from one parent; others, such as cystic fibrosis, require both parents to carry the affected gene.

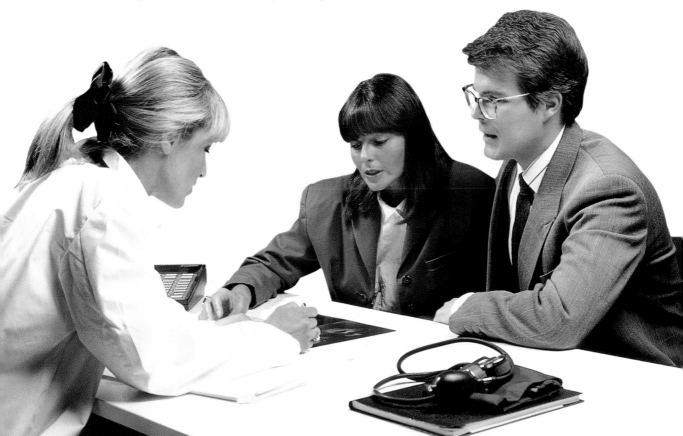

EATING AND DIET

The best way to make sure that you will eat well during pregnancy is to make healthy eating a habit before you conceive.

A well-balanced diet is always important, but never more so than before you conceive and during pregnancy. Women who eat well are more likely to produce healthy babies and to recover quickly after childbirth. They also suffer fewer complications, such as anaemia, pre-eclampsia (see pp. 126–27 and 143) and premature labour. A healthy diet may influence the baby's development and growth rate.

Good food gives your body the minerals and vitamins it needs to function well. Aim for a low-fat, high-carbohydrate diet based on fresh whole foods – plenty of fruit and vegetables, whole grains, moderate amounts of lean meat, and low-fat dairy products.

To make sure your diet is well balanced, follow the food pyramid guide (right). Originally developed by the Australian Nutrition Foundation, the pyramid divides foods into three levels: eat most, eat moderately, and eat in small amounts. Exact quantities of foods are not usually specified, but since women need higher levels of many nutrients during pregnancy, amounts are suggested here to ensure an adequate diet. Nutrients needed in larger quantities include protein, the B group of vitamins, vitamin C and many minerals. Essential fatty acid requirements may also increase, and many women find they need extra fibre to prevent constipation.

FOODS TO AVOID

A good diet minimizes empty kilojoules – "junk" food, such as sweets, carbonated drinks, snacks that are heavy on fat and salt, over-refined foods and sugars – from your diet. Such foods add kilojoules without providing significant nutrition.

Doctors recommend cutting your intake of caffeine – tea, coffee and cola drinks – as well. Experts believe that too much caffeine may

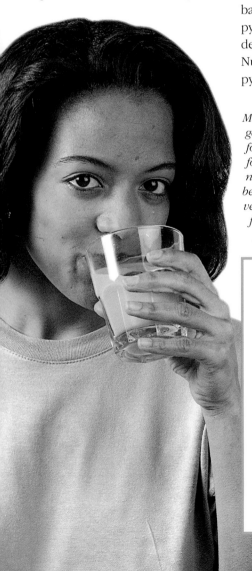

Make sure you get as much natural goodness as possible by eating fresh foods. Processed and prepared foods are generally lower in nutrients and fibre. Vitamins can be destroyed in cooking, so cook vegetables lightly and eat some raw fruit and vegetables – or drink fresh juice – every day.

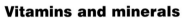

Vitamins and minerals

A healthy diet should provide all the vitamins and minerals your body needs (see pp. 36–37). But studies indicate that in the three months before and after conception, extra folate – one of the most important B group vitamins – is especially important. Increasing the amount of folate in your diet can significantly reduce the risk of having a baby with one of the birth conditions known as neural tube defects (NTDs): principally, spina bifida and anencephaly.

You can increase your intake of foods rich in folate by eating more of the following:
- Leafy green vegetables – such as spinach, broccoli, Brussels sprouts – green beans and cauliflower.
- Wholemeal bread, cereals and pasta. Choose folate-fortified cereals and wholemeal bread.
- Citrus fruits and avocados.
- Pulses, such as kidney beans, chick peas and lentils.
- Milk, yoghurt and cheese.
- Yeast extracts.

increase the risk of miscarriage, while tannins inhibit your ability to absorb iron from food.

PREGNANCY AND WEIGHT

It's best to start your pregnancy at, or close to, your normal weight. Avoid crash diets. They do nothing to establish good eating habits and can leach essential nutrients from your body and even stop ovulation. If you need to lose weight, do it slowly and allow your body to stabilize before conceiving. Your dietitian or doctor can provide a plan for healthy weight loss.

If you suffer from an eating disorder, such as anorexia nervosa or bulimia (binge eating followed by self-induced vomiting), seek help before trying to conceive. Such illnesses impose enormous stress on the body and may decrease your ability to conceive.

If you are underweight or exercise so intensely that your periods are irregular or have ceased, get professional advice before trying to conceive.

The food pyramid:
recommended quantities for pregnant women

Fats, oils and sugars
Eat in small amounts

Cheese, yoghurt, milk: 2 to 4 servings – 30 g cheese; 250 ml milk, or 150 g yoghurt
Eat moderately

Meat, fish, eggs, pulses, nuts: 2 to 4 servings – 90 g meat or fish, 1 egg
Eat moderately

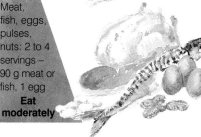

Fruit: 2 to 4 servings
Eat most

Vegetables: at least 3 to 5 servings
Eat most

Bread, cereals, rice and pasta: 6 to 11 servings – one slice of bread, half a cup of cooked rice or pasta
Eat most

If you find it difficult to take in enough folate from food, ask your doctor's advice about taking a supplement in tablet form: an additional 400 mcg (micrograms) each day has been shown to reduce the incidence of neural tube defects by as much as 50 to 70 percent. One caution: *never* take more than the recommended dose.

Foods rich in folate often contain other vitamins and minerals, too: leafy vegetables and citrus fruits contain vitamin C, for example, and wholemeal bread is rich in some B vitamins.

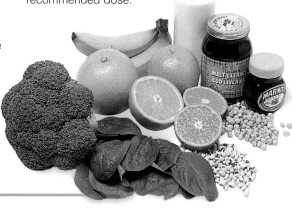

This version of the food pyramid shows the balance of different foods pregnant women should aim to eat each day. Carbohydrates should make up at least 55 percent of your kilojoule intake, and fats no more than 20 to 25 percent. Many proteins and foods rich in minerals, such as red meat and cheese, are also sources of fat.

FITNESS

Conception is the start of some of the most important work your body will ever do, so start getting into shape.

A fit body produces more energy and uses it more efficiently than an unfit one. Aerobic exercise – any form of exercise that increases your heart rate – helps all your organs and cardiovascular system work better.

Women who exercise before conception and during pregnancy can maintain their fitness throughout pregnancy. Keeping muscles toned and strengthened helps a woman to carry the extra weight associated with pregnancy more comfortably and to cope better with labour and delivery by providing greater support to her back and legs.

Bicycling and walking outdoors are enjoyable ways of getting yourself fit for pregnancy, and they can include your partner. Regular activity three times a week does you far more good than a frantic burst once a week.

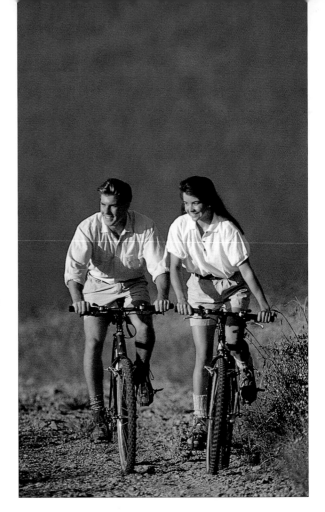

Exercises

As little as 10 minutes twice a day spent doing simple exercises for your legs (below), arms and shoulders (centre), and lower back, shoulders and thighs (far right) can increase your overall level of fitness. Start with one set of each exercise. After a few weeks you should be able to do each set twice before moving on to the next exercise.

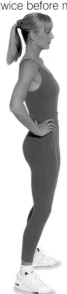

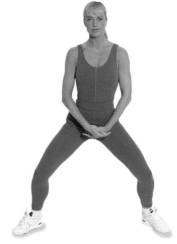

Lunges
1 Stand with your feet hip width apart and toes pointing forwards. Bend your knees slightly. Pull your stomach in and tilt your pelvis forwards.

2 Breathe in as you take a step forwards with your right foot. Lower your left knee to within 15 cm (6 in) of the floor. Keep your right knee behind your toes.

3 Hold for a count of 6, then breathe out as you stand up. Do this 6 to 8 times. Repeat the entire exercise, using your left leg.

Arm swings
1 Stand with your feet more than shoulder width apart. Turn your toes out at 45 degree angles. With your back straight and stomach pulled in, cross your hands in front of your hips. Slowly bend your knees to the position shown.

Exercise also improves the circulation, which enhances the supply of oxygen to the baby and reduces the likelihood of varicose veins, haemorrhoids and fluid retention in the mother. Exercise burns kilojoules, too, helping to prevent excessive weight gain and making it easier to get your figure back after the birth. Exercise also helps you to sleep well.

Always consult your doctor before starting an exercise regime. If you have a history of miscarriage, premature labour or other problems, your doctor may advise you not to exercise vigorously and suggest alternative activities. Intense workouts – training for a marathon, for example – may depress your fertility (see pp. 28–29).

GETTING STARTED

If you do not usually exercise, start by making minor changes in your daily routine that will help to increase your baseline fitness. Using the stairs rather than the lift at work and in shops, running up the stairs at home, and walking up escalators all increase your heart rate, oxygenate your body, burn fat and improve overall muscle tone.

Change your approach to travelling: make one journey a week by bicycle instead of car, walk to the railway station, or get off the bus or train one or two stops early and walk the rest of the way. Modify your usual weekend stroll by running or jogging in five-minute bursts, alternated with brisk walking.

DEVISING A PLAN

Spend 20 minutes on organized exercise at least two or three times a week. Vary the exercise; you are less likely to get bored if you try different activities. Good aerobic forms of exercise include:

- Swimming;
- Brisk, steady walking;
- Jogging;
- Bicycling (on an exercise bike or outdoors);
- Rowing (an indoor rower is as effective as a boat on water);
- Exercise classes, such as step, slide, low-impact aerobics or calisthenics;
- Tennis or other racquet sports.

Weight or resistance training in a gym provides good cardiovascular activity and targets particular muscles to improve tone. For the best all-round fitness, alternate weight training with two or three sessions of aerobic activity each week.

Schedule your exercise. If you have a regular day or a class, you are more likely to stick to it. You may also find that exercising with a friend provides extra motivation. After three or four weeks, you should start to feel stronger and more energetic; after six to eight weeks, you'll look more toned. To keep up your motivation, monitor your progress by noting how far you walk or swim without starting to feel breathless. You should see a gradual improvement over the weeks and months.

Look after yourself when you exercise. Eat well, avoid overheating, and follow the general guidelines on pp. 42–43.

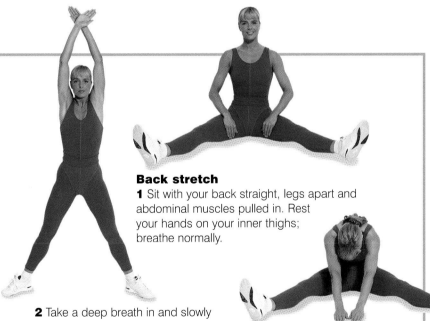

Back stretch
1 Sit with your back straight, legs apart and abdominal muscles pulled in. Rest your hands on your inner thighs; breathe normally.

2 Take a deep breath in and slowly swing your arms out to your sides and up over your head. As you do so, straighten your knees and stand upright.

3 Breathe out as you swing your arms back to the start position. Repeat 10 times, keeping a flow of movement.

2 Relax your shoulders, then lift from your waist and bend forwards from your hips to place your hands on the floor. When you feel mild tension in your groin, lower back and back of thighs, hold for 8 to 10 seconds. Repeat 6 to 8 times.

TOBACCO, ALCOHOL AND DRUGS

Some risks to health are unavoidable, but others are within your control. Such controllable risks include the use of tobacco, alcohol and other drugs.

All drugs, including tobacco and alcohol, carry some degree of risk for your baby's health while you are pregnant, and the use of certain drugs may make conceiving itself more difficult. You and your partner should review your intake of tobacco, alcohol and other drugs before you try to conceive.

STOPPING SMOKING

Cigarette smoking is the major cause of illness and premature death in the Western world. It reduces the efficiency of your lungs, inflaming the bronchi and making you more susceptible to bronchitis. It increases your risk of developing cancer of the mouth, throat and lungs. Nicotine also makes the heart beat faster and work harder, increasing the risk of heart attacks. Even "passive smokers", those who inhale the smoke of others, are at some risk.

Smoking has also been linked to fertility problems, because the chemicals in tobacco interfere with hormone levels. Nicotine has been found in concentrated levels in the dividing fertilized egg and may be responsible for abnormal cell division.

Smoking during pregnancy has been shown to increase the risk of miscarriage and premature delivery and can also affect the baby's development. Smokers are more likely to have low birthweight babies, who in turn are more likely to suffer illness and perinatal death (death during or soon after birth). Sudden infant death syndrome (SIDS), or "cot death", is more common among babies of smokers.

Doctors strongly recommend that you stop smoking completely before you start trying to conceive. Your doctor can probably direct you to a good,

Partners and alcohol

Alcohol affects the production of testosterone, the male hormone connected with the formation and maturation of sperm. Moderate and heavy drinkers may produce sperm that are abnormally formed, lacking a tail, or with a tail that is too small for adequate movement. Such men also have lower sperm counts and sperm functioning – and thus lower fertility – than men who drink only occasionally.

In addition, alcoholic fathers have a higher risk of producing babies with foetal alcohol syndrome (FAS). These babies are small, which makes them vulnerable in the early weeks of life, and may suffer serious mental and physical defects.

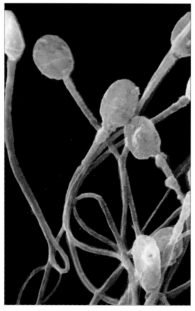

Healthy sperm

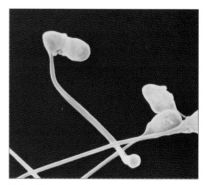

Unhealthy sperm

Alcohol reduces the number of healthy sperm that reach the ejaculate. The sperm levels of men who drink can be increased by cutting out alcohol at least three months before conception is planned.

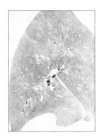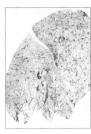

The lungs of a non-smoker (left) are clear and a healthy pink. In addition to nicotine and carbon monoxide, cigarette smoke contains sticky tars that adhere to the delicate tissue of the lungs (right) and impair their functioning.

local support group. Experiences of former smokers differ; some people have achieved success by cutting down gradually, while others have found it most effective to stop the habit "cold turkey".

If you've tried one way before and failed, try another. Some former smokers have found it helps to set a "giving-up-smoking-day" in the near future, at a time when they can arrange to be under less stress and know they will be prepared.

Nicotine patches and chewing gum are sometimes prescribed for smokers who want to stop but can't do it without help. These are not recommended for use in pregnancy, so if you are planning to become pregnant, avoid them or stop using them before there is a chance of conceiving.

Complementary therapies, such as acupuncture and hypnotism, have helped some people to give up.

ALCOHOL CONSUMPTION

Heavy drinking can have serious effects on your health, increasing the risk of liver damage, disorders of the digestive system and certain cancers. It can also affect fertility by disrupting a woman's

A Case in Point
A Smoker's Story

MARGARET, 32, STARTED SMOKING CIGARETTES AT UNIVERSITY.

"Everyone else smoked, and it seemed like the thing to do. Soon it became a need, not just a social habit, and when I felt particularly tense and anxious, I went through two packets a day.

"Then I met Bill, a non-smoker. He loved me but hated my smoking and the smell of tobacco that clung to my clothes and hair. I knew smoking was affecting my health, but I couldn't give up, even though I did attend a group with others who wanted to stop.

"When we married and decided to have children, I became desperate to give it up. I knew the risks associated with smoking during pregnancy, and I didn't want to do anything that might endanger my baby. As a last resort, I went to a hypnotist. I was sceptical, but, amazingly, after

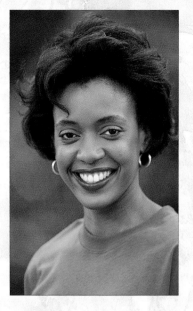

several sessions it worked. Four years later, I still haven't had a cigarette – but I do have a healthy two-year-old son and a thriving three-month-old daughter. Giving up smoking was the best gift I could have given my children."

menstrual cycle and decreasing a man's sperm count (see p. 13).

If you drink alcohol during pregnancy, your baby drinks with you, because the alcohol enters the foetal bloodstream. Many women worry about drinks they had when they were unaware that they were pregnant. An occasional drink usually does no harm, but regular or binge drinking can be dangerous. The best way to reduce the risks to your baby is to stop drinking altogether before you conceive.

If you find you can't stop drinking, ask your doctor's advice or seek out a support group such as Alcoholics Anonymous.

HARD DRUGS

Cocaine, heroin and other hard drugs, as well as cannabis in all its forms, have demonstrated harmful effects on a woman's fertility and a man's sperm. For example, cannabis contains THXC, a hormone-like chemical which accumulates in a man's testicles. Regular use lowers sperm count and affects sperm formation.

Hard drugs increase the risks of miscarriage, early delivery and birth defects. Cocaine crosses the placenta, reducing blood flow to the foetus and inhibiting growth. Taking any of these drugs during pregnancy puts your baby's health at great risk.

HAZARDS AND POLLUTANTS

No matter where you live or what you do, you will be exposed to some potentially harmful elements in your daily life. But you can minimize the dangers.

Pregnancy and childbirth in the developed world are safer today than ever before in history, and the vast majority of babies are born healthy. Nevertheless, chemical and other dangers exist in your home and work environment, and you should be aware of them, especially if you are planning a pregnancy.

AROUND THE HOME

In some areas, water contains high levels of pollutants, particularly from lead. If you live in an old house, it is worth having your water tested. In the meantime, use filtered or bottled water for drinking.

Many cleaning products contain toxic chemicals. When cleaning your home, wear rubber gloves so that you do not absorb such chemicals through your skin. Read the labels and avoid using products that warn that they may be toxic. Never mix chlorine-based products with those containing ammonia, because the combination produces potentially lethal fumes. Use any strong-smelling products, such as polishes, only in well-ventilated areas.

Insecticides can also contain potentially harmful chemicals. Stick to natural methods of pest control in your house and garden, and avoid going outside if someone else is spraying insecticide. If you live near agricultural land that is regularly sprayed, stay inside with the windows closed during the

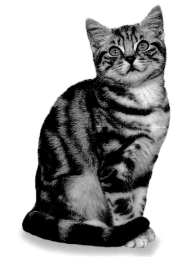

If you own a cat and are planning a pregnancy, you can ask your doctor for a blood test to check your immunity to toxoplasmosis. Many cat owners have had the infection and so are immune.

spraying and have your drinking water tested.

Cat and possum faeces contain an organism that causes toxoplasmosis, a disease that can affect a developing foetus, resulting in a premature or low-birth-weight baby. It can also cause fever, jaundice or eye problems in the baby. If you are pregnant or planning a pregnancy, do not handle cat faeces or the litter tray. (If there is no one else to clean the

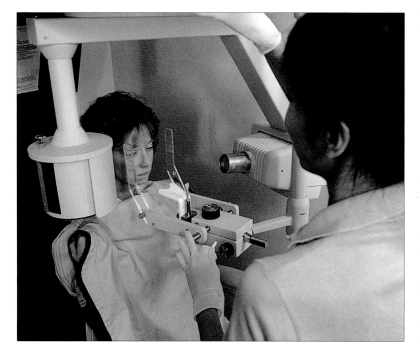

If you are, or think you might be, pregnant, avoid X-rays unless refusing one puts your health in danger. If you do have an X-ray, insist on wearing a protective lead-lined apron over your abdomen. Radiation is expressed in rads. Embryo and foetal damage occurs only at high doses – more than 50 rads; most modern diagnostic equipment delivers a dose of less than 5 rads.

litter tray, wear disposable gloves to do this.) Wash your hands after touching a cat. Make sure that the cat stays away from all surfaces where food is eaten or prepared. Wear gloves when gardening – even if you don't have a cat yourself – since cat and possum faeces may have contaminated the soil in your garden.

Lambs and sheep can harbour *Chlamydia psittaci*, an organism that can cause abortion in ewes. For this reason, avoid contact with lambs and milking ewes.

AT WORK

If you work with computers, consider the latest studies on the potential hazards before you become pregnant (see box, right).

Work that involves strenuous activity or heavy lifting can slightly increase the risk of miscarriage and early delivery. If you work with potentially toxic substances – such as dry cleaning fluids or photographic or printing chemicals – you should check on safety procedures. Speak to your employers if you are in any of these circumstances. They may be legally required to offer you an alternative position (see also pp. 118–19).

Health workers are exposed to risks from the chemicals used for sterilization, gases used in anaesthesia, infections carried by the people in their care and radiation from X-ray equipment. Women working with X-rays should ask about monitoring their daily exposure to make sure it does not exceed safe levels.

If you work with small children, it is vital to have your immunity to childhood diseases confirmed (see pp. 12–13).

Are VDUs safe?

A visual display unit (VDU) emits a low and continuous level of radiation. In theory at least, this can be harmful to the reproductive system of both men and women, as well as to a foetus in very early pregnancy. But while we know that radiation is potentially harmful, we also know that the human race has always lived with natural forms of radiation.

Since the mid-1980s, studies around the world have indicated a higher risk of miscarriage, stillbirth and birth defects among women who work with VDUs. Yet other research seems to refute these studies, or at least question them.

Until more definite information becomes available, the safest approach if you are pregnant or planning a pregnancy is to limit your exposure time. No problems are associated with those women who use a VDU for less than 20 hours a week. You should also follow the more general safety measures common to all VDU users for maximum well-being: take regular breaks and get up and stretch your legs; make sure that your chair has a backrest that supports your lower back and that the keyboard and monitor are at appropriate heights; and sit a minimum of 75 cm (30 in) from the computer screen and its hard drive.

If you are worried about the effects of radiation from your VDU, ask your employer and your doctor about protective devices. An apron over your body or a filter over the screen may reduce the amount of radiation reaching your body.

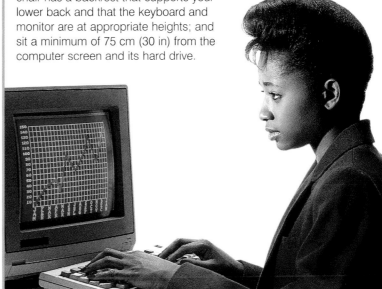

PARTNERS: YOUR RISKS IN THE WORKPLACE

If you work with hazardous materials or in an area where pollution is high, your fertility may be affected. Studies have shown that environmental or workplace materials and chemicals affect sperm. In some cases, these hazards have been linked with infertility, miscarriage, birth defects and stillbirth.

Although you are unlikely to be able to change jobs or conditions at will, you can help minimize possible damage. Be sure to follow strictly all safety procedures and wear appropriate protective clothing whenever necessary.

STRESS

A degree of stress adds excitement to life and helps you perform more effectively. It also helps you recognize danger and other threats to your well-being.

If you feel exhilarated and challenged by your life, you are experiencing the positive aspects of stress. But too much stress can adversely affect your mental and bodily functions.

YOUR BODY AND STRESS

Excess stress shows itself in physical symptoms in many areas of the body. Most commonly, stress causes tension headaches, tightening of the neck and face muscles and backache. Tension can also reduce the appetite and produce stomach upsets, indigestion and, in extreme cases, irritable bowel syndrome and stomach or duodenal ulcers.

Acute stress raises the heart rate and blood pressure. Chronic stress increases fatigue and affects the immune system, reducing resistance to infection. Skin tone diminishes, and a pasty appearance, along with itching and rashes, may occur. Hair may lose its lustre and even start to fall out. In addition, stress can lead to depression and disrupted sleep patterns.

Especially important to people hoping to conceive, stress lowers the libido in both sexes and may affect fertility. A woman who is highly stressed may ovulate irregularly; a man's production of viable sperm may decline. Stress can also create a disastrous psychological cycle: not getting pregnant when you want to can produce stress, which in turn makes conception more difficult. Research has shown that the stress induced by infertility is similar to that experienced by people coping with life-threatening illnesses, such as heart disease and cancer.

ARE YOU STRESSED?

The way you live and react to the various situations you face daily can affect your stress levels. Consider your working life. If you find it hard to turn off from work, or feel guilty about taking a couple of days off, for example, you may be under too much stress. Do you sleep well, or do you often lie awake at night worrying about work, your family, your health, money and other concerns? That, too, is a sign that you may be under stress. People who are stressed typically feel unwell, and are quick to anger. They may also depend on alcohol or other drugs to enjoy life.

If you are stressed, consider practising some or all of the stress-relievers suggested here. If stress symptoms are extreme, talk to your doctor about getting professional help.

REDUCING STRESS

The first step in reducing the stress in your life is identifying the cause. If you are doing too much, either at home or at work, try to delegate or eliminate some of your responsibilities. Listing in order of importance a manageable number of tasks for the day can help to reduce stress. It will also give you a feeling of achievement and of being in control of the situation if you cross each task off your list as you complete it.

Take time away from pressure and activity, without feeling guilty about it. Relax in a warm bath or get under a refreshing shower. Devote some planned time to listening to music or indulging in an activity you enjoy. Participate in a favourite sport or just go for a long walk. You will come back refreshed and better able to fulfill the demands of a busy life.

Share your problems with your partner or, if you find you simply worry each other, talk things over with a family member, a friend or a professional counsellor.

WHOLE BODY RELAXATION

You can use the breathing techniques outlined on pages 56 and 57 as an instant stress-beater. Then proceed with the following general relaxation techniques which will also help to relieve tension in your body:

Once a day, spend 10 minutes or more on focused relaxation. Find a quiet spot and lie with your head on a comfortable support. Close your eyes and imagine yourself in a peaceful place – a tropical island, perhaps, or beside a gently flowing river.

Contract and relax every part of your body. Starting with your toes, tense for a count of four, then relax. Move upwards through your calves, thighs and torso to your head, and don't forget your fingers. Stay in this state, making sure all your muscles are relaxed and repeating the exercise for any areas that still seem tense. At the same time, concentrate on your imagined place – the aim is to prevent worrying thoughts from entering your mind. Walk around your island, have a swim in your river. Hear the sounds of your beautiful place. Give yourself over to the sensation of tranquillity.

FEELING THE BENEFITS

Learning to master stress will help you to cope better with the irritations and problems of life and prevent them from robbing you of happiness or health. If you are relaxed, you will experience fewer minor aches and pains, sleep better, be less tired, less dependent on artificial stimulants and more efficient. As a delightful bonus, your health, looks and lovemaking will improve. Most important of all, you will get far more enjoyment from life and you will be more fun to be with.

Relaxation time is never wasted or self-indulgent, though you may be tempted to view it that way. Rather, it is a vital and revitalizing life skill that will help you, not only as a new parent, but in all areas of daily living.

Relaxation techniques

If you can cope with minor irritations as they happen, you are well on the way to reducing stress. This quick and easy sequence is an instant stress-reliever that you can do almost anywhere – at home, in the office, in the car or in the shower.

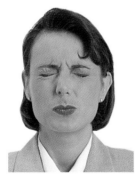

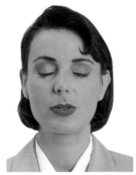

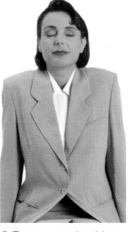

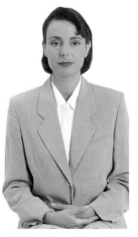

1 Scrunch up your face by frowning hard, pursing your lips and closing your eyes tight. Hold for a count of four.

2 Relax your face, feature by feature, slowly and gently.

3 Tense your shoulders, bringing them up towards your ears and holding them there for a second or two.

4 Relax them, then "roll" them – five times forwards, five times backwards.

COMMON QUESTIONS BEFORE CONCEIVING

Q *Should we arrange a blood test before we try to conceive?*

A In certain circumstances a blood test may be desirable. It enables you to determine your immunity to diseases that may harm your baby if you contract them in pregnancy – chickenpox and German measles, for example. A blood test is essential if you or your partner have reason to suspect that either of you has an underlying disease, such as HIV. If you are concerned about inherited conditions, a blood test can provide valuable information (see also pp. 12–13).

Q *I have rhesus negative blood, and my partner is rhesus positive. Does this mean we will have problems?*

A The baby in a first pregnancy will not be affected, but the rhesus factor (see below) poses a threat in subsequent pregnancies. Your doctor will order periodic blood tests to determine whether there is any threat to the baby's well-being. If necessary, injections that contain anti-D immunoglobulin can be administered to counter rhesus haemolytic disease and prevent harm to the baby.

Q *I get occasional headaches that I treat with aspirin or paracetomol. Are these safe to use in pregnancy?*

A The occasional tablet of either of these drugs is absolutely safe to take. Many women have taken over-the-counter medicines before they knew they were pregnant, and the medicines did not affect their pregnancies or babies. But any medication you take will cross the placenta, so many doctors advise you to avoid all but the most essential medication both before you conceive and in pregnancy.

The rhesus factor

If your red blood cells contain a substance known as rhesus factor, you are rhesus, or Rh, positive. If a woman who is Rh negative conceives a baby by a man who is Rh positive and the baby, in turn, is Rh positive, the woman may become sensitized to the Rh positive blood at the time of delivery. If a subsequent baby is also Rh positive, the mother's body recognizes the baby's "foreign" blood and produces antibodies that attack the baby.

First pregnancy

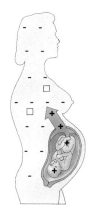

Rh positive blood from the baby enters the mother's bloodstream.

After first baby

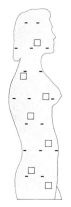

Antibodies develop in the mother to combat Rh positive blood and remain afterwards.

Subsequent pregnancies

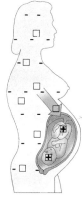

Antibodies enter subsequent Rh+ baby's blood, causing rhesus haemolytic disease.

— Rh negative

+ Rh positive

☐ Antibodies

⊞ Rhesus haemolytic disease

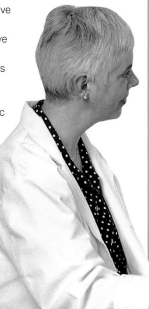

Q *My sister claims she conceived her much-wanted son by timing conception to get a boy. Is that possible?*

A Some people believe that the closer to ovulation intercourse takes place, the better chance there is of the baby being a boy. Male sperm are stronger swimmers than female sperm, but they are not as long-lived. Their chance of survival to conception decreases if ovulation takes place a day or two after intercourse.

Other people say that a diet low in sugar and high in salt and potassium will produce a boy, while a diet containing plenty of calcium and magnesium will result in a girl. And douching with baking soda – an alkali – before intercourse is said to increase the likelihood of conceiving a boy, and with white vinegar a girl.

None of these methods has had proven success. Some families produce more children of one sex than the other. There is no evidence that this is due to any factor other than chance.

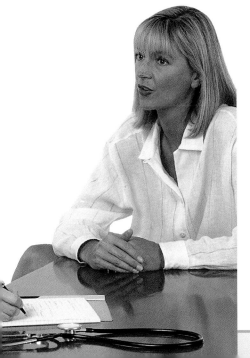

The family tree of genes

The characteristics of the mother and father are passed on to a baby in chromosomes, which contain many genes. Birth defects and inheritable diseases can also be passed on in the same way.

The baby inherits two versions of each gene – one from each parent. Sometimes the genes are identical. But if they differ, one may be dominant and the other recessive, making the baby a carrier of a trait, but not affected by it. If a recessive gene matches a similar one farther down the family tree, the child will inherit the characteristic. This is how the colour of hair and eyes and incidence of diseases such as diabetes "skip" a generation.

How genes affect eye colour

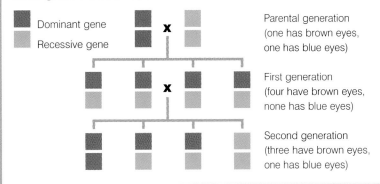

■ Dominant gene
■ Recessive gene

Parental generation (one has brown eyes, one has blue eyes)

First generation (four have brown eyes, none has blue eyes)

Second generation (three have brown eyes, one has blue eyes)

Q *Are twins inherited? My mother was a twin, I have an aunt who had identical twins and a cousin who had triplets.*

A Yes – and no. The tendency for a woman to produce more than one egg per ovulation does seem to run in families, so fraternal twins or triplets – who develop from separate eggs – are more likely to happen if there is a history of multiple births in the mother's family. Identical twins, however, arise from a single fertilized egg that then splits. No evidence exists that this has anything to do with heredity.

A visit to a doctor before you conceive provides an opportunity to talk through any concerns. It will also give you the chance to determine whether you are going to be happy in his or her care once you are pregnant.

Q *I am 35, and, ideally, I'd like to wait a year or so before I conceive. As an older mother, what can I expect from pregnancy and childbirth?*

A As you get older fertility declines, so it may take you longer to become pregnant. But once you conceive, the major difference between you and a younger mother is an increased risk of Down's syndrome and other chromosomal abnormalities. These risks increase gradually during your fertile years.

Among older mothers, slightly higher risk exists of miscarriage, diabetes and cardiovascular disease, as well as the need for caesarean section. However, once a chromosomally normal pregnancy is established, your chances of a successful outcome are very high.

How Your Body Works

In the years during which a woman is able to have children, her body is subject to a rhythm of hormonally controlled changes – the menstrual cycle.

A woman's body starts preparing for conception before she is born. At birth, a girl's ovaries contain all the eggs (ova) that she will release during the years in which she is capable of having children. But the eggs lie dormant in her body until puberty. At the onset of puberty, her body produces hormones that stimulate her breasts to enlarge, her pelvis to widen, and hair to grow on her underarms and pubic area. About a year after these changes, when she has reached about 47 kg (7 stone) and her body fat makes up approximately 25 percent of her total weight, the menstrual cycle begins.

THE MENSTRUAL CYCLE

The onset of menstruation, known as menarche, marks the beginning of a woman's fertile years. Menopause, when periods cease – usually between the ages of 45 and 55 – marks their end.

In 95 percent of women, the menstrual cycle lasts an average of 28 days, but doctors consider the normal range to be anywhere from 22 to 35 days.

At the beginning of the cycle, the uterus's lining, or endometrium, is thin and the ovaries are inactive. Then the pituitary gland releases follicle-stimulating hormone, which causes a follicle containing an egg to ripen in one of the ovaries (usually alternating between the ovaries each month). The cells of the follicle then secrete the

The female reproductive system

The delicate female reproductive organs are surrounded and protected by the bones of the pelvic girdle in the lower torso.

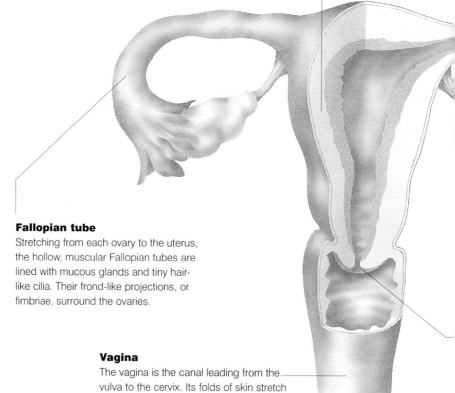

Uterus
The uterus, or womb, is the muscular cavity in which a fertilized egg is implanted and grows.

Fallopian tube
Stretching from each ovary to the uterus, the hollow, muscular Fallopian tubes are lined with mucous glands and tiny hair-like cilia. Their frond-like projections, or fimbriae, surround the ovaries.

Vagina
The vagina is the canal leading from the vulva to the cervix. Its folds of skin stretch when needed to allow the baby to exit during childbirth.

hormone oestrogen, which causes the endometrium to thicken in preparation for a fertilized egg. About 14 days before the onset of menstruation (halfway through a regular cycle), the follicle ruptures, releasing a mature egg. This is called ovulation. The egg travels along the Fallopian tube.

If it is fertilized (see pp. 62–63), it embeds itself in the rich lining of the uterus; if it is not fertilized, it dies, and the uterus sheds its lining in a menstrual period. Bleeding generally lasts three to five days, although seven days is not uncommon. The cycle then begins again.

Your partner

A man produces sperm from puberty onwards; sperm production results from the influence of the sex hormone testosterone and of gonadotropins secreted by the pituitary gland. These hormones are released continuously, rather than cyclically like their counterparts in the female body.

The reproductive organs – the testes, epididymis, vasa deferentia, and penis – produce, store and eject the sperm that may eventually fertilize an egg in a woman's body.

Sperm, which form constantly, take 100 days to mature fully. During this period, the original cells produced in the testes divide so that they contain only half the normal complement of chromosomes (see pp. 62–63). As they develop, they leave the testes and travel along the spermatic duct to the epididymis. There they continue to mature, and grow the whip-like tail that will eventually propel them through the female reproductive tract. After another growing and maturing stage, they pass into the vas deferens, where their development is completed. Once fully matured, they measure about 0.05 mm ($\frac{1}{500}$ in) in length.

During ejaculation, sperm are released from the penis. If ejaculation does not take place, mature sperm are reabsorbed by the body and new ones are produced. Each ejaculate contains about 300 million sperm, or 100 million per 1 ml ($\frac{1}{200}$ oz) of semen. Although only one sperm is needed to fertilize an egg, men who have a sperm count of less than 20 million per 1 ml ($\frac{1}{200}$ oz) may have difficulty fathering children.

The male reproductive system

Ovary

Ovaries contain eggs and produce the hormones oestrogen and progesterone. There are two ovaries, each about the size of a small grape and located on each side of the womb.

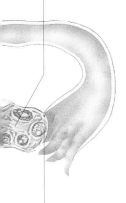

Follicle

The follicle is a small ball of cells within the ovary that holds an egg.

Cervix

During pregnancy, the neck of the womb, called the cervix, remains tightly closed until the onset of labour, when hormones influence the womb to start contracting, causing the cervix to open.

Vas deferens

The two vasa deferentia – there is one vas deferens for each testis – conduct the sperm from the testis to the urethra.

Urethra

The urethra, the tube connecting bladder and penis, carries sperm and semen during ejaculation, and allows urine to leave the bladder.

Penis

The penis is the external male sexual organ through which sperm must travel in order to reach and fertilize an egg. During sexual arousal, the veins of the penis fill with blood and the penis becomes hard and erect.

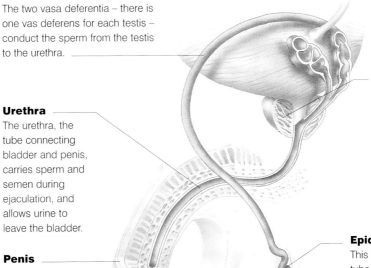

Prostate gland

The prostate produces secretions that form part of the seminal fluid.

Epididymis

This long, flat, convoluted tube links the testes to the vas deferens.

The testes

Contained by a skin sack called the scrotum, the testes manufacture sperm. They hang outside the body, where they are able to maintain the slightly lower temperature that is better for sperm production.

TRYING TO CONCEIVE

Your chances of having a baby sooner rather than later are excellent: three out of four couples conceive within six months of having regular unprotected sex.

If you and your partner have followed the advice on lifestyle given earlier in this chapter (see pp. 12–23), you are giving yourselves the best chance of conceiving and having a healthy child. This is important for *both* of you: about a third of all cases of infertility are attributable to some problem in the man.

WHEN DO I OVULATE?

Ovulation is essential to conception. Ovulation occurs about 14 days before a period is due, regardless of the length of your cycle, so keeping a note of the average length of your menstrual cycle may help you pinpoint when you ovulate.

Some women experience abdominal pain at ovulation; all women have certain changes in their vaginal secretions. The mucus becomes thinner, more slippery and more copious when ovulation occurs. If you note your secretions each day of the month, you will be able to anticipate ovulation by the changes that occur.

The body temperature sometimes falls immediately before ovulation, then rises after ovulation takes place. To detect this change, take your temperature each morning before you get out of bed and before having anything to eat or drink. You should keep a chart for several months if you want to identify a clear and consistent pattern.

The making of an egg

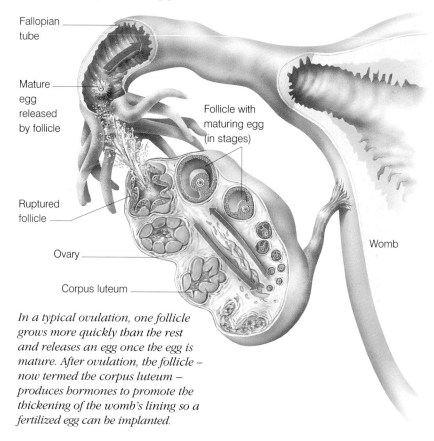

Fallopian tube

Mature egg released by follicle

Follicle with maturing egg (in stages)

Ruptured follicle

Ovary

Corpus luteum

Womb

In a typical ovulation, one follicle grows more quickly than the rest and releases an egg once the egg is mature. After ovulation, the follicle – now termed the corpus luteum – produces hormones to promote the thickening of the womb's lining so a fertilized egg can be implanted.

Finally, you can use a home fertility test kit, available from a chemist. This detects in a sample of your urine the increase in luteinizing hormone, or LH (see p. 66), which happens about 24 to 36 hours before ovulation.

WHEN WILL I CONCEIVE?

Once you have learned to pinpoint the time of ovulation, you will be better able to plan conception by having intercourse during the most fertile part of your cycle.

Having intercourse as close to ovulation as possible – the day before or the day itself – is ideal. If you are not certain of the day, make love at least once every 48 hours for three or four days on each side of the most likely date. Once an egg is released from the ovary, it remains fertile for 12 to 24 hours. But sperm can live inside a woman's body for two or three days, so it is possible for an egg to be fertilized by a sperm that is already in the Fallopian tube at the time of ovulation.

The position in which you have intercourse can improve the chances of your partner's sperm reaching the unfertilized egg. The missionary position – particularly if you put your legs on your partner's shoulders – allows deep penetration and the sperm is ejaculated as close as possible to the neck of the womb. If you have an orgasm, your cervix "dips" into – and is bathed in – semen, which increases the chances of sperm reaching their destination. More sperm will remain in your body if you lie on your back with a cushion under your buttocks for about 20 minutes after intercourse.

FACTORS AFFECTING OVULATION

Having a regular menstrual cycle of around 28 days is a good sign that you are ovulating. Lengthy menstrual cycles – over 35 days – and shorter ones – under 21 days – may indicate a problem.

Weight can have a bearing on fertility, as well as on general health. If you are very underweight or exercise excessively, you may not ovulate or menstruate. Women who are seriously overweight – that is, 20 percent heavier than average for their height and build – may ovulate erratically and are prone to such problems as high blood pressure (hypertension).

Age can be another factor: the steepest decline in female fertility happens after the age of 35, and the rate speeds up after you turn 42. The eggs you produce at this time may be less than perfect: they don't fertilize as easily, or they don't implant after fertilization.

FOR YOUR PARTNER

A man cannot check his own fertility, but he can improve it. Sperm thrive best at less than body temperature, so keeping the testicles cool by wearing loose pants can increase the number of viable sperm.

The drop in temperature before ovulation is about 0.2°C (0.5°F); the rise at ovulation about 0.5°C (1°F). If you want to know when you ovulate, take your temperature each day using a special fertility thermometer (available from chemists). This has more precise gradations than a standard thermometer.

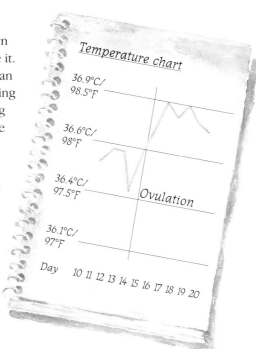

Temperature chart

36.9°C/98.5°F

36.6°C/98°F

36.4°C/97.5°F — Ovulation

36.1°C/97°F

Day 10 11 12 13 14 15 16 17 18 19 20

A Case in Point
Facing Infertility

LISA, 38, HAD NEVER DOUBTED HER ABILITY TO BECOME A MOTHER.

"*Rick and I married when I was 34. I stopped using contraception on our honeymoon, but after 18 months still wasn't pregnant. We grew anxious, so my doctor suggested we see a specialist. She found that my ovulation was irregular, though Rick's sperm count was normal. I was shocked. Although Rick was supportive, I felt responsible.*

"*Our doctor suggested fertility treatment, which involved self-administered hormone injections. It became a shared concern that brought us closer together. After four months I hadn't conceived, so it was suggested we try in-vitro fertilization. Two failed attempts later I had become so tense that the clinic advised us to 'rest' for six months. They also suggested we see a counsellor to work*

through how we would cope if we didn't have a child.

"*Attending the sessions was the first step to accepting that we might remain a couple but not become a family. Incredibly, halfway through the rest period, I conceived naturally.*

"*Now we have a baby son, and couldn't be happier. I'll never dismiss infertility casually again.*"

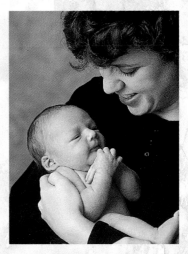

WHEN YOU CAN'T CONCEIVE

Even when they have done everything possible to improve their chances of conceiving, some couples require medical intervention to have a baby.

Knowing when to seek help for a possible fertility problem can be difficult. The decision depends largely on your health and age. If you suspect you might have a problem – you don't menstruate, have fibroids or have been treated for them or for endometriosis, or a sexually transmitted disease – see your doctor sooner rather than later. If you are a young, healthy couple in your 20s, you can try unsuccessfully for more than a year and still have high hopes of conceiving without help. If you're in your mid-30s or older, seek help if you have been trying unsuccessfully to conceive for at least six months.

IDENTIFYING THE PROBLEM
You or your partner may have a problem that makes you infertile; or you may both have minor problems that combine to prevent conception. Seek help as a couple and treat this as something to tackle together.

Your doctor will ask questions about your health and medical history, and about the frequency and timing of sexual intercourse. If he or she can identify nothing that indicates the source of the difficulty, you may be referred to a specialist for tests. These are likely to include the following: a sperm count for your partner; a close look at the formation of the sperm and the way they move; blood tests to check your hormone

Why can't I conceive?
The causes of infertility in women are more diverse than in men. Investigations work by a process of elimination, so if your partner is found to be fertile, your reproductive system will be checked area by area.

Fallopian tube

In the ovaries
Endometriosis and other infections can result in the scarring and malfunctioning of the ovaries.

In the womb
Surgery for fibroids sometimes weakens the womb; fibroids or polyps can alter its shape; congenital defects or exposure to certain drugs and hormones while in your mother's womb may affect the ability of your womb to sustain life.

Womb

Cervix

Vagina

levels; a hysterosalpingogram (see right); a laparoscopy (see right); and a test to examine your cervical mucus after intercourse to check the activity of the sperm.

The most common cause of infertility in women is blocked Fallopian tubes (responsible for about 50 percent of cases). In a

further third of cases, hormonal problems are to blame: if you are not producing enough oestrogen or progesterone, you may ovulate infrequently, or your womb's lining may not thicken sufficiently to nurture a fertilized egg.

Your partner may have too few – or no – sperm in his ejaculate.

In the Fallopian tubes

The scars from pelvic inflammatory disease (PID), endometriosis or an ectopic pregnancy can cause blockages of the Fallopian tubes; the tubes can also be damaged by surgery.

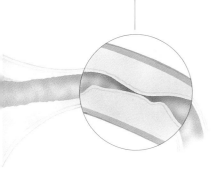

Womb lining

In the cervix

Infection, such as chlamydia, can cause you to develop allergic reactions to your partner's sperm, causing you to produce antibodies to neutralize them; your cervical mucus may be too thick to allow sperm through or so thin that it does not encourage sperm to move past the cervix.

His sperm may be damaged and unable to make the journey to the egg or to fertilize it successfully if they get there.

If no medical problem can be identified, psychotherapy may help to pinpoint a stress-related cause, and GIFT (see p. 33) may be recommended.

Understanding the jargon

Your specialist should explain the purpose of any tests that are suggested to you. The most common procedures relating to fertility are outlined here.

Tubal investigation

A tubal investigation checks the condition and function of the Fallopian tubes. This may involve a laparoscopy, hysterosalpingogram or both.

Laparoscopy

To detect ovarian cysts, endometriosis and other conditions affecting the reproductive organs, a small cut – about 12 mm (½ in) long – is made near your navel, then the tubelike laparoscope is inserted. Light from the laparoscope gives the surgeon a view of your ovaries, womb and Fallopian tubes.

Hysterosalpingogram

In this procedure, a dye is injected through the cervix. The dye should pass through the womb into the Fallopian tubes. If it does not, one or both of the tubes may be blocked.

Sperm count

A sperm count is the most basic test for men. Only one sperm is needed to fertilize an egg, but unless sperm are present in the seminal fluid in sufficient quantity – 50 to 150 million per ml $\frac{1}{300}$ oz) – problems with conception can occur.

Acrosome reaction test

The acrosome, in the head of the sperm, contains enzymes that enable it to break down the egg wall and allow fertilization to occur. A test to check whether your partner's sperm can penetrate one of your eggs may be carried out if a sperm count proves normal.

The laparoscope gives an excellent view of the ovaries (white), womb (orange) and Fallopian tubes. Video pictures are often recorded for reference. A laparoscopy done in the second half of the menstrual cycle can also reveal whether ovulation has taken place.

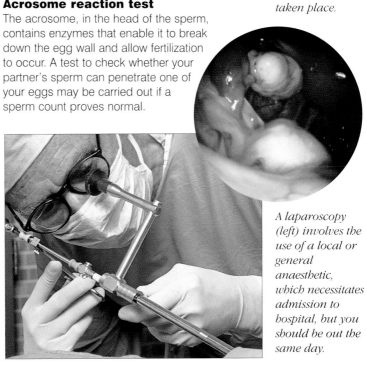

A laparoscopy (left) involves the use of a local or general anaesthetic, which necessitates admission to hospital, but you should be out the same day.

TREATING INFERTILITY

Infertility treatment is one of medicine's great success stories. In the 20 years since the first test tube baby was born, thousands of couples who had given up hope of conceiving have become parents.

Once the most likely cause of your inability to conceive has been established, you may be offered treatment. Remember, however, that no treatment guarantees success. Before you begin, consider together how vital a baby really is to you. Under what circumstances, and after how many courses of treatment, will you call a halt? Counselling has helped many couples to work through how they might feel if they were unable to become birth parents.

YOU AND YOUR PARTNER

If your problem is related to ovulation – you are not ovulating or you ovulate irregularly – fertility drugs in the form of injections or pills may be suggested. Taken at a certain point in the month, these stimulate a menstrual period. You will then be checked to see whether this in turn stimulates ovulation and, if so, advised on when to have sexual intercourse.

Hormonal imbalance that inhibits either ovulation or the implantation of a fertilized egg

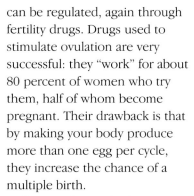

can be regulated, again through fertility drugs. Drugs used to stimulate ovulation are very successful: they "work" for about 80 percent of women who try them, half of whom become pregnant. Their drawback is that by making your body produce more than one egg per cycle, they increase the chance of a multiple birth.

Surgery (increasingly laparoscopy combined with laser surgery) can sometimes be used to clear endometrial scars and other small blockages of the Fallopian tubes. In cases where the tubes themselves are damaged – if they do not contract to help the egg on its way from ovary to womb, or if the tiny hairs that line them and also help the egg on its journey are damaged – surgery probably will not be an option.

A low sperm count can sometimes be raised by hormone treatment, and a blockage in the vasa deferentia or epididymis can be cleared by surgery. But if the problem is in getting sperm to the right place – if you have hostile cervical mucus, for example (see pp. 28–29) – artificial insemination by your husband or partner (AIH) may be offered. This involves your partner ejaculating sperm into a container, and a sample being injected directly into your womb. Intra-uterine insemination (IUI) is often used in conjunction with fertility treatments that encourage the production of more than one egg, thereby increasing the chances of conception.

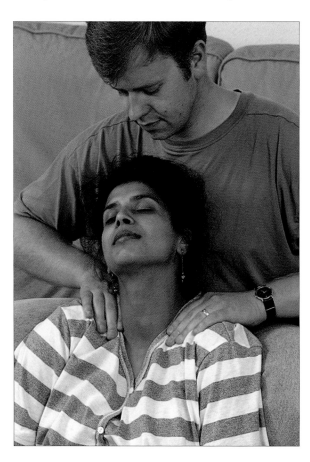

Facing the challenge of infertility can bring a couple closer, but is also sometimes the cause of couples drifting apart. For the sake of a strong, supportive relationship, it is important not to place blame. Tests and treatments need not take over your life. Be sure to keep up other interests – careers, friends, hobbies – and continue to talk and listen to each other.

Other options include in-vitro fertilization (IVF) and gamete intrafallopian transfer (GIFT), as described at right.

OUTSIDE HELP

Most fertility treatments involve using your eggs and your partner's sperm. But if a problem exists with either one of them, other options may be suggested.

If there is little possibility of your partner's sperm fertilizing one of your eggs, you may wish to consider artificial insemination using donor sperm (DI). Donors are carefully screened for sexually transmitted and genetically carried diseases and are matched physically as closely as possible to the "father". The sperm are then injected into the woman's vagina or womb. Success rates can be as high as 70 percent.

Women whose ovaries fail prematurely, or who are born with ovaries that do not function, may be able to have a baby through the use of a donated egg, fertilized with their partner's sperm, using a procedure similar to that of IVF. A general shortage of donor eggs may make this treatment harder to obtain.

COMPLEMENTARY THERAPIES

A number of complementary therapies have been successful in treating infertility. If you find the conventional treatment intrusive or embarrassing – as many people do – or want to avoid surgery or drugs, you may choose to consult a homeopath or acupuncturist. Keep your doctor informed at all times and never stop taking any conventional medication without discussing it with your doctor first.

IVF and GIFT

In IVF (in-vitro fertilization), fertilization takes place in a laboratory dish. The resulting embryo is then placed into the woman's womb, where, if all goes well, it implants and continues to develop as in a conventional pregnancy.

If you opt for IVF, you will be given hormone treatment to make you ovulate to order and produce several eggs at a time. These eggs are removed and then fertilized with your partner's sperm. Sperm may be gathered from several ejaculations to get a higher effective concentration, then washed to remove any unhealthy sperm. Sometimes a number of eggs are fertilized and up to three embryos are put into the womb; "spare" embryos are frozen and can be used for another attempt, if anything goes wrong or to offer you the chance of a second baby at a later date.

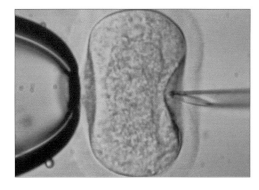

In gamete intrafallopian transfer (GIFT), the egg and sperm are obtained as in IVF, but are then inserted into the Fallopian tube so that fertilization takes place inside your body. This method more closely resembles natural conception. GIFT is often successful when the problem is in the man's sperm, or the cause of infertility is not known.

There are a number of factors to consider before trying IVF or GIFT. Most importantly, neither process guarantees success. Centres with considerable experience and expertise have a 30 percent or higher success rate with IVF, up to 35 percent with GIFT. The average couple tries IVF three or four times before conceiving and bearing a child, and some need more attempts. The costs of treatment vary, but can be high, especially if several attempts are necessary.

Treatment is physically and emotionally demanding and stressful. There is an increased likelihood of multiple pregnancy, with attendant risk to mother and foetuses. (Up to a quarter of mothers who have successful IVF treatment carry more than one baby.) The early stages of your pregnancy will be monitored more closely than if you conceive "naturally". Once the first couple of months have passed, however, your pregnancy stands an excellent chance of progressing smoothly to the birth of a normal, healthy baby.

In IVF, your partner's or donor's sperm are gathered and then placed in a dish alongside the egg. In some clinics the egg's outer membrane may be pierced, although not ruptured, by a microneedle containing the sperm. Fertilization takes about 18 hours, and the cell starts to divide 12 hours later.

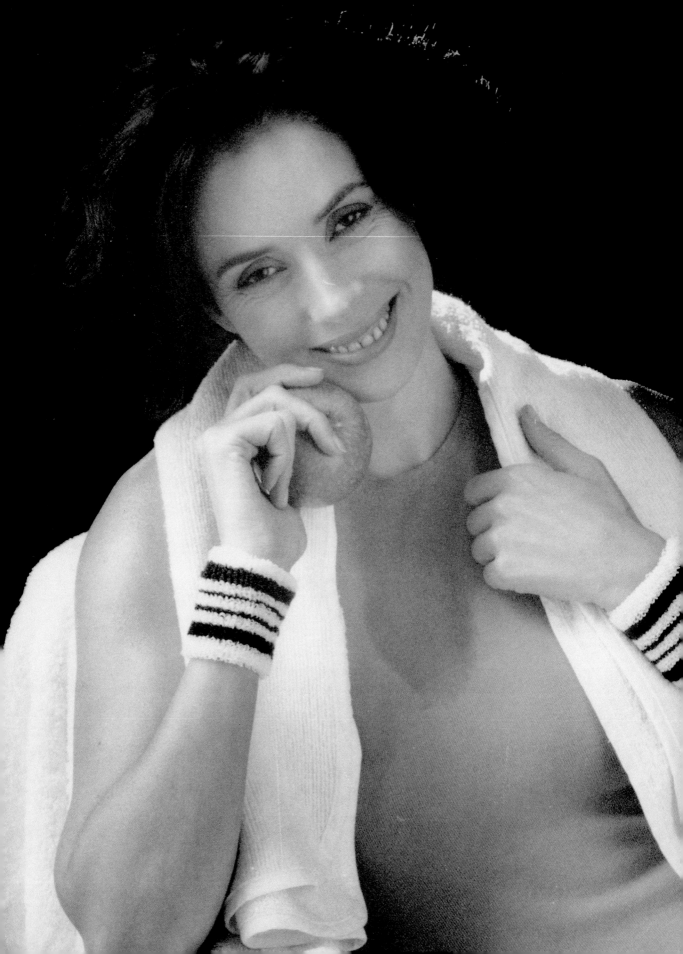

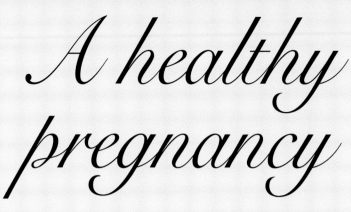

A healthy pregnancy

PREGNANCY IS A TIME to pay special attention to your health, diet and fitness. In these months:

- *Your body will make extra demands as you nurture the new life inside you*

- *Eating well and staying fit will help you to prepare for labour and birth, and for the enormous challenges of early parenthood*

- *You may need to modify how you do simple, everyday tasks, such as lifting, to avoid straining your muscles*

- *You will probably learn relaxation techniques and instant stress-beaters to help you through labour and beyond.*

This is a time to live well, not just for today, but to give you the vitality you need for the demanding and rewarding days ahead!

EATING WELL IN PREGNANCY

A healthy diet during pregnancy nourishes your baby as well as you. You don't have to eat "for two", but you must have enough of all the necessary nutrients.

During pregnancy, your body needs a healthy diet, with more of most nutrients. You need extra energy to maintain your fitness for the nine months during which your weight will increase considerably, and to meet the extra demands on your major organs. You also need sufficient nutrients to feed the new person growing inside you.

Your body does what it can to help you. Metabolic changes ensure that you get better value from the food you eat. Most women need to add only about 800–1200 kilojoules (200–300 calories) a day to the 6000–8000 kilojoules (1500–2000 calories) that are normal for most women.

A BALANCED DIET

A healthy, balanced diet should provide a daily supply of all the nutrients your body needs.

Protein forms the building blocks of new body tissue. Good sources of protein include fish, meat, eggs, milk, cheese, nuts, pulses and grains.

Unrefined carbohydrates are vital for health and energy. Most of your carbohydrate intake should come from starchy foods, such as potatoes, brown rice, wholemeal bread, pasta, flour and cereals. Refined carbohydrates, found in sugar, soft drinks, cakes, biscuits and sweets, add kilojoules but few nutrients.

Vitamins assist the functioning of many bodily systems and processes, including the immune system. Fresh fruits and vegetables are good sources of vitamins and should be eaten raw, steamed, stir-fried or microwaved whenever possible: boiling can reduce the vitamin content. Other vitamin-rich foods include fish and meat, milk, cereals and wholemeal bread.

Minerals are also vital to the body's functioning. Calcium helps to build strong bones and teeth, and iron is necessary for healthy, iron-sufficient blood. Your need for both of these minerals increases during pregnancy. You also require tiny quantities of several other minerals, including iodine, magnesium and zinc. Small amounts of many minerals are found in grains, fruits and vegetables. Iron is found in red meat, fish, pulses, wholemeal bread and dark-green vegetables. Calcium is present in dairy products, some soy products, some fish, and leafy green vegetables.

Essential fatty acids are necessary for development and growth. The best sources are fish or other seafood, linseeds and canola oil.

Recommended daily intakes (RDIs) of vitamins and minerals

The average pregnant woman needs the amounts listed of these important vitamins and minerals daily. If you don't do so already, check labels to make sure you are getting what you need, but do not exceed the recommendations, particularly of vitamin A..

Calcium	1100 mg
Phosphorous	1200 mg
Magnesium	300 mg
Iron	22–36 mg
Zinc	16 mg
Vitamin A	750 mcg
Vitamin E	7 mg
Vitamin C	60 mg
Vitamin B	
Thiamin	1.0 mg
Riboflavin	1.5 mg
Niacin	15 mg
Vitamin B_6	1–1.5 mg
Folate	400 mcg
Vitamin B_{12}	3 mcg

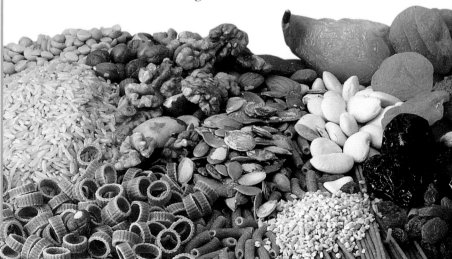

EATING WELL IN PREGNANCY

Fibre aids digestion and helps to prevent constipation. Fibre-rich foods include wholemeal flour, wholemeal bread and pasta, beans and some breakfast cereals.

You should also increase your fluid intake during pregnancy. Your increased blood supply (see pp. 96–97) needs liquid to sustain it, and your baby's body is made up largely of water. A minimum of 2 litres (8 cups) of liquid a day is recommended, consisting mainly of water, fruit and vegetable juices, skimmed milk, fruit and herbal teas, weak tea and decaffeinated coffee (see p. 14).

HEALTHY SNACKS

Throughout your pregnancy, you will probably find that you are hungrier than usual. Try to eat a good breakfast – cereal, fresh fruit or fruit juice, yoghurt, eggs, or toast made with wholemeal bread. If you need a snack to restore flagging energy levels, opt for bread, yoghurt, dried or fresh fruit or wholemeal crackers. If you don't normally eat between meals, two such snacks a day will provide all the extra kilojoules you need.

Follow the guidelines set out in the food pyramid on page 15, and read the labels on packages when choosing products.

If organic fruits, vegetables and grains are available in your area, choose them over non-organic varieties. Organic produce is grown in soil certified as free of chemical residues from pesticides.

Special diets

If you eat well, you should not need vitamin or mineral supplements, except folate (see pp. 14–15). However, if you eat a restricted range of foods – whether for reasons of health, religion or choice – you must make sure that your body is receiving all the nutrients it needs.

Vegetarian

It is commonly believed that because they don't eat meat or fish, vegetarians miss out on protein, iron, calcium and vitamin B_{12}. But, in fact, these nutrients are present in dairy products, beans, nuts, seeds, grains, pulses, peanut butter, soy foods (such as tofu and tempeh) and vegetables. Vegetarians who eat plenty of these foods and follow the guidelines given on pages 14–15 should have no dietary problems during pregnancy.

Vegan

A diet that excludes all meat, fish, eggs and dairy products can lead to nutrient deficiencies. Vitamin B_{12} occurs naturally only in animal products, although it is sometimes added to foods such as some soy beverages. Check the labels of the foods you buy, and consider taking a supplement.

Vitamin D is found in dairy products and in fish-liver oils, but is mainly manufactured by the body after exposure to sunlight.

Although calcium is found in many foods (see below), it is most concentrated in dairy products. Again, you may need a supplement or a calcium-fortified soy beverage.

Gluten-free

If you are sensitive to gluten (a protein that occurs in many cereals, especially wheat), you need to avoid breads, pasta, baked goods and many other cereal foods (unless they are labelled gluten-free). Lentils and pulses, potatoes and brown rice are good alternative sources of carbohydrate.

Lactose-free

Some people find lactose – a carbohydrate present in milk – indigestible. Some can tolerate it in cheese or yoghurt, but not in milk. If this applies to you, you still have a ready source of calcium. But if you can't take lactose in any form, it is important to find your calcium elsewhere: in fortified soy milk; in bony fish, such as sardines or salmon (you have to eat the bones); in some green vegetables, such as Asian greens and broccoli; in dried fruit, tahini, almonds and tofu. In some states, calcium-enriched, lactose-reduced milk is available. If you are not sure that you are getting enough calcium, your doctor may advise a supplement.

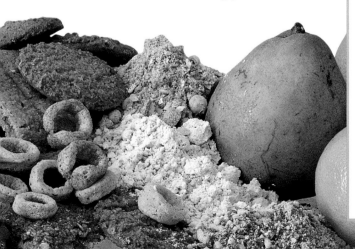

MODIFYING YOUR DIET

There's no need to become over-anxious about what you eat during pregnancy, but some risks are known to be avoidable, so it's wise to take a little extra care.

Indigestion and heartburn tend to be facts of life during pregnancy. They are caused by hormonal changes in your digestive tract; by the relaxation of all your muscles, including those of your stomach, which allow acid from the stomach to flow back into your oesophagus; and by your expanding uterus pressing against your stomach. None of this does any harm to your baby, but it can be uncomfortable for you. You can minimize these discomforts by modifying your eating habits.

HEALTHY EATING HABITS

During pregnancy, eat smaller meals – little and often is a sensible rule. Doing so ensures that your stomach acids have something to digest, without your feeling uncomfortably full.

Keep food simple – avoid anything too rich or spicy, such as hot curry or chilli, or cream or wine sauces. Buy fresh foods whenever possible, and steam, bake or roast fish or meat rather than frying it. Similarly, bake potatoes instead of frying them. Avoid processed meats (such as

sausages or bacon) and chocolate, both of which commonly cause indigestion. Choose foods low in fat, salt and refined sugar.

You can make similar choices when you feel like eating out. Most restaurants are fine when you are pregnant, but some are better than others. For example, at some fast food restaurants, all the food offered is high in fat.

Asian food is usually a good choice, but check to make sure that no monosodium glutamate is used. Pasta and pizza are also fine, but choose the simpler sauces and toppings. Ask for salad dressings to be served separately,

---

Smoking and drinking in pregnancy

Smoking during pregnancy harms your baby. The best advice is to give up – preferably several months before you try to conceive. Babies born to smokers are at greater risk of premature birth and cot death in babyhood, and of respiratory problems and developmental and growth delays in childhood.

Smoking raises the levels of carbon monoxide in the mother's bloodstream. As a result, oxygen is transported less efficiently to the foetus. Nicotine constricts the blood vessels on the mother's side of the placenta, which impairs the general functioning of the placenta. This impedes the baby's growth, and for some babies, the resulting low birth weight is literally a matter of life and death.

The more you smoke, the greater the risk. If you can't give it up, cut down. If you become pregnant before you have got

round to giving up, it is better to stop smoking at any stage of your pregnancy than not to stop at all.

If you drink while you are pregnant, the alcohol reaches your baby's bloodstream as well as your own. However, opinions differ on the level of risk attached to light or moderate drinking.

Continuous heavy drinking is the cause of foetal alcohol syndrome – a group of symptoms that include distinct facial characteristics, low birth weight and impaired mental ability. Lower levels of alcohol intake are also associated with early miscarriage and with difficulties in becoming pregnant. Research to determine a safe level of alcohol consumption, if any, is impossible to carry out. The best advice is simply to abstain from drinking when you are pregnant.

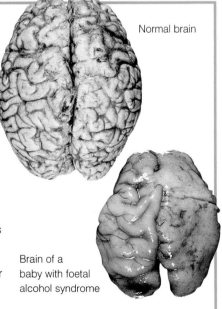

Normal brain

Brain of a baby with foetal alcohol syndrome

The brain of a baby whose mother drinks heavily during pregnancy is smaller than normal, and its cortex (outer layer) has fewer folds and poorly organized cells. Connections between the cells are impaired, resulting in mental deficiency.

and use only a small amount.

Many restaurants now serve fruit teas as well as coffee: try one of these at the end of your meal.

FOODS THAT MAY HARM

Foods that harbour organisms that can affect your health or that of your baby are rare. But by paying attention to your diet and avoiding certain foods, you can reduce the risks still further.

Listeria is a bacterium that can occur in certain foods and can cause listeriosis, a disease characterized by flu-like symptoms that may lead to premature birth or miscarriage. During pregnancy you should avoid the following:

- unpasteurized milk
- cream cheeses
- soft, mould-ripened cheeses (including Brie, Camembert, Danish blue, blue Stilton)
- soft ice cream from machines
- fish and meat pâtés stored unwrapped at a deli counter
- pre-cooked or pre-roasted poultry
- cook-chill foods.

Listeria is less likely to be present in foods that have been prepared, stored and sold in hygienic conditions. Food that has been left out in warm temperatures and in contact with the air carries the most risk. Heat-treated foods, such as canned meats and pasteurized or sterilized milk and other dairy products, are safe, because this processing kills the bacterium. Pasteurized milk and cheese and hard ice cream sold in blocks or tubs are fine.

Salmonella does not cross the placenta, so it cannot harm your baby, but it can make you feel very ill, with severe nausea, vomiting and diarrhoea. Avoid undercooked poultry.

The organism that causes toxoplasmosis may be present in uncooked or undercooked meat or fish, and in cat and possum faeces (see pp. 20–21). Most people are immune to toxoplasmosis, and a mother's immunity protects her unborn baby. However, if you catch it while pregnant, your baby is at risk. The effects can range from jaundice to blindness or mental disabilities.

A blood test can determine whether you are immune to toxoplasmosis. Wash and peel fruits and vegetables, and if you are not immune to toxoplasmosis, eat them cooked whenever possible. Unless you are immune, you should also avoid eating raw meat and fish (including sushi).

Although pregnant women were once advised to eat liver for its iron and vitamin A content, excessive quantities of vitamin A may be toxic to the unborn child. Pregnant women should avoid eating liver and all other offal, since they often contain very high levels of vitamin A.

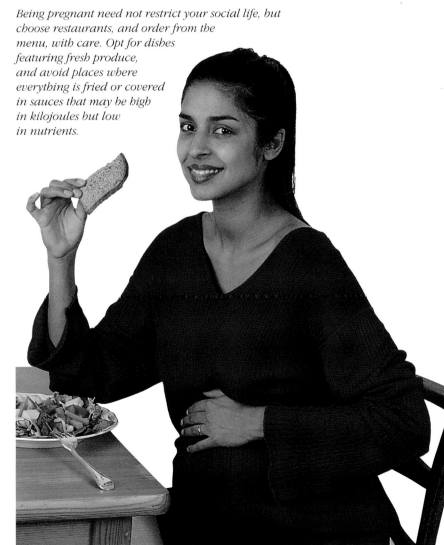

Being pregnant need not restrict your social life, but choose restaurants, and order from the menu, with care. Opt for dishes featuring fresh produce, and avoid places where everything is fried or covered in sauces that may be high in kilojoules but low in nutrients.

LIVING WITH CHANGES

Throughout pregnancy, your growing and changing shape makes it important to alter the way you perform a number of everyday tasks and movements.

The most obvious sign of advancing pregnancy is the change in your shape. The placenta produces a hormone called relaxin that makes the joints of the spine and pelvis more flexible, in preparation for birth. This allows your centre of gravity to shift as your uterus grows and becomes heavier, thrusting your abdomen forwards. Your chest pushes forwards as well, and your bottom tends to thrust outwards to help you to balance. Because of this, the small of your back takes a good deal of additional stress, which can lead to slouching and backache.

Take steps to strengthen your back so that it is able to tolerate the extra pressure put on it. If your spine was not well aligned before you became pregnant, the chances of backache during pregnancy are increased.

Adjusting the way you stand, sit, lie and move can reduce discomfort, avoid chronic aching, and prevent some long-term problems. Experiment with what is most comfortable. It may take you some time to adopt new, more supportive postures, but they should eventually become automatic.

STANDING
You can learn to recognize good posture and strengthen your back by standing with your back against a wall. Your shoulders and buttocks should touch it.

Changes in your spine

To compensate for your altered centre of gravity, your spine's normal curves are exaggerated: backwards at the chest and forwards in the lumbar region to balance the weight of your abdomen.

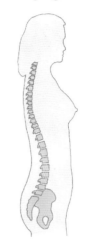

Non-pregnant   **Pregnant**

Upper spine curves outwards.

Lower spine curves inwards.

Keeping your shoulders relaxed, try to touch the wall with the small of your back. You will feel your bottom tucking in as a result, and your spine will straighten. Now walk away from the wall and relax a little so that you aren't so rigid. Whenever you have to stand, try to recreate this relaxed but upright posture.

SITTING
You will feel more comfortable, and protect your back, if you sit with your spine well supported. In later pregnancy, a small cushion tucked into the small of your back will help. If your job involves sitting at a desk or in one position for a long time, roll your shoulders one way and then the other to release tension. If possible, sit in a high-backed chair that supports your upper back. At home, sitting on the floor with your back against the

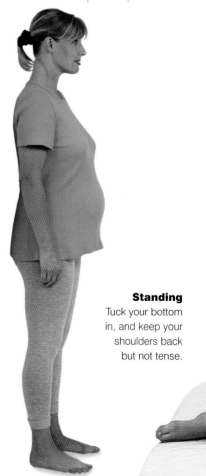

Standing
Tuck your bottom in, and keep your shoulders back but not tense.

wall strengthens the spine and combats a tendency to slouch.

LYING DOWN

It won't hurt your baby if you lie on your stomach all the way through pregnancy, but most women find that it becomes increasingly uncomfortable as pregnancy progresses. Lying on your stomach can also lead to backache if you have a very soft mattress that allows your abdomen to sink into the bed and your back to arch. Instead, try lying on your side, with your upper leg drawn up. You might like to place a pillow between your legs, under your upper knee. If you prefer to lie on your back, make sure your head is

supported with one or two pillows. Some doctors recommend that you do not lie on your back after about 20 weeks, because the pressure of the uterus on major blood vessels can decrease blood flow to the uterus.

LIFTING

To avoid pain and injury when picking something up, use your legs instead of your back. Bend at the knees and then lift. You should feel the strain in your thighs, not your back.

If you need to bend to carry out a task – making a bed or dressing a toddler, for example – kneel on the floor or take up a squatting position.

My back aches...

Backache is one of the most common afflictions during pregnancy. Paying attention to your posture (see opposite) helps you to avoid aches and pains and can relieve any aches that have already started.

You can get relief with some simple exercises, too.

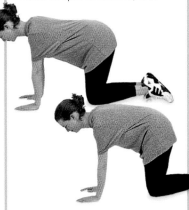

1 Get down on all fours, with your arms straight and your back level: imagine that you are balancing a tray on your back. Then tip the tray off by contracting your abdominal muscles, tucking in your bottom, and pushing the small of your back upwards. Flatten your back again and repeat six to eight times. Hold each position for five seconds.

2 Stand facing a wall with one foot in front of the other. With your arms folded and elbows touching the wall, lean forwards and rest your head on your arms. Tuck your bottom in. Hold for a count of five, then straighten up. Repeat six to eight times. Repeat with the other foot forwards.

3 Rolling each shoulder forwards five times, then back five times can relieve pain in the upper back. (Heavy breasts can add to backache – make sure that your bra provides enough support.)

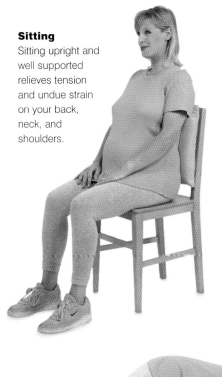

Sitting
Sitting upright and well supported relieves tension and undue strain on your back, neck, and shoulders.

Lifting
Bending from your knees to lift keeps you from shifting your center of gravity even farther forward.

Lying
Lying on your side relieves pressure on your back and does not constrict any major blood vessels.

ANTENATAL EXERCISES: YOUR BACK

Gentle exercise during pregnancy will make you feel more fit and energized, improve your circulation, keep you supple and prepare your body for birth.

The exercises on the following pages concentrate on potential problem areas and help to avoid or relieve constipation, backache, circulatory problems and other common discomforts. Because the exercises stretch and tone your muscles, they will help to prepare you for labour and birth.

During pregnancy, also try swimming, yoga (see pp. 52–53), walking and aerobics classes designed for pregnant women. For more vigorous exercise, such as tennis and jogging, seek the advice of your doctor.

● Always warm up with some gentle exercises before you start anything vigorous.

● Don't allow yourself to get overheated or overtired; exercise enough to feel your muscles working, but not so much that they will hurt for a week.

● Finish as you began, with gentle exercise and a few minutes of relaxation. Stopping abruptly can make you feel dizzy or sick.

● Wear loose, comfortable clothing that allows you to move and stretch easily but does not constrict you around the waist.

● Don't exercise on an empty or a full stomach. The first may make you faint, the second nauseous.

● Exercise on a level floor that has some "give".

● Always tell a class instructor that you are pregnant.

Back stretch

This exercise gives a good stretch from the back of your thighs, up through your spine, and towards the small of your back.

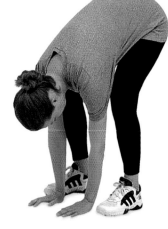

1 Stand with your feet wider apart than your hips and bend your knees slightly.

2 Slowly bend at the waist, very loosely and gently like a rag doll, and relax your shoulders and arms so that they feel loose and floppy.

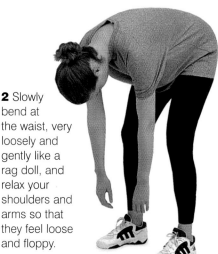

3 Keeping your knees bent, place your hands flat on the floor in front of you. If you can't reach the floor, get your hands down as far as you can.

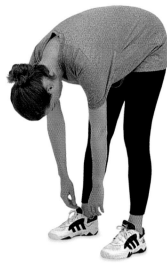

4 Slowly and gently straighten your legs, but do not lock your knees. Your hands will probably come off the floor a little. Feel the stretch, but don't allow it to become uncomfortable. Hold this position for five seconds.

5 Bend your knees again, and relax your shoulders and arms (left). Slowly roll up.

6 Repeat the entire sequence five times.

Lumbar tilt

This exercise strengthens and tones the whole of the back as well as the abdominal muscles.

1 Lie on your back. Bend your knees and keep your feet flat on the floor. Stretch your arms out to the side. Breathe slowly and regularly.

2 Push the hollow of your back into the floor so that your back is straight.

3 When you can feel the stretch in your back and across your stomach, hold the position for five seconds, then release.

4 Repeat five times.

Thigh raises

Thigh raises give a gentle, thorough stretch of the spine and thighs.

1 Lie on your back with your knees bent, and your feet flat on the floor and slightly apart.

2 Place your hands underneath your right thigh. Breathe in as you draw your knee towards your chest.

3 Hold for three

4 Breathe in as you slowly lower your leg to its starting position.

5 Repeat steps 2 to 4 with your left leg.

6 Repeat steps 2 to 4 with both legs: put a hand under each thigh, parting them as you bring them up so that they are on either side of your abdomen.

7 Work five complete repetitions: right leg, left leg, both legs.

Shoulder lifts

You'll need a chair to help you do this exercise. Choose one with a hard, straight back that's easy to grasp.

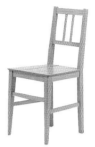

1 With your feet together and your arms relaxed and hanging by your sides, stand very tall, with your bottom tucked in. The chair should be an arm's length in front of you, with its back towards you.

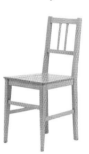

2 Breathe in as you stretch your arms up. Feel your body stretch up, too.

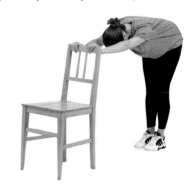

3 Bend over at the waist and hold on to the back of the chair with both hands. Keep your head, neck and spine in a straight line. Take four deep breaths.

4 Unbend slowly and return to the starting position. Repeat five times.

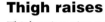
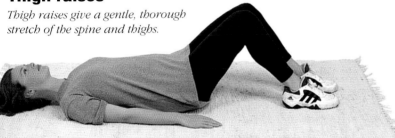
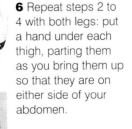

ANTENATAL EXERCISES: PELVIS AND ABDOMEN

Exercising the pelvic floor during and – just as important – after pregnancy prepares the muscles for birth and helps to prevent later problems.

The pelvic floor is made up of a supporting sling of muscle tissue underneath your bowel, bladder and uterus. There are three openings in the pelvic floor – the urethra, the vagina and the anus. Pregnancy hormones make the muscles and ligaments here (as everywhere else in the body) more elastic in preparation for all the stretching they will do during labour. The weight of the baby, the increased size of the uterus, the displacement of other abdominal organs and the process of birth itself, however, can stretch the muscles too much, with a consequent weakening and loss of tone. Exercise can keep these muscles in good shape and help to avoid such post-pregnancy problems as stress incontinence (leakage of urine when laughing, sneezing or running) and even prolapse of the uterus (the uterus dropping into the vagina).

The muscles of the abdomen also stretch as your baby grows. These muscles carry almost all the extra weight of pregnancy, so they need to be strong. Exercising will keep them toned. Strong abdominal muscles also help to support the spine, preventing backache, and may help to reduce the post-childbirth "tummy sag" most women experience to some degree after pregnancy.

Pelvic-floor exercises

The more pelvic-floor exercises you do, the better. Do them sitting down, standing up or lying in bed. Aim for four or five sets of 10 or 12 exercises each day. Practise them after childbirth, too.

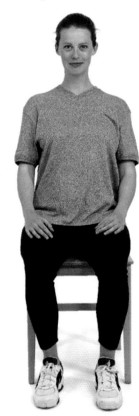

1 Imagine you are trying to hold back a stream of urine, and tighten your muscles to prevent leaking.

2 Breathing normally, hold this for a count of four.

3 Relax slowly.

4 Repeat 10 to 12 times.

If your pelvic-floor muscles are weak, you may find the exercises difficult at first, but you will improve with practice. Think of your pelvic-floor muscles as a lift you can take from the ground floor up to the third floor. Raise the muscles to the first floor and hold; then to the second and hold; and then up to floor three. Hold as long as you can at each level.

Once you have mastered the technique, do these exercises as often as you can. Practise every time you wash your hands; write the letter P on post-it notes and put them around the house – every time you see a P note, do a set of exercises. Repeat a set while you are on the phone.

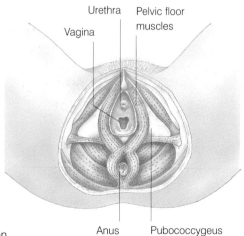

Urethra Pelvic floor muscles
Vagina
Anus Pubococcygeus

The pelvic-floor muscles form a figure eight that supports the pelvic girdle. Deeper layers of muscles support the bladder and the uterus. The largest muscle, the pubo-coccygeus, stretches from the front of the pelvis to the base of the spine.

Pelvic lift

This exercise tones and stretches the abdominal muscles.

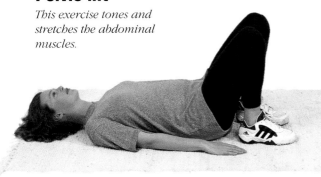

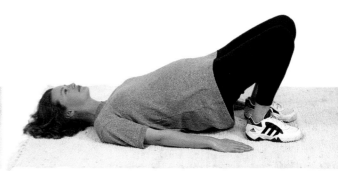

1 Lie on your back, with your arms at your sides, palms to the floor. Bend your knees and bring your feet close to your bottom. Clench your buttocks together.

2 Breathe in as you lift your pelvis off the floor. Hold for four seconds, breathing out slowly.

3 Return to the starting position. Repeat four times.

Abdominal stretch

This exercise is a little more difficult. Don't strain or stress yourself – if it causes discomfort, stop. Do only one or two repetitions at a time.

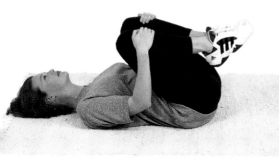

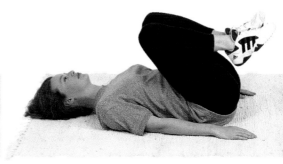

1 Lie on your back, with your arms at your sides. Bend your knees and pull them towards your chest with your hands.

2 Put your hands on the floor, palms down. Breathe in.

3 Breathe out as you straighten your right leg and lower it slowly to the floor. Breathe in, then breathe out as you straighten your left leg and lower it to the floor.

4 Return to the starting position and repeat.

Warning

Strenuous abdominal exercises done while lying on your back (such as sit-ups) should be discontinued after four to five months of pregnancy.

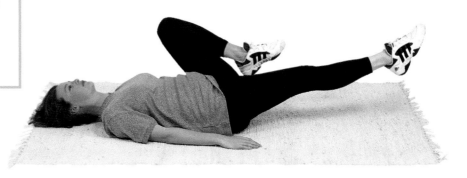

ANTENATAL EXERCISES: ARMS AND UPPER BODY

Keeping your arms toned and strong will help to relieve the aching that heavier breasts can cause in the shoulders, neck and upper back.

The arms and upper body are often neglected in exercise programmes, because they take less stress than other parts of the body. But a strong and supple upper body can help to relieve heartburn and improve your breathing, circulation and lung capacity – all of which have to work harder during pregnancy.

Arm circles

This exercise tones the whole of the arm and the muscle tissue across the back of the shoulders. It can also double as a warm-up at the beginning of any exercise session.

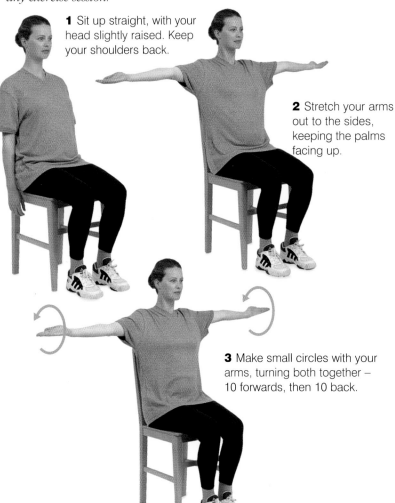

1 Sit up straight, with your head slightly raised. Keep your shoulders back.

2 Stretch your arms out to the sides, keeping the palms facing up.

3 Make small circles with your arms, turning both together – 10 forwards, then 10 back.

Shoulder stretch

This stretch can be difficult at first, but if you keep practising you will notice that you become more supple. Don't force yourself or stretch to the point of pain.

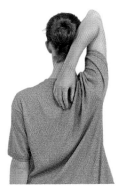

1 Stand up straight and raise your right arm above your head. Bend your elbow, letting your hand drop down behind your back so that it rests between your shoulder blades.

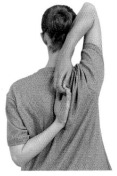

2 Bend your left arm and slide your left hand up your back, palm facing outwards. Try to reach your right hand with your left. If you can't, hold a cloth or a sock in your right hand and try to reach that. Feel the stretch. Breathing normally, hold the position for five seconds.

3 Repeat using opposite hands (you may find that one arm stretches more readily than the other – that's normal). Repeat twice on both sides.

Back stretch

This exercise will help to relieve the tension in your shoulders that is common in pregnancy. Shoulders take some of the strain as your posture changes and your breasts enlarge.

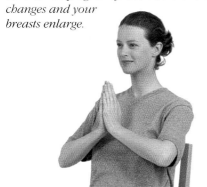
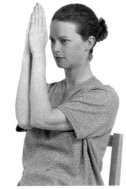
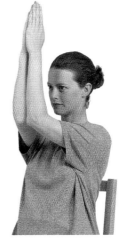

1 Sit up straight and hold your palms and fingers together. Point your fingers upwards.

2 Keeping your hands in this position, raise them slowly. Bring your elbows together as you breathe in slowly.

3 Raise your hands until you can no longer keep your elbows together and can feel the stretch in your upper arms and back. Hold for a count of five. Breathe out as you lower your hands to the starting position. Repeat four more times.

To relieve neck tension

Tension and aching often occur in the neck during pregnancy. This exercise loosens you up and is a good one to include in a warm-up.

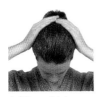

1 Sit and let your head fall forwards on to your chest. Gently press your hands on the back of your head to feel the stretch in your neck. Hold for a count of five.

2 Gently raise your chin to tip your head backwards. Feel the stretch in your throat. Hold for a count of five.

3 Bring your head to the upright position, then lean it towards your right shoulder. Feel the stretch in the left side of your neck. Hold for a count of five.

4 Repeat towards your left shoulder.

To relieve heartburn

This exercise helps to relieve heartburn and tightness in the chest.

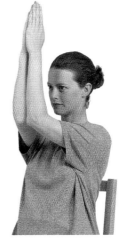

1 Kneel about 30 cm (12 in) away from a wall, with your knees apart.

5 Turn your head to the right and look over your right shoulder. Hold for a count of five.

6 Repeat over your left shoulder.

7 Make small circles with your head, five times one way, then five times the other.

8 Repeat the whole sequence twice.

2 Raise your arms and lean forwards so that your palms rest against the wall. Breathe normally and keep your arms straight. Hold for a count of 10 if you can; if you can't, hold for a count of five and gradually increase. (Note: You should feel no stretch in your back. You should feel it all in your shoulders and arms.)

ANTENATAL EXERCISES: LOWER BODY

Exercising your legs, ankles and feet improves your overall strength and suppleness and helps you to avoid a number of the common discomforts of pregnancy.

Paying attention to your lower body may help to prevent varicose veins; it can also relieve and prevent constipation, cramps and aching due to swelling, and improve overall circulation and energy levels.

Keeping your feet raised at night (by putting a pillow or a couple of thick books under the foot of the mattress) and for periods during the day will also alleviate these problems.

Foot circles

This exercise can be done when you are sitting at a desk or just relaxing. Do it as often as you can, especially if you experience cramp.

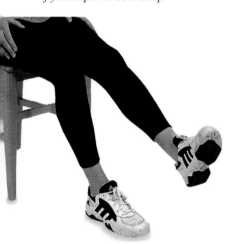

1 Lift one foot off the floor and circle the ankle several times, first one way, then the other. Don't move your knee.

2 Repeat with the other foot.

Calf stretch

Strong, supple calf muscles will help to minimize fatigue and prevent cramps in the lower leg.

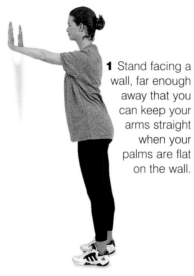

1 Stand facing a wall, far enough away that you can keep your arms straight when your palms are flat on the wall.

2 With your feet apart and flat on the floor, move your body towards the wall as you bend your arms, breathing out as you go. Hold for a count of five.

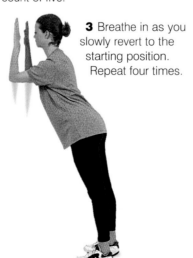

3 Breathe in as you slowly revert to the starting position. Repeat four times.

Thigh stretch

This exercise concentrates on strengthening and toning your thighs, but is also beneficial to overall suppleness and to blood circulation.

1 Repeat the calf stretch but raise one knee towards the wall as you lean towards it. Keep your spine straight and your other foot flat on the floor throughout.

2 Repeat with the other leg, then repeat twice more with each leg.

Stair stretch exercise

Do this stretch every time you climb the stairs. Take off shoes with high heels before you start.

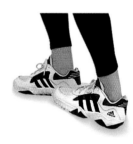

1 Stand on a stair. Keeping your back straight, move one heel back and let it drop below the edge. When you can feel the stretch in your calf, hold for a count of five. Repeat five times, then repeat using your other heel.

Leg extensions

This leg exercise helps to tone your abdominal muscles, too.

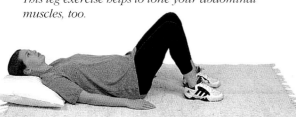

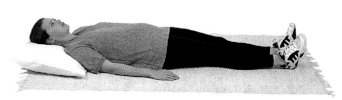

1 Lie on your back, with your head and shoulders supported by a pillow or cushion. Bend your knees and place your feet flat on the floor and slightly apart.

2 Slide both legs down slowly so that they are straight out in front of you.

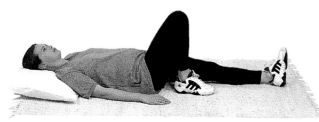

3 Bring first your right knee, then your left, back to the starting position. Don't arch your back: it must stay firmly on the floor. Ask a friend to check that you are doing this correctly.

4 Repeat the sequence five more times.

Squats

Squatting is really a whole-body stretch, although you will feel it in your thighs and groin at first, and then in your lower legs. It is excellent for increasing flexibility in the pelvis and relieving constipation, and it can also become a restful position over time. Some women choose to give birth in this position because it widens the pelvic outlet so effectively. If the full squat is too difficult for you, or if you have varicose veins in your legs, vulva or rectum, practise a supported squat, using a low stool or a large book.

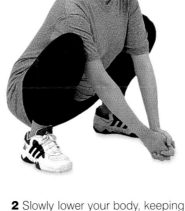

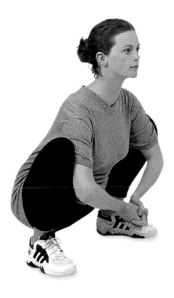

1 Stand up straight with your feet about 60 cm (2 feet) apart.

2 Slowly lower your body, keeping your back straight. Clasp your hands together and use your elbows to press your knees apart. Hang on to something (or someone) to keep your balance, if necessary.

3 Hold this position for as long as it is comfortable. Build up from a couple of minutes a day to as long as you can. You need daily practice to develop this skill and to retain your suppleness.

RELAXATION

Quiet times, spent listening to music or reading a book, allow you to tune in to your baby, away from the other distractions of your life.

Relaxing your body and your mind during pregnancy does more than create a sense of well-being. It allows physical recuperation and helps to prevent the tension that can lead to high blood pressure. It also gives parts of your body that may ache (back, legs, abdomen) a rest from the extra weight and effort of holding you and your baby upright. Because it sharpens your mental faculties and releases natural painkillers, it can be of particular help in managing your labour.

A relaxed body is closely linked to a relaxed mind. Stress and worry can manifest themselves as headache or backache, while physical pain or exhaustion increase worry and stress (see pp. 22–23).

Throughout your pregnancy, try to find a little time every day to devote to yourself. By doing this, you will feel more able (and willing) to devote time and

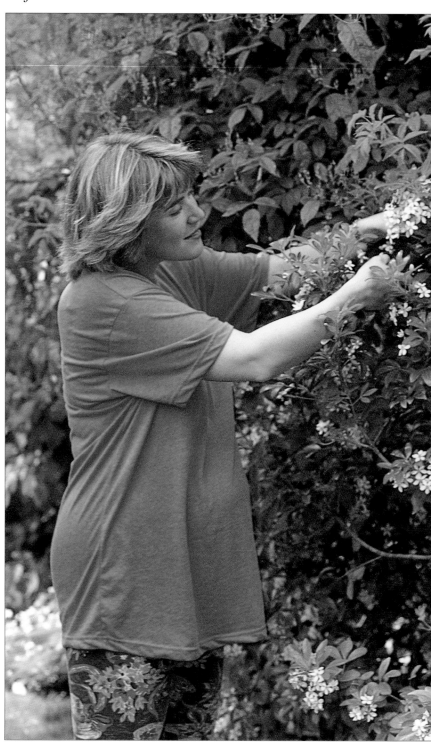

If you had a relaxing hobby before you became pregnant, keep it up. Gardening is a great relaxer: you are surrounded by beauty, out in the fresh air, and can enjoy moving at your garden's pace.

energy to your work, your partner and your daily routine. Try to get plenty of sleep. Ask other people to help with such tasks as shopping that you may find difficult as your pregnancy advances. If your work situation is so stressful that you are finding it hard to cope, talk to your employer about starting your maternity leave early or working part-time for a while.

PRACTISING RELAXATION

Relaxation techniques are simple. The challenge lies in taking the time to practise them. Relaxation doesn't have to be done at exactly the same time and in the same place each day, of course, but if you try to make it a matter of routine, you are more likely to keep it up and to notice the gap in your life when you don't manage to fit it in. Perhaps you can get up 15 or 20 minutes earlier than usual in the morning. Or make time for relaxation as soon as you come home from work or immediately after your bath or shower.

The technique described on pages 22–23 will work well throughout your pregnancy. If in the later stages you feel more comfortable lying on your side, do so. Always end your relaxation session slowly and gently, yawning, stretching and shaking your limbs if you want to.

You can adapt this technique to everyday situations and use it whenever you need to calm down. Any time and anywhere that you feel tense, concentrate on breathing slowly and rhythmically, in through your nose and out through your mouth. Let the tension come out

---

> ## Partners: how you can help
>
> Because you know your partner well and care about her well-being, you may be quicker to spot the signs of stress than she is herself. You may be more aware than your partner that her work or daily tasks are putting her under pressure; you will notice that your partner is more tired – or, perhaps, more short-tempered – than usual; you will spot a tense frown. If you give your partner a massage (see pp. 58–59), you will feel tension across her neck and shoulders, where the muscles are almost literally tied up in knots.
>
> Above all, be available to discuss any problems, and help with domestic chores or other children so that your partner has more time to rest. Encourage her to relax. If you can make time to do relaxation exercises with your partner, so much the better: it will mean that she is more likely to do them. It will be of direct benefit to you as well.

---

of your shoulders by contracting and then releasing them, and clench and unclench your fingers and hands. If you need to talk, do so in a deliberately softer, slower voice. This quick relaxation technique is very helpful during labour and birth, and in the early weeks of motherhood, especially if you have a crying or sleepless baby. It helps to prevent the spiralling of tension between mother and baby that can make trying situations harder to deal with.

TRAINING FOR LABOUR

Relaxation techniques play an important part in preparing you for labour. Tension in one part of the body indicates that there is tension elsewhere. If your neck and shoulders are tense, or if you are clenching your teeth or your fists, your birth canal is likely to be taut as well. Make sure your partner is aware of this; if he works on relaxing tension in your upper body, you will be free to concentrate on relaxing your abdominal muscles.

Antenatal instructors generally teach relaxation techniques. They also explain what you should expect from labour, thereby reducing the element of fear, which is perfectly natural in women expecting their first baby. Fear, of course, causes the body to tense, making delivery more difficult and producing a cycle of fear–tension–pain–more fear.

One of the most popular (though controversial) techniques was pioneered by Dr Fernand Lamaze (see p. 75). This method teaches a woman how both to reduce pain and to use breathing techniques and various forms of diversion to alter her perception of pain, effectively conditioning her not to notice the full intensity of labour. The body responds usefully and positively to labour contractions, without the complication of excess tension.

Critics who object to the idea of a woman's distancing herself from labour pain believe that she should listen to and respond to her body. They suggest that the Lamaze method does not give a full birth experience, but it has proved effective for a large number of women.

YOGA

Yoga practitioners hope to unite the physical, mental and spiritual facets of their being. Many women have found it to be of great benefit in pregnancy.

Yoga is more than a way of exercising. It is an overall approach to the health of body and mind. Yoga practitioners aim to achieve heightened awareness, peace and well-being by means of certain physical postures combined with relaxation. Many of the postures, or *asana*, gently stretch the muscles of the body in a way that is completely safe for pregnant women. The breathing and relaxation techniques of yoga promote a peaceful, calm outlook. In addition, yoga provides an excellent way to relieve many of the discomforts of pregnancy, including stress incontinence, varicose veins, cramps, heartburn, constipation and backache. Because it promotes peace of mind, increases suppleness and emphasizes controlled breathing, practising yoga can also make childbirth much easier.

If you are a beginner at yoga, you will find it helpful to have a teacher. Tell him or her that you are pregnant before you begin. If you already practise yoga, ask for advice on what you can and can't do during pregnancy. Very little is likely to be ruled out, although some of the more advanced positions that need great suppleness and flexibility may not be advisable. Of course, anything that causes undue strain should be avoided.

The positions shown here briefly introduce what you will learn if you practise yoga regularly; they are perfectly safe to do during pregnancy and are most effective if they are performed every day. You can do them whether or not you go on to practise yoga more extensively.

Wear loose, comfortable clothes for these exercises. Begin each session with at least five minutes of relaxation (see pp. 22–23).

Spine stretch

Doing this exercise each day helps to increase the flexibility of your pelvis and keeps the muscles of the pelvis and thighs supple and well toned. Suppleness in these areas is of great benefit during labour and birth.

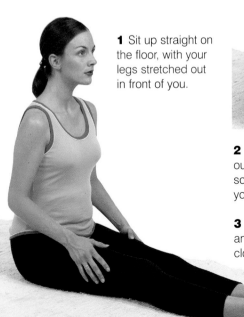

1 Sit up straight on the floor, with your legs stretched out in front of you.

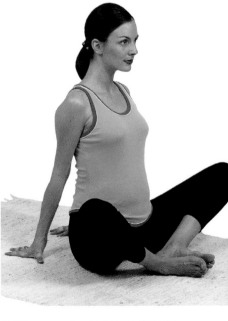

2 Bend your knees, then lower them outwards towards the floor. Place the soles of your feet together and pull your heels towards your body.

3 Place your hands around your ankles and slowly bring your heels closer to your body. Don't strain.

4 When your heels are as close to your body as you can get them, rest your palms on the floor behind you. Feel your spine stretch upwards. Retain this pose for about two minutes, then slowly relax, breathing deeply two or three times.

Knee bends

This posture strengthens your legs and improves the flexibility of your thighs and upper body.

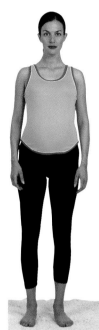

1 Stand up straight, looking ahead and breathing slowly and regularly.

2 Place your feet more than shoulder width apart. Turn your right foot slightly inwards towards your body, and point your left foot outwards.

3 Raise your arms to shoulder height and stretch your hands and fingers out to the sides.

4 Bend your left knee so that your knee makes a right angle and your thigh is almost parallel to the floor (but don't extend your knee farther forward than your toes). Without twisting your body, turn your head and look at your left hand.

5 Breathe regularly in this pose for a minute. Then, as you breathe in, straighten your left leg and lower your arms.

6 Repeat steps 2 to 5, bending your right knee and looking at your right hand.

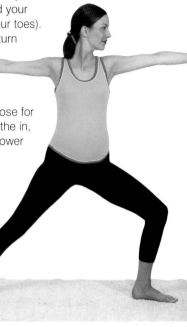

Knee sits

This position is a particularly effective one for relieving constipation and digestive problems.

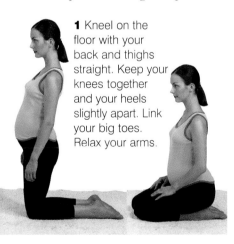

1 Kneel on the floor with your back and thighs straight. Keep your knees together and your heels slightly apart. Link your big toes. Relax your arms.

2 Gently and slowly lower your bottom to sit between your heels. Rest your hands on your thighs. Breathing slowly and evenly, relax the muscles of your abdomen. Hold this position for two minutes. Relax, then repeat.

Pelvic rock

This exercise helps to relieve backache during pregnancy and is particularly effective if you do it daily.

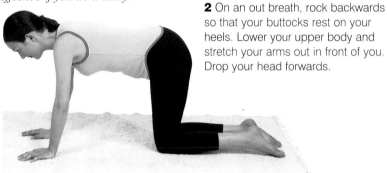

1 Kneel on all fours with your back and arms straight. Breathe regularly.

2 On an out breath, rock backwards so that your buttocks rest on your heels. Lower your upper body and stretch your arms out in front of you. Drop your head forwards.

3 Breathe in as you rock forwards, keeping your hands in the same place. Straighten your legs, and allow your arms to straighten.

4 Continue to rock backwards and forwards for as long as it feels comfortable. Keep movements slow and gentle.

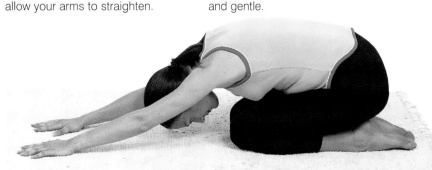

COMPLEMENTARY TECHNIQUES

Complementary exercise and relaxation techniques can enhance your fitness, prepare your body and mind for birth, and relieve pregnancy discomforts.

These suggestions offer you a brief introduction to a number of therapies and techniques that some pregnant women have found helpful. If you want to explore any of these further, you can find a qualified practitioner, join a class, or read more in a book devoted to the subject.

ALEXANDER TECHNIQUE

This method of retraining and improving posture and body movement was developed 100 years ago by an Australian actor, F. Matthias Alexander. It has been used successfully to relieve such conditions as stress, respiratory disorders, arthritis, backache and disorders of the digestive tract.

In pregnancy, the Alexander technique can help you to make adjustments to your posture when you sit, stand and lie down; it can alert you to when your posture is poor; it can also help you to tune in to your body's needs so that during labour you will be more aware of what might make you more comfortable.

You cannot learn the Alexander technique at home or practise it yourself; you need to find a qualified teacher. One of the organizations listed on pages 218–19 will be able to recommend one in your area. Lessons are offered on a one-to-one basis, and your teacher will identify improvements you may make in the way you hold your body. One lesson, for example, might teach you how to lie with your spine, neck and head in line.

T'AI CHI

This Chinese system of flowing, relaxed movement is sometimes described as "meditation in motion". The discipline includes breathing techniques, correct balance and proper alignment of the body, and is believed to raise physical and spiritual awareness. Proficient practitioners speak of the sensation of calm, wholeness, and peace they experience. Groups practising T'ai chi often choose an outdoor setting – they are a familiar sight in parks all over the world.

T'ai chi is very gentle. Its effectiveness depends on relaxed, slow movements. Because T'ai chi requires little physical effort, it is suitable for all stages of pregnancy and for all levels of fitness. T'ai chi's therapeutic use to relieve stress and anxiety may be its greatest benefit during pregnancy.

T'ai chi should be learned with a teacher, and watching others can be helpful.

According to Chinese philosophy, T'ai chi harmonizes yin and yang – the active and passive aspects of the cosmos. This ancient Chinese art of flowing, rhythmic and deliberate movement is reputed to improve the ability to relax.

MEDITATION

Meditation, in its many forms, is closely related to yoga (see pp. 52–53) and brings about a state of inner calm. Having a teacher, at least at first, can help you to develop basic techniques. You will learn to induce a meditative state – emptying your mind of all extraneous thoughts and distractions – by using breathing techniques, chanting, repeating a sound, humming or focusing on a special object. You'll be encouraged to set aside a quiet time to meditate every day to gain the greatest benefit from it.

Practitioners believe that meditation helps you to develop greater sensitivity to your own needs and to those of others. They claim that it can also foster an accepting, positive attitude – all of which can be of enormous benefit during pregnancy and labour.

ACUPRESSURE

Some women have found acupuncture helpful during pregnancy, labour, and birth. For those who find the idea of needles off-putting, acupressure serves much the same purpose. Using fingers instead of needles, this treatment stimulates specific pressure points linked to what in traditional Eastern medicine are called the "meridians" – pathways through the body that are linked to the functioning of the various organs.

Acupressure can relieve a variety of problems, from stress to digestive complaints to pain. You can learn to practise a simple form of acupressure on yourself, applying pressure to certain

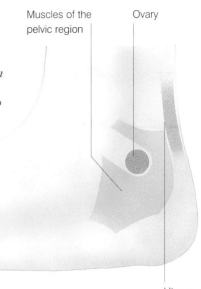

Acupressure applied to an area of the foot affects a specific part of the body: the left foot influences the left side of the body, and the right foot, the right side of the body. In addition to promoting relaxation, pressure applied to specific points can help to relieve problems in the associated areas, such as backache.

Muscles of the pelvic region

Ovary

Uterus

points on the temples, for example, to relieve a headache or to the wrist to combat nausea.

SHIATSU

This ancient Japanese therapy involves many of the elements of acupressure. It is believed to promote a healthy mind and body by stimulating the flow of the body's natural energy through the meridians.

In Japan shiatsu is regarded as a healer of specific ailments or disorders, as an aid to diagnosis, and also as a preventative technique that encourages all-round good health. Although you can learn to treat yourself with shiatsu, you should seek professional advice if you are in any doubt about what you are doing. Practitioners advise against applying pressure to certain areas during pregnancy. Most of the techniques are quite safe, however, and can help to relieve some of the aches and minor discomforts of pregnancy and help you to approach labour in good health.

VISUALIZATION

Visualization therapy uses the power of the imagination, aiming to combat negative feelings and physical conditions or discomforts with positive mind pictures. Combined with relaxation, visualization induces a calm, receptive, stress-free state (see pp. 22–23 and 50–51).

Some women find that a similar technique can help them to prepare for birth and parenthood. Antenatal classes sometimes encourage participants to close their eyes and imagine themselves giving birth. They visualize themselves opening up without effort, relaxed and happy as the baby is born. The women are then asked to visualize themselves holding the baby, getting to know the baby, loving the baby. Reflecting on the happy, positive emotions you experience during these visualizations can help you to discover and explore anxieties and doubts, and to become more confident about the challenges that lie ahead.

BREATHING TECHNIQUES

Learning to breathe differently may sound difficult, but certain breathing techniques can become second nature, given time and practice.

With the exception of those who suffer from asthma or a similar disorder, most of us are not conscious of how we breathe most of the time. In order to learn therapeutic ways of breathing, however, we have to become aware of what we are doing.

When you breathe, you take air into your lungs. The oxygen in the air passes through the walls of the lungs and into the bloodstream, then circulates throughout the body, nourishing the internal organs. When you are pregnant, it also passes through the walls of the womb into the placenta, where it supplies oxygen to your growing baby. The bloodstream carries the waste product carbon dioxide away from the organs (and your baby) back to the lungs so that you can breathe it out. During this process the diaphragm moves up and down, massaging the internal organs and muscles. Irregular breathing causes movements of the diaphragm that are also irregular and not performing their function properly. Breathing too fast often means inhaling before the last breath is properly exhaled, leaving stale air in the lungs and impeding the flow of oxygen to the rest of the body – and to your baby.

During exercise, you can make the most of your movements or stretches by breathing out during the movement that requires the most effort. Breathe in through the nose, and out through the mouth. Don't hold your breath at the same time that you are contracting a muscle – this can impede blood flow and cause dizziness. Keep your breathing moderately deep and regular.

When relaxing, concentrate on your breathing. Again, breathe in through the nose and out through the mouth. As you inhale, imagine that you are breathing in calmness and peacefulness. As you exhale, think of breathing away all the tension in your body. Breathe slowly and deeply.

BREATHING DURING LABOUR
Controlled breathing is sometimes taught as a technique for managing the pain of contractions in labour. Breathing regularly helps you to avoid the tendency to tense up with fear or discomfort – which then increases pain (see pp. 50–51). To prepare for childbirth, you can learn different ways of breathing and practise them so that you are confident and prepared when labour begins. None of these techniques is intended to take

---

Getting it right

It is easier to practise breathing techniques when you know you are doing it correctly.

1 Sit in a relaxed position. Hold a feather about 15 cm (6 in) away from your mouth. For level 1 breathing, the feather should flutter slightly but remain upright as you breathe out. For level 2, the feather should move more rapidly, as well as bend slightly but perceptibly away from you. For level 3, the feather should clearly bend away from you.

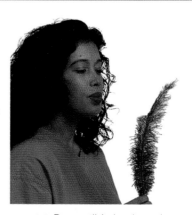

Level 2 Perceptible backward curve

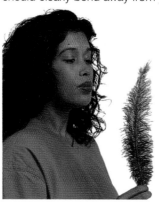

Level 1 Slight flutter

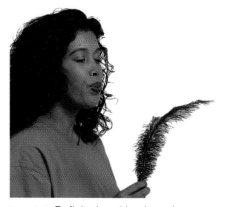

Level 3 Definite bend backwards

your mind off labour. Instead, they offer you a way to work with your body and adapt as the demands upon it change.

● Level 1: Relax and start breathing in. When you breathe out, make a little more of an effort than you would normally, and imagine all the air in your lungs being emptied out. Breathe in and out again in the same way, keeping a slow, regular, gentle rhythm. Breathe this way between contractions.

● Level 2: Use this as you feel a contraction coming. Breathe a little more quickly, and don't empty your lungs as you exhale. Continue breathing quickly, without emptying your lungs completely through the peak of the pain. As you feel the contraction ending, revert to slower breathing so that when the contraction is over, you are at level 1. Signal the end of the contraction with a long breath out.

● Level 3: During transition (see pp. 180–81) or towards the end of the first stage of labour, your contractions may be intense, requiring all your strength and concentration. Quick, shallow breathing will help. Breathe in quickly and blow out, then breathe in quickly again. (This is not the same as panting.) Some women find it helps to vocalize on the breath out – say "hoo hoo" as you do so, to maintain rhythm and concentration.

Hyperventilation

When you breathe out too much carbon dioxide – which sometimes happens when you panic or feel out of control – you start to hyperventilate, or overbreathe. You may feel faint or dizzy as a result.

Hyperventilation is not unusual in labour, and it is worth recognizing its signs and knowing how to deal with it. You can get your oxygen levels back to normal by cupping your hands over your nose and mouth and taking a few breaths; or breathe into a paper bag. Making a conscious effort to relax will also help. You may find it helpful if your partner breathes normally with you.

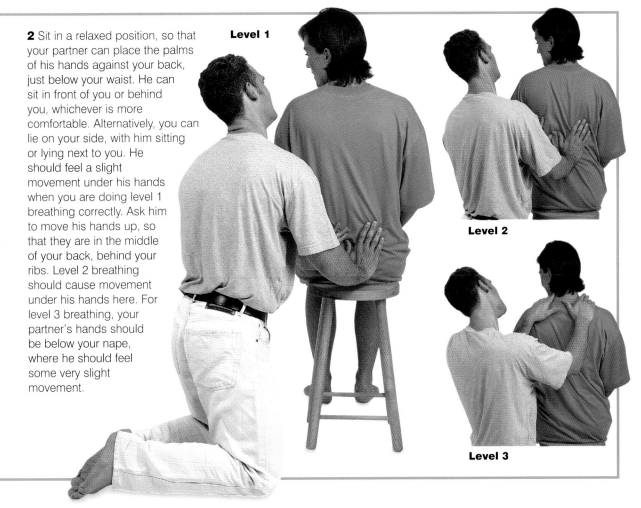

2 Sit in a relaxed position, so that your partner can place the palms of his hands against your back, just below your waist. He can sit in front of you or behind you, whichever is more comfortable. Alternatively, you can lie on your side, with him sitting or lying next to you. He should feel a slight movement under his hands when you are doing level 1 breathing correctly. Ask him to move his hands up, so that they are in the middle of your back, behind your ribs. Level 2 breathing should cause movement under his hands here. For level 3 breathing, your partner's hands should be below your nape, where he should feel some very slight movement.

Level 1

Level 2

Level 3

MASSAGE

Whether you visit a professional masseur or ask your partner to give you a massage, massage can stimulate, refresh, relax and comfort.

In addition to being immensely pleasurable, massage has definite therapeutic benefits. It improves circulation, alleviates digestive and elimination problems, helps with minor aches and stiffness, and encourages sleep.

If your partner is not confident about giving you a massage, you have the option of visiting a professional or inviting a masseur into your home. Massaging a partner, though, is a wonderfully intimate thing to do. The basic techniques are not difficult to learn: use the exercises here to guide you. You will get better as time goes by; ask each other what feels good, and note the effects on your body and mind the next day.

Use a light lotion or vegetable oil, perhaps including a few drops of essential oil (see Aromatherapy, opposite). This will prevent the masseur's hands from pulling or dragging on your skin and will leave your skin smooth and soft.

MASSAGE TECHNIQUES

Different techniques use different movements of the hands.
● Effleurage: stroking over a large area, using firm, slow movements.
● Percussion: chopping in short, quick movements (this should be avoided during pregnancy, except on the legs).
● Friction: rubbing in circular movements with one or more fingers, the thumbs or the heels of the hands.

● Pétrissage: grasping and squeezing, to stimulate the blood circulation and relax the muscles.

A MASSAGE SESSION

Lie on your side. Bend your lower leg slightly, and draw your upper leg up to a 90° angle, bending at the knee; place a cushion under the bent knee. Place other pillows or cushions around you to aid in your comfort – under your head, abdomen or shoulders. Have the masseur kneel or lie beside you.

If you don't have time for a whole body massage, don't hurry the movements. Focus on fewer areas instead.

MASSEURS: WHAT YOU CAN DO

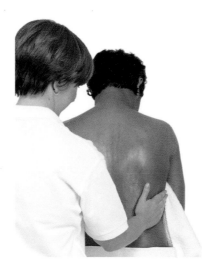

1 Start with the back, and use effleurage on either side of the backbone. Move from the waist to the shoulders and back again, covering the sides of the back. Repeat several times.

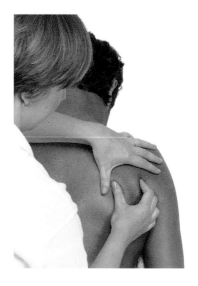

2 Grasp and squeeze the flesh of the back all over, starting from the spine and working towards the side, first on one side and then the other.

3 Now circle the pads of your fingers all over the back. Don't be afraid to press quite firmly, but ask the person receiving the massage to tell you if it becomes uncomfortable.

4 Repeat the same sequence of techniques on the buttocks.

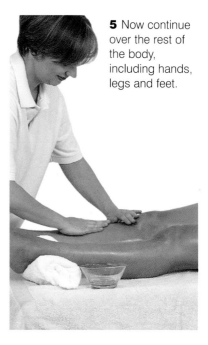

5 Now continue over the rest of the body, including hands, legs and feet.

Self-massage

This is a useful skill that you can use before and after pregnancy, to ease tension and energize yourself at any time.

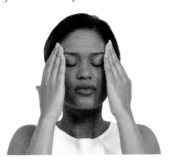

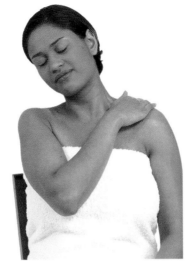

Face

Massaging the face is a gentle way to relieve headaches. Use a mild oil to avoid stretching the skin. Place your hands over your face and stroke slowly out towards your ears. Imagine any aches and tension being smoothed away as you stroke.

With your eyes closed, move your hands up your cheeks. Make small circles over your forehead with the tips of your fingers. Smooth your fingers up and across your brow.

Neck and shoulders

Relieve stiffness and aching in these areas by stroking down one side of your neck, over your shoulder and down your arm to your elbow. Repeat several times, then do the same on the other side.

Legs

You can ease any aches in your legs by rubbing oil into them, using smooth movements from ankle to thigh. Firmly and methodically squeeze and release the flesh on your thighs and then your calves. Then stroke each leg again. (See p. 48 for a useful exercise that helps to prevent cramps.)

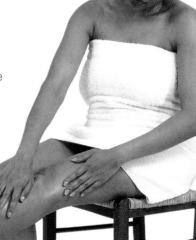

6 The abdomen can be massaged gently. Using the flat of your hand, apply light circular strokes. First work around the navel, then work outwards from it, concentrating on keeping your movements flowing and rhythmic.

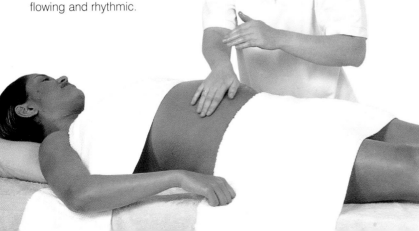

Aromatherapy

Using essential oils will make your massage more pleasant and relaxing. However, most aromatherapists recommend a weaker solution of essential oil during pregnancy than at other times to allow for increased skin sensitivity. Use five drops of essential oil to every two tablespoons of carrier oil.

It is also important to use a vegetable oil, such as almond, jojoba or sesame (mineral oils should be avoided during pregnancy).

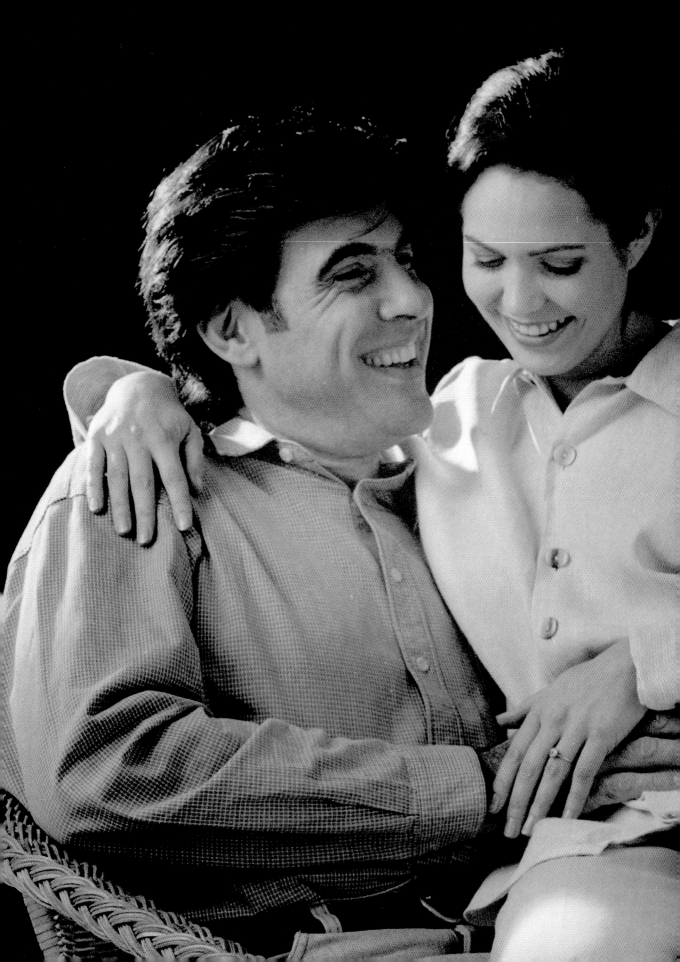

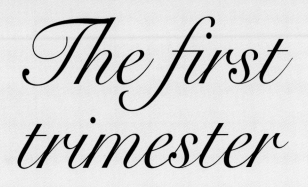

The first trimester

DOCTORS USUALLY *divide pregnancy into three trimesters of three months each. During the first three months of your pregnancy, you will experience:*

- *The excitement of learning that a new life has begun*

- *Physical changes as your body prepares to nurture your unborn baby*

- *Hormonal shifts that aid the formation of your baby's major organs*

- *Mood swings – from elation to panic or depression – as your mind and body adjust to your new role.*

This is also the time to choose the medical practitioner who will guide your antenatal care and to start thinking about where and how you would like to give birth.

CONCEPTION

Conception occurs when a sperm fertilizes an egg. A few days later, this rapidly dividing ball of cells implants in the lining of your uterus and pregnancy begins.

For conception to occur, sexual intercourse usually has to take place within 36 hours of ovulation (see pp. 26–27). Although millions of sperm escape from a woman's body because of gravity, and millions more simply die, about 2000 from each ejaculation succeed in their journey up the vagina. They pass through the cervix and uterus into the Fallopian tubes. Meanwhile, when the egg is released at ovulation, the Fallopian tube helps it travel with the movement of fine, hair-like cilia and contractions of the tube itself.

The egg may attract the sperm by releasing chemicals that act as a magnet. Numerous sperm may reach the egg, but only one releases enzymes to dissolve the egg's outer layer and penetrate it. The surface of the egg closes behind the successful sperm so that no others can enter. The nuclei of the egg and sperm fuse.

THE SEX OF YOUR BABY

It is at this stage that the sex of your baby is established. At the moment of fertilization, each

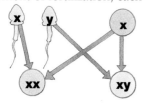

Sperm contain X or Y chromosomes (left), and eggs, only X. Two Xs will result in a girl, but if an X and a Y are joined, the baby will be a boy.

From fertilization to conception

Fertilization takes place in the upper part of the Fallopian tube about an hour after intercourse. Over the following few days, the resulting cell moves down the Fallopian tube to the uterus, dividing every 12–15 hours as it travels. When it reaches the uterus, it comprises about 100 cells, and it implants in the soft, spongy lining of the uterine wall. Conception has now taken place.

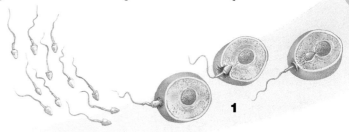

1 Fertilization
The fusing of the nuclei of egg and sperm forms a new cell of 46 chromosomes: 23 from the sperm, 23 from the egg.

2 Cell division
The new cell divides immediately in two and begins to move down the Fallopian tube. The cells, called blastomeres, continue to divide, becoming smaller with each division.

parent contributes one sex-determining chromosome, an X or a Y. Because women carry only X chromosomes and men carry both X and Y, the man's contribution determines the baby's sex. If the sex cell of the sperm is an X, the baby will be a girl; if it is a Y, the baby will be a boy.

THE PROCESS OF CONCEPTION
The fertilized egg travels from the Fallopian tube to the uterus. Cell division starts at fertilization and continues throughout the journey.

Conception takes place when the bundle of cells, now technically known as a blastocyst, implants in the uterine wall (see above).

Occasionally, the blastocyst implants not in the uterus but in a Fallopian tube. This situation, known as an ectopic pregnancy, often causes pain and bleeding. It's important to see your doctor immediately if such symptoms appear. The pregnancy will eventually miscarry, but without medical intervention, the tube may rupture, which can be life-threatening.

4 Implantation

The cluster of more than 100 cells – now called a blastocyst – hollows out a site on the wall of the uterus and becomes implanted. This process can cause slight bleeding, which you may interpret as a very light period.

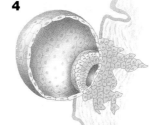

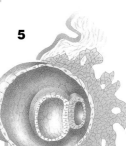

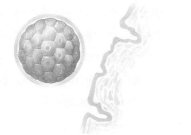

3 Arrival in the uterus

About 60 hours after fertilization, the cluster of cells, or morula, contains 8 to 16 blastomeres and reaches the uterus.

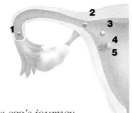

The egg's journey from the site of fertilization to implantation takes between five and seven days.

5 Conception

At the site of implantation, the outer layer of cells obtains nourishment from your bloodstream; this part of the outer layer will develop into the placenta.

More than one... or two

About 1 in every 80 pregnancies results in twins. As recently as 15 years ago, the figure was about 1 in 100 pregnancies. The increase is usually attributed to fertility treatments – particularly to the use of drugs to stimulate ovulation. Such treatment aside, women are more likely to have twins if they become pregnant after the age of 35. Afro-Caribbean women are twice as likely as those of European descent to have twins. And women with a family history of twins may inherit the tendency (see pp. 24–25).

About two-thirds of twins are non-identical, or fraternal. These occur when two eggs are released at ovulation and fertilized by separate sperm. Fraternal twins are no more alike than any other pair of siblings.

Identical twins result from the chance splitting of one fertilized egg into two. Always the same sex, identical twins share identical genetic make-ups.

Larger multiple births of identical and fraternal babies occur in the same way as twins do. Despite fertility treatments, these are rare: for example, only 1 in 800 pregnancies results in triplets and perhaps 1 in 8000 results in quadruplets.

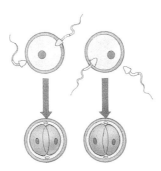

Fraternal twins develop when two separate eggs are fertilized, each by one sperm.

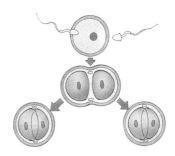

Identical twins develop when one sperm fertilizes one egg, which then splits into two.

ARE YOU PREGNANT?

If you have been trying to become pregnant, you'll be watching for signs. If your pregnancy is unplanned, some of the signs may go unnoticed.

The most obvious indication that you are pregnant is, of course, a missed period, although you may have one or more other signs.

A HOME TEST KIT

You can buy a pregnancy test kit from a chemist to use at home. Accurate from the first day of your missed period, the test checks for the presence in your urine of human chorionic gonadotropin (HCG), a hormone secreted only when you are pregnant. Since it is often most abundant first thing in the morning, kits usually recommend that you use the first sample of urine that you pass in the morning.

If you follow the instructions carefully, you can expect quick, accurate results. Occasionally, a test may give a "false negative" result, indicating that you are not pregnant when actually you are. This happens if there isn't enough hormone present to register a result. If you still don't have your period in a week's time, try the test again. A hydatiform mole (see p. 91), not a true pregnancy, is the only likely cause of a "false positive".

AT YOUR DOCTOR'S

If you're not sure of the results of a home test, doctors, hospitals, pregnancy advisory services and women's health clinics offer testing. Urine tests – the same as those you can do at home – are statistically more accurate

The telltale signs

Taste changes
The hormonal changes that sometimes contribute to pregnancy sickness may also make certain foods distasteful to you in early pregnancy.

Breast changes
Raised levels of progesterone may make your breasts feel full, heavy and tender as they prepare to produce milk. Your nipples may darken slightly in colour.

Pregnancy sickness
High levels of HCG, the relaxation of the muscles of your digestive system, increased stomach acid, and sensitivity to smell may contribute to nausea and vomiting (see pp. 84–85).

Fatigue
All your baby's major organs and the placenta are forming. The demands being made on your body may make you feel very tired.

Sensitivity
You may have a heightened sensitivity to smells, probably due to hormonal changes. Such odours as cigarette smoke or cooking smells may make you feel quite sick.

Frequent urination
Pregnancy hormones – relaxin, in particular – relax all your muscles, including those of the bladder. Increased blood flow through the kidneys causes an increase in urine production. There are also more fluids in your body because of the increased activity of your tissues and organs.

Vaginal discharge
Hormonal changes often cause an increase in vaginal discharge.

when done by professionals (they do more of them). Alternatively, you may be offered a blood test, which measures the precise amount of HCG in your bloodstream. This can be useful in dating a pregnancy accurately since the amount of HCG varies throughout pregnancy.

When you are one or two months into your pregnancy, your doctor can gently perform a pelvic examination. To the expert, the uterus will feel larger and somewhat softer than usual.

A POSITIVE RESULT

Consult your doctor as soon as you have a positive test result. He or she can guide you through your antenatal options – the care you can expect, tests you may want to make sure the baby is developing properly (see pp. 100–101), and any changes you should make in your lifestyle, diet and exercise regime. If your pregnancy is planned, you have probably been following the advice given in Chapter 1; if not, now is the time to start taking care of yourself and your unborn baby.

Estimated date of delivery

January	1	2	3	4	5	6	7	8	9	10	11	12	13	14	15	16	17	18	19	20	21	22	23	24	25	26	27	28	29	30	31
October	8	9	10	11	12	13	14	15	16	17	18	19	20	21	22	23	24	25	26	27	28	29	30	31	*1*	*2*	*3*	*4*	*5*	*6*	*7*

February	1	2	3	4	5	6	7	8	9	10	11	12	13	14	15	16	17	18	19	20	21	22	23	24	25	26	27	28
November	8	9	10	11	12	13	14	15	16	17	18	19	20	21	22	23	24	25	26	27	28	29	30	*1*	*2*	*3*	*4*	*5*

March	1	2	3	4	5	6	7	8	9	10	11	12	13	14	15	16	17	18	19	20	21	22	23	24	25	26	27	28	29	30	31
December	6	7	8	9	10	11	12	13	14	15	16	17	18	19	20	21	22	23	24	25	26	27	28	29	30	31	*1*	*2*	*3*	*4*	*5*

April	1	2	3	4	5	6	7	8	9	10	11	12	13	14	15	16	17	18	19	20	21	22	23	24	25	26	27	28	29	30
January	6	7	8	9	10	11	12	13	14	15	16	17	18	19	20	21	22	23	24	25	26	27	28	29	30	31	*1*	*2*	*3*	*4*

May	1	2	3	4	5	6	7	8	9	10	11	12	13	14	15	16	17	18	19	20	21	22	23	24	25	26	27	28	29	30	31
February	5	6	7	8	9	10	11	12	13	14	15	16	17	18	19	20	21	22	23	24	25	26	27	28	*1*	*2*	*3*	*4*	*5*	*6*	*7*

June	1	2	3	4	5	6	7	8	9	10	11	12	13	14	15	16	17	18	19	20	21	22	23	24	25	26	27	28	29	30
March	8	9	10	11	12	13	14	15	16	17	18	19	20	21	22	23	24	25	26	27	28	29	30	31	*1*	*2*	*3*	*4*	*5*	*6*

July	1	2	3	4	5	6	7	8	9	10	11	12	13	14	15	16	17	18	19	20	21	22	23	24	25	26	27	28	29	30	31
April	7	8	9	10	11	12	13	14	15	16	17	18	19	20	21	22	23	24	25	26	27	28	29	30	*1*	*2*	*3*	*4*	*5*	*6*	*7*

August	1	2	3	4	5	6	7	8	9	10	11	12	13	14	15	16	17	18	19	20	21	22	23	24	25	26	27	28	29	30	31
May	8	9	10	11	12	13	14	15	16	17	18	19	20	21	22	23	24	25	26	27	28	29	30	31	*1*	*2*	*3*	*4*	*5*	*6*	*7*

September	1	2	3	4	5	6	7	8	9	10	11	12	13	14	15	16	17	18	19	20	21	22	23	24	25	26	27	28	29	30
June	8	9	10	11	12	13	14	15	16	17	18	19	20	21	22	23	24	25	26	27	28	29	30	*1*	*2*	*3*	*4*	*5*	*6*	*7*

October	1	2	3	4	5	6	7	8	9	10	11	12	13	14	15	16	17	18	19	20	21	22	23	24	25	26	27	28	29	30	31
July	8	9	10	11	12	13	14	15	16	17	18	19	20	21	22	23	24	25	26	27	28	29	30	31	*1*	*2*	*3*	*4*	*5*	*6*	*7*

November	1	2	3	4	5	6	7	8	9	10	11	12	13	14	15	16	17	18	19	20	21	22	23	24	25	26	27	28	29	30
August	8	9	10	11	12	13	14	15	16	17	18	19	20	21	22	23	24	25	26	27	28	29	30	31	*1*	*2*	*3*	*4*	*5*	*6*

December	1	2	3	4	5	6	7	8	9	10	11	12	13	14	15	16	17	18	19	20	21	22	23	24	25	26	27	28	29	30	31
September	7	8	9	10	11	12	13	14	15	16	17	18	19	20	21	22	23	24	25	26	27	28	29	30	*1*	*2*	*3*	*4*	*5*	*6*	*7*

The chart above will help you calculate the day on which your baby is "due" – your estimated date of delivery, or EDD. Find the first day of your last menstrual period on the top line; the date below it is your EDD. The dates printed in italic at the end of each EDD line indicate the start of the following month.

Keep in mind, however, that only 5 percent of babies arrive on their due date. It is often easier to think of your baby arriving any time from two weeks before to two weeks after the due date. Twins are almost always born early.

REPRODUCTIVE HORMONES

Hormones are chemical messengers that stimulate parts of the body to perform certain functions.

Produced by the endrocrine glands, hormones are chemical substances that the bloodstream transports to the cells or tissues they will affect. Along with your nervous system, hormones control the functions of your organs. Among their numerous responsibilities is the vital role they play in every aspect of reproduction: regulating the menstrual cycle, supporting the pregnancy, triggering labour, assisting with delivery and stimulating the production of breast milk.

The pituitary gland, at the base of the brain, produces eight hormones that control all the body's other hormone-producing glands, including the ovaries. Among the pituitary hormones are the gonadotropins, which stimulate the gonads (the ovaries and the testes), causing sexual development and enabling reproduction.

Most female hormones – principally oestrogen (an umbrella term that refers to several different hormones) and progesterone – are produced in the ovaries.

The pituitary gland is responsible for controlling other hormone-producing glands and organs, including the ovaries (1), parathyroids (2), thyroid (3), pancreas (4) and kidneys (5).

How hormones affect your body

When you aren't pregnant ...

During your fertile years, if you are in good health, your body is regulated by the menstrual cycle, which is orchestrated by a number of hormones.

The part of the brain adjoining the pituitary gland, called the hypothalamus, triggers the pituitary gland to secrete follicle-stimulating hormone (FSH). FSH travels in the bloodstream to an ovary and instructs it to prepare an egg for ovulation. Several cells gather around the egg, forming a ball-like structure, called a follicle, within the ovary. The fluid produced by the follicle cells is rich in oestrogen hormones.

A number of follicles begin to develop, but eventually one develops faster than the others and makes its way to the surface of the ovary. In response to the high levels of oestrogen in the bloodstream, the pituitary gland produces luteinizing hormone (LH). The surge of LH causes the follicle to release its egg and also transforms the burst follicle into the corpus luteum. The corpus luteum is then stimulated by the hormone luteotropin to produce progesterone.

If a fertilized egg does not implant in the wall of the uterus, levels of oestrogen and progesterone fall; it is this drop in hormones that causes the uterine lining to shed – which is your period.

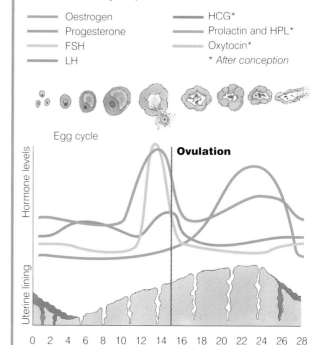

▬ Oestrogen	▬ HCG*	
▬ Progesterone	▬ Prolactin and HPL*	
▬ FSH	▬ Oxytocin*	
▬ LH	*After conception*	

Egg cycle

Hormone levels

Ovulation

Uterine lining

0 2 4 6 8 10 12 14 16 18 20 22 24 26 28

At conception ...

When a developing fertilized egg embeds in the wall of your uterus, it triggers the production of the hormone human chorionic gonadotropin (HCG). This hormone prevents menstruation. At the same time, the corpus luteum continues to grow and produce progesterone. Progesterone, together with oestrogen synthesized by the ovarian follicle, helps to sustain the pregnancy and build up the nutritious lining (endometrium) of the uterus.

The progesterone influences other parts of your body, too. For example, your breasts begin to prepare for lactation. The areolae enlarge and darken, and Montgomery's tubercles become more prominent – these will lubricate the nipple during breast-feeding (see p. 106). The breasts themselves swell, as tissue in which milk will be produced and stored is created. These changes are responsible for the soreness or tenderness most women feel in their breasts during pregnancy.

Reactions to the hormones may cause early pregnancy sickness and even mood swings.

During pregnancy ...

From the 10th week on, the placenta takes over the task of nourishing the developing foetus and creates high levels of progesterone, which continue to inhibit ovulation. Progesterone also relaxes your blood vessels – so that they can carry a greater volume of blood, which helps your heart and lungs cope with the demands of pregnancy – and the smooth muscle of such organs as the uterus, bladder and intestines.

The placenta also secretes relaxin, which causes your soft connective tissues and ligaments to relax. Production of prolactin and human placental lactogen (HPL), milk-making hormones, are triggered by the pituitary gland and the placenta. Oestrogen and progesterone delay milk production.

Your adrenal glands release extra cortisone, which may reduce allergic reactions common to disorders like asthma. Levels of the hormones adrenaline, noradrenaline and endorphin also rise, increasing the rhythm of the heart rate and breathing rate, and making the digestive system work more quickly. They also account for mood swings, as they heighten the "fight or flight" mechanism.

At childbirth ...

The hormone oxytocin stimulates your uterus to begin contracting in order to help push the baby out. Doctors may use synthetic oxytocin to induce labour or to speed it up if contractions are weak or slow.

Once the placenta has been delivered (see pp. 192–93), levels of progesterone and oestrogen quickly fall, and prolactin and human placental lactogen (HPL) can begin their work.

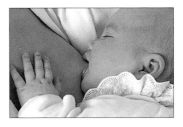

When the baby begins to suck, the action sends impulses to your pituitary gland. This releases more oxytocin, which acts as a stimulant. Tiny contractions in the cells that store milk in your breast push the milk out. In the early days, oxytocin also causes contractions of the uterus as you breast-feed your baby; these contractions are responsible for "afterpains".

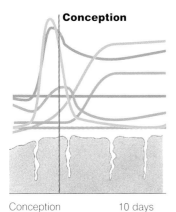

Conception

Conception   10 days

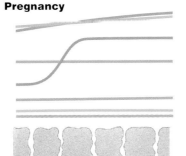

Pregnancy

10 days   9 months

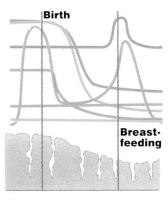

Birth

Breast-feeding

Birth   Breast-feeding

THE EMOTIONAL IMPACT

Physical changes are only half the story of pregnancy. The emotional impact and its effect on you and your relationships can be just as important.

Q *I always looked forward to being a mother. Now that it's finally about to happen, I'm scared. I can't believe that I will ever be good enough. Is my lack of confidence normal?*

A It's not at all uncommon to be shaken by the enormous responsibility of parenthood. Sometimes, a lack of confidence may be a reaction to your own experiences of being parented – good or bad. You may think your parents were great and believe that you'll never be as good as they were. Or the memory of an unhappy childhood that's been largely forgotten can re-emerge, with old resentments and hurts taking centre stage – perhaps for the first time.

Talk to your partner, to friends who are parents, and to your own parents. You may find that the impending baby brings the generations closer and your present feelings subside as you gain insight into what your parents felt, and feel, about you.

Reading some books on parenting, joining antenatal classes, and asking the experts about anything that bothers you will boost your confidence in your ability to be a mother.

Q *I feel negative about my pregnancy and guilty because I don't relish the thought of having a baby. Will I always feel this way?*

A Not all women welcome the thought of having a baby. Even when the pregnancy is planned, women may have second thoughts once it's actually confirmed. But the powerful hormonal changes that are happening to you now are preparing you – almost despite yourself – to meet the needs of your new baby. Once he or she arrives, you will almost certainly be overwhelmed by feelings of love and protectiveness for this tiny person whom you and your partner have created and who depends entirely on you.

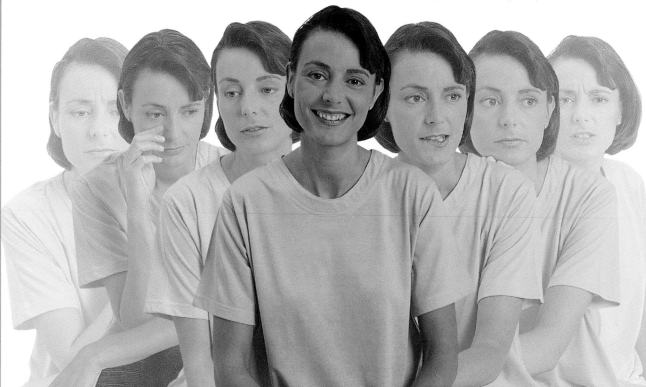

Q *After years of fertility treatments, my wife and I have just learned that she is pregnant. Our families and friends are overjoyed. I'm relieved that the ordeal of "trying for a baby" is over, but now life has returned to normal and I feel deflated. Is pregnancy really this ordinary?*

A It can be. Many couples who have taken a long time to conceive (even those who have not needed help) find that their focus has been so fixed on becoming pregnant that they cannot see past this stage to the pregnancy itself, or beyond that to becoming parents.

It may also be that you are feeling unsure of your own role. Your emotions have been wholly engaged as you and your partner have tried to conceive and have watched for signs that you have succeeded. Now that it has happened, your partner may seem to need you less. But she still needs your support. Remain involved in the pregnancy by accompanying her to antenatal classes, clinic appointments, and testing. Talk to each other about the baby and your life together after the birth. Your excitement should return as the birth nears.

Most women are thrilled at the prospect of becoming a mother. But it is completely normal to have some misgivings as well – you are, after all, taking on responsibility for the health and well-being of a new person. Share your concerns with those around you, especially your partner.

Q *I feel very up-and-down, and some days I lose my temper with my husband for no obvious reason. There are times when I become incredibly moved by a news item on TV and find myself crying. I have been told that my moods are governed by my hormones and that things will settle down in time. Is this true?*

A It's perfectly normal for your hormones to produce marked ups and downs during pregnancy. Elation at the thought of being a mother can make the highs higher, and fatigue and sickness may make the lows seem even lower. You can offset this by making sure you get enough rest and eat well. Avoid caffeine, chocolate and other quick, sugary fixes – although they lift your mood temporarily, they also worsen the lows.

Exercise regularly, by walking, swimming or continuing a modified form of aerobics class two or three times a week. Exercise triggers the release of endorphins, sometimes referred to as the "happy hormones".

Above all, even if you don't feel like making love, stay in close touch with your partner. Talk through your feelings with him and make the most of the fact that, right now, it's still just the two of you.

While mood swings are a normal part of pregnancy, depression is not. If you feel unable to cope with the lows for more than a week or two, talk to your doctor. He or she may recommend that you seek more specialized help.

Q *We wanted a baby, but not quite yet. We've just taken on a large financial commitment. We're now worried about the cost of having a child. Is it really as expensive as we're told?*

A Babies' needs are very basic: food, shelter, warmth and love. It's true that as they grow, children add expenses, but most parents manage to grow into the demands. Don't allow worries over possible future financial problems to dominate your pregnancy now. Use these months to seek out inexpensive equipment and clothing (see pp. 136–39), and don't be ashamed to accept hand-me-downs from friends and family.

Q *I didn't realize that child care in my area is so expensive. Neither of us can afford to give up work, and I am really concerned that we won't be able to manage.*

A For most working parents, the biggest outlay after having a baby is child care. And this is the one area where you can't – and won't want to – cut corners, unless you have a trusted relative who is willing to help. Some of the different kinds of child care are detailed on pages 120–23. Read them all, then consider which is best for you and for your baby. It is important to consider all your options, including one parent leaving a job. It may be that you need less than you think you do once you eliminate the hidden costs of pursuing a career.

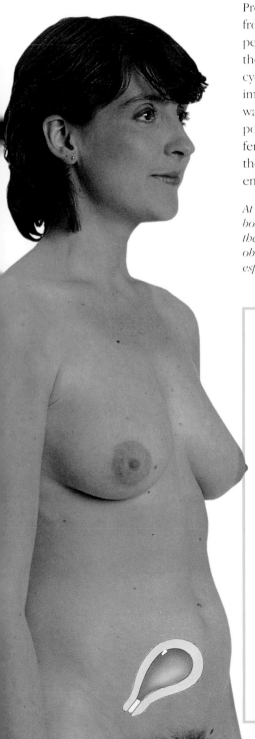

FOR YOU

Pregnancy is usually counted from the first day of your last period. The first month includes the portion of the menstrual cycle that took place before implantation, when your body was preparing your womb for a potential pregnancy. After fertilization, hormones prevent the lining of the womb – the endometrium – from starting to

At the end of the first month, your body and womb are likely to remain their normal size. It will not be obvious that you are pregnant, especially in a first pregnancy.

break down, as it would in a normal menstrual cycle. While the ball of cells (blastocyst) is dividing and travelling down the Fallopian tube (see pp. 62–63), hormones cause the endometrium to thicken in readiness for implantation. Once implantation occurs, hormones suppress ovulation (see pp. 66–67).

You may not be aware that you are pregnant, but especially if you have been trying to conceive and are watching for indications that you may be pregnant, you may notice some of the early signs (see pp. 64–65).

Total weight gain

Some women start to gain weight right from the start of pregnancy and by the end of the first three months may have put on 1 kg (2 lb) or more – particularly on the hips, breasts and thighs. Your body requires extra fat to sustain you during pregnancy and breast-feeding.

Depending on your build and whether you were underweight when you conceived, you are likely to gain a total of 10–16 kg (22–35 lb). Most of this weight accumulates in the second half of pregnancy, although it's common to gain no more than 250 g (½ lb) in the last few weeks.

Nowadays, less emphasis is placed on weight gain than in previous years. It used to be thought that pregnant women should be encouraged to control their weight strictly. We now know

that some women naturally gain more than others. Moderate, steady weight gain, a healthy diet and a good level of fitness may help to prevent many discomforts, such as varicose veins and backache.

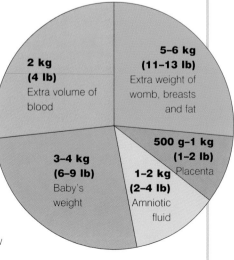

2 kg (4 lb) Extra volume of blood

5–6 kg (11–13 lb) Extra weight of womb, breasts and fat

3–4 kg (6–9 lb) Baby's weight

500 g–1 kg (1–2 lb) Placenta

1–2 kg (2–4 lb) Amniotic fluid

FOR YOUR BABY

Five to seven days after the egg is fertilized (see pp. 62–63), the blastocyst reaches the womb and becomes embedded in the lining of the womb. By this time it is known as an embryo.

The embryo secretes its own protective substances, which help to change your immune system so that your body will accept the baby. The baby's genetic make-up – half from you and half from your partner – would otherwise produce antibodies in your body.

The outer cells of the embryo start to reach out in the following week, attaching themselves to your blood vessels and forming the first links with your system. This begins formation of the chorionic villi, which will become the placenta. Your body's response to fertilization is to produce human chorionic gonadotropin (see pp. 66–67), which circulates around your body, appearing in your blood and urine.

The inner cells of the embryo then divide into three layers – each one containing the beginnings of a different part of your baby.

26–27 days
The organs, limb buds, and a head with a mouth and eyes appear.

21 days
Somites, or sections of tissue, form. These will be the nerves and muscles of the embryo.

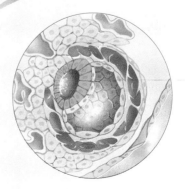

12–15 days
The chorionic villi form, and the shapes of the umbilical cord and the baby start to appear.

5–7 days
The blastocyst embeds itself into the uterine wall.

Actual size
This incredibly complex organism is about the same size as the period at the end of this sentence. It is contained in a gestational sac which is about 6 mm (¼ in) in diameter.

APPROACHES TO CHILDBIRTH

As modern society increasingly comes to accept childbirth as a natural process, you will find a growing number of options available for giving birth.

Doctors have learned how to eliminate most of the pain associated with childbirth. Every day they use technological intervention in problem deliveries to save thousands of babies who might otherwise not have survived. But until recently, such advances turned childbirth into an impersonal procedure in many hospitals, and mothers and fathers had little say in how the birth was managed.

Today most doctors accept that you have choices that allow you to decide how much medical intervention you want during labour and the birth itself. Many women have a more positive experience when they have a say in their care, including how and where to give birth (see pp. 80–81). Studies have shown that these women feel more fulfilled in the birthing process and suffer from less depression afterwards, regardless of whether their labour was easy or problematic, long or short.

The time to start thinking about childbirth is in the early stages of your pregnancy. You'll need time to research the possibilities. Consider whether to use the public hospital system, a private hospital, a private obstetrician, who may deliver in either, or even an independent midwife. Although you cannot decide everything in advance, you may find it helpful to talk matters over with your partner, medical advisers, family and friends (see pp. 132–33 for advice on making a birth plan).

As you consider various approaches to childbirth, keep in mind those issues that are most important to you.

A MANAGED BIRTH

Some mothers feel safer and less anxious if their birth is closely managed and controlled by their carers, with technical support readily available. You may know in advance that you want medication for pain relief (see pp. 172–73). Or you may be advised to have a particular kind of pain reliever if your baby's birth is being induced (see pp. 168–69).

Your doctor may recommend a caesarean before you go into labour for a variety of reasons. If your baby assumes a footling breech or transverse presentation, for example, surgery may be advisable (see pp. 166–67). Doctors also encourage medical intervention when mothers have certain medical conditions, such as hypertension, kidney disease or active genital herpes.

NATURAL CHILDBIRTH

This is an umbrella term that refers to giving birth without medication and intervention from doctors and nurses. In its strictest interpretation, this approach rules out such procedures as induction, acceleration of labour, artificial rupture of the membranes, continuous electronic foetal monitoring, use of forceps or vacuum extraction, or caesarean section. Natural childbirth relies on support and encouragement from the doctor or midwife, and your birthing partner. Breathing and relaxation techniques may help you to manage the pain and eliminate the need for medication.

If natural childbirth appeals to you, treat it as an ideal. If unforeseen complications arise, however, or your labour is painful or prolonged, you should be prepared to seek the advice of your carers.

ACTIVE CHILDBIRTH

This is a form of natural childbirth, but it is often taught as a separate method to couples. Active childbirth involves moving around in the early stages of

The days when partners anxiously paced a waiting room or corridor while women gave birth are long gone. Birthing is now recognized as a family experience, and your partner will be encouraged to be at the birth. He may support you physically, by massaging or rubbing parts of your body that are tense; or mentally, by reminding you of breathing techniques, for example; or emotionally, by cheering you on and praising your efforts.

labour, which may increase the speed with which the cervix dilates. It also alleviates the tension that can build when you are sitting or lying down simply waiting for the next contraction. When contractions become stronger, your partner or a birth companion supports you physically – for example, in a squatting position. Delivering a baby while lying flat on your back has real disadvantages: it inhibits the supply of oxygen to the baby and it requires that you push against gravity, instead of letting gravity help you deliver the baby.

The room used for active childbirth is typically equipped with chairs, beanbags and furniture of different heights. These allow a labouring woman to find a variety of comfortable positions and to keep moving for as long as she wants.

PSYCHOPROPHYLAXIS

Made widely popular in the West through the work of Fernand Lamaze (see p. 75), this technique was first practised in Russia. Psychoprophylaxis prepares the mind for labour and birth, using breathing exercises that help reduce and distract from the pain. Some teachers of antenatal classes combine this training with relaxation techniques that suppress pain, prevent fear-induced tension, and aid the birthing process. Critics of this approach argue that it is

better for a woman to work with her body and actively use the pain of contractions to help labour along.

WATER BIRTH

Many women find relaxing in a bath of warm water a good way to cope with labour contractions, a factor that led some women to stay in the water throughout labour and delivery.

Many mothers who have tried a water birth have found it a positive, loving way to bring their baby into the world. If you think you would like a water birth, check whether the hospital you choose has the facilities. If you want a home birth, pools are available to hire (look in the small ads in pregnancy and parenting magazines for suppliers). Check that your midwife has delivered a baby this way before and can give you the support you need.

WHICH IS BEST FOR YOU?

Many hospitals are equipped to deal with most types of birth and will be able to accommodate your preferences.

Your health and that of your baby must be the determining factors in any decisions you make. If you are healthy and the pregnancy is normal, you will have the most freedom of choice. A woman who has developed a condition such as pre-eclampsia (see p. 143) or placenta praevia (see pp. 176–77), or who has a history of complications, will be more limited.

Read as much as you can about your options and talk to friends about their experiences, then make your decision.

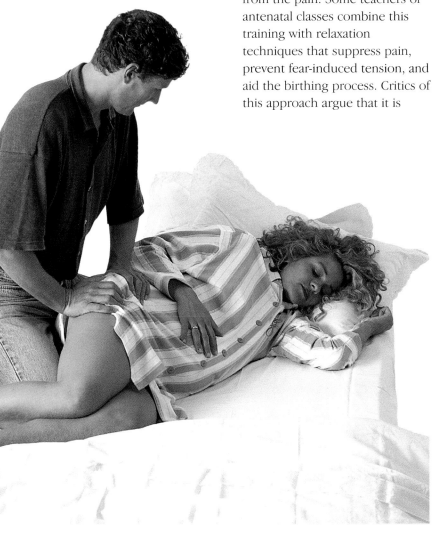

WHO'S WHO IN YOUR CARE

Having a healthy pregnancy and a good birth experience depend on you, your partner and the health-care professionals you choose to assist you.

Depending on where you choose to give birth, various health-care professionals may be involved in your antenatal care. Many women choose "shared care", seeing their GP for some antenatal visits and attending the hospital for others.

YOUR GP

Your general practitioner is interested in all aspects of the health of your whole family: you, your partner and your children.

Your first visit after a positive pregnancy test should be to your GP. If you do not have a GP, now is a very good time to find one. Not all GPs offer shared antenatal care, and you may wish to find one that does, or you can choose to have all your antenatal appointments at the hospital.

To find a GP with a special interest in pregnancy and childbirth, contact your local hospital's antenatal clinic. You could also ask for advice at the local child health clinic, or ask friends who have recently had babies what they thought of their GP.

Before your first visit to the hospital in which you are going to have your baby or – if you plan a home birth – to your GP or midwife, write down those questions relating to the birth that seem most important to you.

A CONSULTANT OBSTETRICIAN

If you have your baby in a public hospital, you will be under the nominal care of a consultant obstetrician. In a pregnancy that is progressing normally, however, you will probably see him or her infrequently. If your pregnancy is considered high-risk (if, for example, you have a history of three or more miscarriages, have diabetes or suffer from heart or kidney disease, or develop severe pre-eclampsia), the consultant will see you at some or all of your antenatal visits, and may be on hand when you go into labour.

A MIDWIFE

Midwives are trained to handle normal pregnancies and deliver babies when labour is unproblematic, as is usually the case. Unfortunately, in most

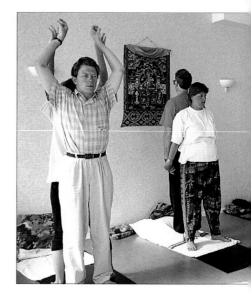

Limbering-up exercises are an essential part of Lamaze training (see box, right). These prepare your body physically for the demands of labour and birth. The mental preparation is equally important. Lamaze classes aim to lessen the perception of pain through breathing exercises.

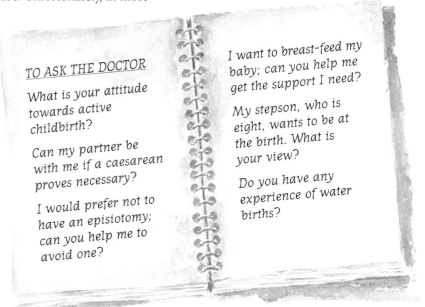

TO ASK THE DOCTOR

What is your attitude towards active childbirth?

Can my partner be with me if a caesarean proves necessary?

I would prefer not to have an episiotomy; can you help me to avoid one?

I want to breast-feed my baby; can you help me get the support I need?

My stepson, who is eight, wants to be at the birth. What is your view?

Do you have any experience of water births?

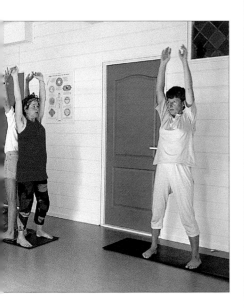

hospitals the midwives in the antenatal clinic and the midwives in the delivery suite are separate teams, and although you may see the same midwife at most of your antenatal visits, you are likely to meet a new one when in labour. If you are having a home birth, your midwife will stay with you throughout your labour and deliver the baby.

Remember that if at any time you are unhappy with any of your carers you can ask to be seen by someone else. You should always be consulted before anyone who you have not seen previously sits in on any of your antenatal appointments.

Innovators in childbirth teaching

Since the 1950s, a wealth of books and videos aimed at presenting alternative ideas about pregnancy and childbirth have been produced. At the time some of these works appeared, they propounded ideas that were largely dismissed by healthcare professionals and parents. But gradually some of the views presented have made their way into mainstream healthcare. Here are some of the names – and the main tenets of their philosophies – that may be mentioned by your doctor or midwife, or at antenatal classes, or that you may find reference to in pregnancy- and birth-related literature.

You do not, of course, have to follow one approach slavishly: many women borrow those elements of the various philosophies that meet their needs best.

Robert Bradley

The "inventor" of so-called husband-coached childbirth in the 1970s, this American doctor promoted a healthy diet and exercise during pregnancy to prepare the body for labour and delivery, and he advocated drug-free childbirth. He believed that this could be achieved if a woman worked with her body, using deep abdominal breathing during labour rather than trying to distract herself from the pain.

Sheila Kitzinger

In her works, Kitzinger focuses on the rights and needs of the mother to have the sort of birth she wants, where she wants. Sceptical about institutional practices, she has written extensively on home birth. Her *Good Birth Guide*, published in the 1980s, evaluated hospital birth from the consumer's point of view and led to changes in hospital practices worldwide.

Fernand Lamaze

Influenced by the British doctor Grantley Dick-Read's *Childbirth Without Fear*, the French physician Fernand Lamaze outlined *accouchement sans douleur* ("childbirth without pain") in the 1950s. He believed that the pain of childbirth was heightened by fear and tension, so he advocated relaxation techniques, training and practice to respond to pain in positive rather than negative ways.

Frederick Leboyer

The French doctor Frederick Leboyer wrote *Birth Without Violence*, first published in the 1970s. Leboyer asked why the birth environment was not geared to the sensitivities of the newborn. He felt that standard obstetrics – which ignored the effect on a baby of bright lights, noise, and separation from his or her mother – could be damaging to the baby. A Leboyer birth takes place in a dimly lit room, and is attended by quiet, respectful carers who support and encourage the mother through the delivery, handle the baby gently and lovingly, and make sure mother and baby share the precious first few hours of the baby's life.

Michel Odent

In *Entering the World*, his most widely read book, the French doctor Michel Odent argued that childbirth should be as technology-free as possible. He advocated active childbirth (see pp. 72–73) and was one of the first obstetricians to recognize the value to some women of labouring in water.

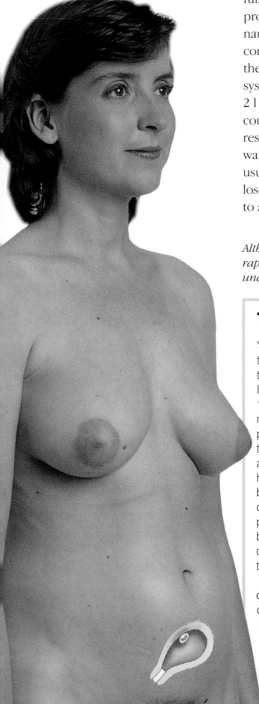

FOR YOU

As the placenta starts to function fully, the surge in hormones it produces may make you feel nauseous and can cause constipation. Pregnancy increases the demands on your circulatory system, which produces an extra 2 l (3 pints) of blood in the course of the 40 weeks. As a result you may feel puffy and want to urinate more often than usual. Sickness may make you lose your appetite and contribute to any feelings of fatigue. Eat well

Although your baby is developing rapidly in your uterus, others may be unable to tell that you are pregnant.

and make getting plenty of rest a priority.

If you are thrilled to be pregnant, you probably want to tell everyone. But early miscarriage is not uncommon (as many as one in six pregnancies ends in miscarriage). If you do not wish the world to be aware of your loss if you do miscarry, tell only your partner and one or two others. On the other hand, some women have been grateful to be able to share their sorrow and valued the support of friends at the loss of a pregnancy. By the end of the third month you can announce your news with confidence.

The placenta

Your baby's life-support system, the placenta, develops during the second month of pregnancy. It is fully functioning by 10 to 12 weeks, collecting oxygen and nutrients from your bloodstream, processing them, and passing them on to the baby. It also acts as a filter, straining out some hazards before they reach your baby. Some of your immunities to disease cross the placenta to protect your baby, and all of your baby's waste, including carbon dioxide, returns across the placenta to your body for disposal.

The placenta develops from the chorionic villi. The chorion is the outer surface of the sac holding the embryo; the finger-like villi grow out of the chorion. On one side the villi burrow into the uterine wall to receive

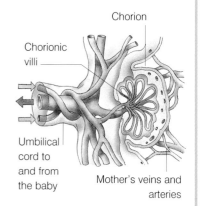

Chorion

Chorionic villi

Umbilical cord to and from the baby

Mother's veins and arteries

nourishment from you. The chorion becomes the outer surface of the placenta, and the villi, on the opposite side, flatten out. As the structure grows, it becomes more complex. It reaches its full thickness of about 2.5 cm (1 in) by the 16th week but continues to grow in diameter. It weighs about 500 g (1 lb) and is 20 cm (8 in) across at delivery.

FOR YOUR BABY

Between the 7th and 11th weeks of pregnancy, the tiny embryo becomes recognizable as a human form. By the eighth week, a distinct head develops, much larger than the rest of the body. The trunk has become straight, but the head still bends forwards to the chest. The tail, which was visible in the first month, shortens and disappears.

The embryonic period is complete by the 10th week after conception; the baby then enters the foetal stage and is referred to as a foetus. Much of the important work of forming the internal organs, the brain and nervous system, and the skeleton occurs in this month.

The embryo contains three layers of cells. The baby's nervous system starts to form when the top layer folds in on itself to make a tube. From this neural tube, the baby's spinal cord and brain will develop.

Major developments of the baby's internal organs take place in the second layer of cells; in the second month the lungs, liver, kidneys and digestive system become well established.

The third layer of embryonic cells becomes the heart. The foetus has its own blood vessels by this time, some of which connect to your blood system in the uterine wall, and it's these that become the umbilical cord, which holds the blood vessels that act as the pathway into and out of the placenta.

Arms and legs
The limb buds have extended to form recognizable arms and legs; slight depressions in the hands and feet show where the fingers and toes will be.

Inside the uterus
The umbilical cord has elongated, and the foetus is floating freely inside the amniotic sac, which protects the baby throughout the pregnancy.

Head and face
The facial features are becoming more obvious: the mouth and tongue have formed; the eyes and nostrils, which formed at the sides of the head, are now at the front; and the ears have moved from the neck towards the head.

Size
At the end of nine weeks, the embryo has doubled its size of just two weeks before. It now measures 16 mm (⅔ in), the size of a small grape.

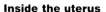

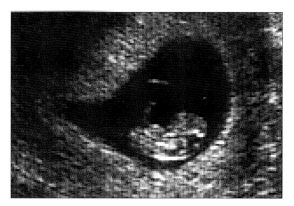

By the eighth week, the embryo's shape has changed. There is a larger, rounded end, which is the head. An ultrasound scan taken at this time will show the heart beating.

THE FIRST ANTENATAL VISIT

Expect the first visit to your doctor after your pregnancy is confirmed to be one of the longest. Many of the tests done at this time will not be repeated.

When you visit your doctor for an initial check-up, he or she will ask questions and carry out several tests to establish your basic health profile. Later your doctor or midwife will use this information as a comparison to gauge how your pregnancy is progressing.

While your doctor or midwife is finding out about you, you can learn more about him or her and about your pregnancy. Don't be afraid to ask any questions that you may have. Nothing that is causing you concern is too trivial to mention at a check-up.

Your doctor will ask you about this pregnancy and any previous ones (including miscarriages and terminations), and he or she will question you about any past history of serious illness, allergies, gynaecological infections and surgery. You may also be asked for information about your parents' and your partner's health, about any illnesses or medical conditions in either of your families, and about alcohol, drug and medication use.

You will then be given a series of tests. Some of these are administered once only; others will be repeated at each antenatal visit. Whenever you have tests, make sure that you understand the procedures and results. Nothing about your antenatal care should be a mystery to you.

ONE-OFF TESTS

Your doctor will perform baseline blood tests, which involves taking a small sample of blood with a syringe. The sample is analysed to identify your blood type, to determine if you are rhesus (Rh) positive or negative (see p. 24), and to check your immunity to rubella (German measles).

Depending on where you live, and sometimes on who your

Recording your pregnancy

Your doctor or midwife will keep a record of your antenatal visits (referred to as your notes), which will include: physical details, as well as information about any previous pregnancies, miscarriages or terminations; a record of any dietary advice or information he or she gives you; the plan for your care throughout your pregnancy; the schedule for such procedures as ultrasound or amniocentesis; your birth plan (see pp. 132–33); and any correspondence between you, the doctor or other health professionals.

Some doctors suggest that you keep these notes yourself. Others simply give you an abridged version to carry with you. This notes such basic information about you as your blood type and some of the readings that are taken at each visit, such as your blood pressure

and the size of your uterus.

You may want to carry these notes with you at all times so that in the unlikely event that you need urgent medical treatment, a practitioner has immediate access to information about your pregnancy.

You may also want to keep your own notebook in which to record more personal information. Jot down questions as you think of them so that you remember everything when you have your check-up. Write down the answers given to your questions as well, to maintain a record of any advice you are offered. Later you can add such information as when you first feel the baby move, hiccup or kick; take notes at your antenatal classes; jot down the names of pieces of equipment that friends have found useful; and write down what you intend to pack in your hospital bag.

First antenatal visit: 6/7

Blood type: O+

Blood pressure: 120/70

Height: 1.73 m (5 ft 8 in)

Weight: 65 kg (10 stone 2 lb)

Height of uterus: 7.5 cm (3 in)

Use your pregnancy notebook as both notepad and diary. It will provide a unique personal record of these exciting months.

doctor is, you may be tested for various sexually transmitted diseases (STDs), including HIV, the virus that causes AIDS. Ask which conditions are being looked for, particularly if you suspect that you are at risk of having contracted an STD.

If you are at risk of having contracted HIV, ask for an opportunity to discuss HIV testing and counselling. If you know you are HIV positive, tell your doctor. You will be monitored carefully and given medication to reduce the risk of transmitting the virus to your baby during delivery.

You may also have a cervical smear to rule out any possible abnormalities of the cervix. If your smear shows an infection, you can be treated so that it will not interfere with your pregnancy. If pre-cancerous cell changes are identified, they can be monitored.

You may be weighed and measured. Being seriously underweight or overweight (generally 20 percent below or above the average weight for your height) may make your pregnancy more difficult. Some midwives will monitor your weight at every visit during your pregnancy; others see no point in weighing an obviously healthy woman.

Your breasts and nipples will be examined. If you have inverted nipples, you may be advised to wear a nipple shield under your bra for a short period each day, increasing the time as your pregnancy progresses. This gently pulls the nipple out so that it will be ready for breast-feeding.

ROUTINE TESTS

At each visit, you will be asked to supply a urine sample, which will

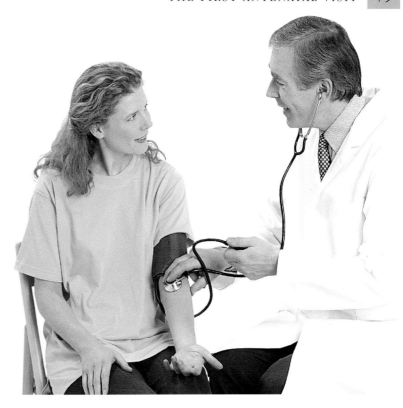

be tested for traces of sugar and protein. A change in sugar level may indicate so-called gestational diabetes. Some women develop diabetes during pregnancy (see p. 143), but providing this is controlled through careful diet or insulin, it will not harm you or your baby. It disappears after the baby is born.

Protein in your urine may be a sign of infection or pregnancy-induced hypertension. Infections of the kidney and bladder may also show up in a urine test.

Your blood pressure will be monitored to check that it stays within the normal range (100 to 140 over 60 to 90). If your doctor tells you that your blood pressure is slightly raised, don't panic. Pregnant women often have a single higher reading, caused by hurry or anxiety. If your blood pressure is higher on two successive visits, your doctor may want to monitor you more closely.

The blood pressure reading taken at your first antenatal visit is an important baseline. Blood pressure usually falls a little during the first few months of pregnancy. This is why you may feel faint or dizzy on occasion. Blood pressure then rises slightly around the seventh month. If you differ from this pattern, your midwife may suggest more frequent antenatal appointments to keep a close watch on your pregnancy.

Your doctor or midwife will feel the outside of your abdomen to gauge how much your uterus and baby have grown. You may also have an internal examination, again to determine the size of your uterus. This provides another indication of how long you have been pregnant and helps alert the doctor early to any internal problem, such as fibroids. He or she will also check for any abnormalities in your pelvis, vagina and cervix that might affect the delivery.

WHERE TO GIVE BIRTH

You will probably enjoy childbirth more if you find your surroundings comfortable and your attendants friendly, helpful and professional.

Q *How can I find out about the policies and practices of different hospitals and what it might be like to give birth in them?*

A Ask your GP, who may recommend a particular hospital to you. And speak to mothers who have had a baby in the past year or so. You can also ring hospitals and simply ask about procedures. From this you should be able to get a good idea of their facilities as well as their general policies on the length of stay, visiting arrangements and so on.

Q *Can I visit the hospital or unit before I choose whether or not to have my baby there?*

A Yes. Phone the hospital and ask when prospective parents can see the labour and delivery rooms and postnatal wards. If such visits are not routine, ask your doctor or midwife to arrange a time for you to go (even a busy unit usually has a free room). Visits are often organized in conjunction with clinic- or hospital-based parentcraft classes, but if you miss the visit, or if your partner is unable to go with you and you want him to see the facilities too, you should be able to arrange an alternative time.

Q *What should I be looking for when I visit?*

A Judge the atmosphere and openness to questions, as well as the overall appearance of the place. Prepare a few questions ahead of time on issues that are important to you.

Ask staff how sure you can be of getting the type of help you may need – assistance with breast-feeding, for example. If they focus on staff availability and other potential variables, you have a strong clue that you may not get the support you want.

Note, too, the attitude of the midwives and nurses? Are they professional, but friendly? Do they listen to your concerns and questions? Do you find their answers informative and reassuring?

Note the layout of the labour and delivery areas. Is there furniture at different heights for an active birth, if you want one? Or is your overriding impression that it is filled with lots of shiny equipment? Forward-thinking units have the equipment, but it is kept out of sight when not in use; the emphasis is on a comfortable atmosphere rather than a stark and clinical one.

Obviously, you want to feel that you will be able to relax in the hospital. But remember that delivering a healthy baby is your priority: room decor should really be a secondary consideration.

Q *After a caesarean that left me depressed for months following the birth of our first baby, I'm determined to avoid surgical intervention this time around. I feel the only way to do that is to have my baby at home. Am I right ?*

A If your caesarean was occasioned by a problem that is unlikely to be repeated (see pp. 176–77), you may well manage a vaginal delivery this time. The majority of obstetricians still prefer women to give birth in hospital after a previous caesarean because of the increased risk of complications, particularly rupture of the scar in the uterus. Discuss your views with a number of obstetricians, so that when you finally make a decision, your wish to avoid surgical intervention if possible is known and respected.

Birthing beds are a popular choice in many hospitals. The head can be raised to support you if you want to sit during labour and delivery and the base can be removed shortly before the birth to allow your midwife to deliver the baby.

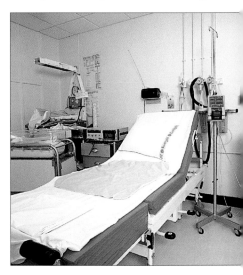

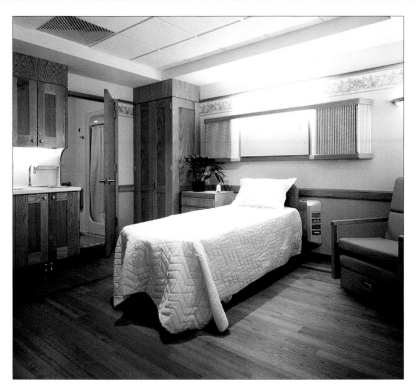

A modern delivery room may look more like a room in a hotel than one in a hospital. Soft lights, sympathetic decor, and "home-like" linens and furniture will help you to relax and feel at home. Such a setup demonstrates hospital policy and attitude: you are not ill; therefore, you need not be treated as a patient. You and your health team are partners in delivering your baby.

Q *Although my hospital has some hotel-style delivery rooms, they don't have enough to go around. Can I insist on having one?*

A Modern delivery rooms offer many of the facilities of a hotel room. You do not have the disturbing experience of being moved to a delivery room when your midwife thinks you are ready to give birth or to a postnatal ward where there are other mothers and babies when you are trying to spend a quiet couple of hours becoming a family. But such rooms are often in limited supply, and most hospitals allocate them on a first-come first-served basis.

Make your wishes known. If, when the time comes there isn't a room available, hospital staff may try to re-create as many of the advantages as they can in a regular set-up.

Q *My partner plans to be with me when our baby is born. It seems so odd that he will be able to stay only a couple of hours, and then have to go home. Why can't fathers stay with their babies?*

A In some hospitals they do, although this is not a common practice, usually for reasons of space. Also, hospital stays for most new mothers and babies are now only 24 to 48 hours, so you won't be apart for long. You will both need to rest. Labour and birth can be lengthy, and both physically and mentally tiring. Your partner should be able to stay for as long as he wants after the birth and visit at any time, but after a few hours you may both feel that you need some sleep.

Going home also allows your partner to make sure everything is ready for your homecoming.

Q *I had several operations when I was in my early teens, which have left me with a dread of hospitals. I want to have my baby at home, but am I being irresponsible?*

A The fact that you have had some bad experiences in hospital should not affect the birth of your baby. The labour and delivery wards are the happiest places in most hospitals, with new parents, excited siblings and grandparents, and masses of flowers and gifts in evidence.

Many healthcare professionals argue that first babies should be born in hospital, although there is no substantial research to support this claim. Hospital birth has been shown to carry certain risks, mainly from untimely or unnecessary intervention and inappropriate use of technology. There is also evidence that women who want to give birth at home and do so are more relaxed and recover more quickly from the birth.

Although a previous bad experience in an unrelated context should not be the major factor in your decision making, remember that you have a right to a home birth and to appropriate care for such a birth, if that is what you want.

FOR YOU

If you have been suffering from pregnancy sickness, you should see a considerable improvement in your symptoms this month. By the 14th week of pregnancy, the placenta has completely taken over hormone production and levels of the HCG drop (see pp. 66–67).

Your breasts will become larger and more tender than they were

A slight, rounded "bump" starts to become more obvious from about this stage of your pregnancy.

(see pp. 106–107), and you may notice some coloration of your face and body (see pp. 96–97). Some women will already have a small but noticeable "bump" in the abdominal area, but the time that it appears and its size vary a great deal. This protrusion is prominent at this stage not because the uterus is enlarging, but because many of the other organs in the pelvic area are being displaced (see pp. 112–13) as the uterus moves slightly farther up.

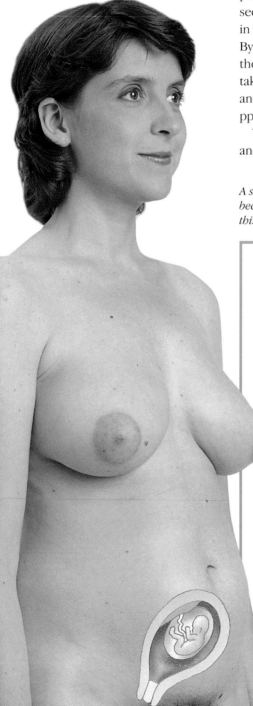

Coping with tiredness

One of the most common effects of pregnancy in the first trimester is tiredness. In fact, you may be more weary at this time than you will be for another four or five months, when the extra weight you're carrying can add to your fatigue. Maintaining some good health habits will help you cope.

Eat a well-balanced diet (see pp. 36–37), including plenty of carbohydrates to keep up your energy. Have meals regularly, and never skip a good breakfast. If you find that you have little appetite, try eating a number of smaller meals or nutritious snacks throughout the day. Avoid stimulating drinks such as tea, coffee and cola, and eliminate alcohol.

Rest when you can. A short nap in the afternoon, or just half an hour relaxing with a book, may revive you for the evening. And accept all offers of help at home.

Change your habits. Try to travel outside of peak hours, to be sure you get a seat on public transport and so that you do not arrive at work tense and stressed. If you find your energy levels flagging, go for a brisk walk in the fresh air.

If you are having trouble sleeping, try to identify the cause. Are you lying awake worrying about the birth, the baby, or financial and other problems? Share your concerns with your partner and get specialist help if necessary.

Spend the evening winding down, and make a conscious effort to relax before going to bed. Read a book, listen to music, watch a favourite film on video. Try a fruit tea or choose a warm, milky drink, perhaps one you enjoyed as a child to help you to sleep. A warm (not hot) bath with a few drops of lavender essential oil added is also relaxing.

FOR YOUR BABY

All the baby's organs and limbs are completely formed by the end of the 12th week, although the baby has months to go before being ready to live outside the uterus. The rest of your pregnancy is devoted to the growth and maturation of the baby.

With the placenta functioning fully, its hormones take over the duties previously performed by the corpus luteum (see pp. 66–67). The umbilical cord carries nutrients from the placenta to the baby, and removes waste products from the baby.

The baby still has plenty of room to move around in the amniotic sac, which is the membrane that surrounds the baby and contains about 100 ml (3½ oz) of amniotic fluid. This fluid supplies the baby with nutrients, maintains a sterile environment at a constant temperature, and protects him or her from blows. Although the baby does indeed move around, rather than just floating or responding to the movements of your body, you will not feel these movements yet (see p. 102).

At this stage the baby begins to move his or her upper lip, which is the first stage in the development of the sucking reflex, and swallows some of the amniotic fluid. The baby also produces drops of sterile urine, which are removed by the regular exchange and refreshing of the amniotic fluid.

Hands
The fingers have separated and the hands are fully developed – with cuticles but no fingernails.

Head and face
The baby has a tiny nose and chin. The eyelids have developed over the eyes. The teeth are present inside the gums. The ears have reached their final position.

Genitals
The external sex organs are now developed enough for the baby's sex to show up on an ultrasound scan if the baby's position allows this.

Skeleton
Complete in structure, the skeleton at this time is made from soft cartilage.

Size
At the end of the 14th week, the baby is about 7.5 cm (3 in) long, the size of a small pear.

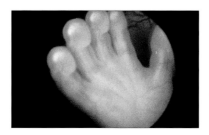

The baby's hand, less than 6 mm (¼ in) in length, is nevertheless fully formed and clearly recognizable.

PREGNANCY SICKNESS

The good news on pregnancy sickness is that half of all women don't have it; even if you do, you can usually expect it to cease by the end of the third month.

The term "pregnancy sickness" covers anything from a slight feeling of nausea in the morning to all-day queasiness and vomiting. Although this has earned it the name morning sickness, only 10 percent of women have it solely in the morning.

WHAT CAUSES IT?

Some experts speculate that the hormone HCG (see pp. 66–67) is responsible for triggering sickness. Since levels of HCG fall after about three months, when sickness usually diminishes, this theory seems plausible. It is also borne out by the fact that women carrying twins – who have greater quantities of pregnancy hormones circulating – suffer from sickness more often than those who are pregnant with single babies.

Stress may also be a cause. Women who are under a great deal of stress, either at home or at work, seem to suffer more. Those who are particularly tired seem to be more prone to sickness – which in turn makes them more tired.

Excess acid in the stomach in early pregnancy, combined with the relaxation of all the body's muscles, including those of the digestive system, may also contribute to pregnancy sickness.

Other triggers are many and various; they include specific smells or tastes that may never have bothered you before; fried or spicy foods, or even a lack of food. You may develop an aversion to coffee or to the smell of cooked vegetables.

HOW TO COPE

Women have found many simple remedies and tips that help them deal with pregnancy sickness.

The most important factor is to eat as well as you can. Have frequent small, bland meals to keep food in your stomach at all times – nibble on a cracker or rice cake before hunger strikes. Eat breakfast if you can, even if you feel worst at this time. Carbohydrates will keep your energy levels up.

When nausea strikes, try a small, sweet snack or a cracker, or

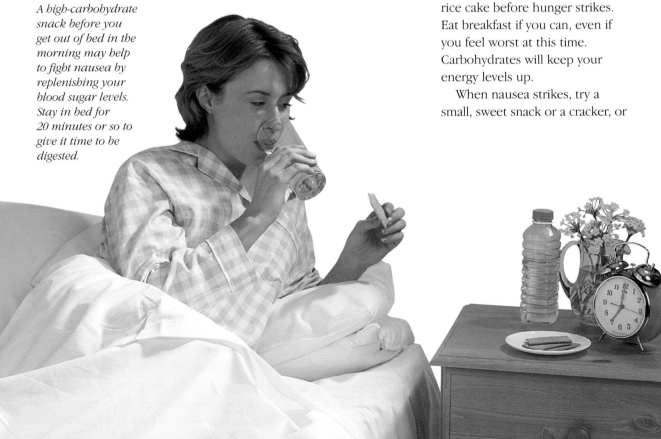

A high-carbohydrate snack before you get out of bed in the morning may help to fight nausea by replenishing your blood sugar levels. Stay in bed for 20 minutes or so to give it time to be digested.

slowly sip a carbonated drink, such as ginger ale or cola (caffeine-free is better than caffeinated). Tradition has it that warm ginger tea relieves any form of sickness. You can also ingest the soothing ginger by sucking on a piece of crystallized ginger or by eating a ginger biscuit.

If you experience severe vomiting, ask your doctor about taking a nutritional supplement to compensate for some of what you are losing. Some women have found that eating foods high in vitamin B_6 can help reduce the severity of pregnancy sickness. Foods with high levels of this vitamin include sesame seeds, raisins, bananas, wheatgerm, tuna and potatoes.

Be scrupulous about dental care, since vomit contains acids that attack tooth enamel. Cleaning your teeth frequently will also help to keep your mouth feeling fresh through bouts of nausea. Keep a toothbrush at work.

WHEN TO SEE THE DOCTOR

Severe pregnancy sickness, known as *hyperemesis gravidarum*, occurs in about 1 in 200 pregnancies and may necessitate medical intervention, including changes in diet, rest, and antacid or anti-emetic medication. Do not treat yourself with drugs to combat nausea (anti-emetics); these should be prescribed by a doctor. In rare cases, this treatment does not control the nausea and hospitalization becomes necessary. There the pregnant woman receives intravenous feeding to ensure that she and the baby receive adequate nourishment.

If you find yourself in this rare situation, remember that pregnant women and their babies invariably recover from severe pregnancy sickness, and treatment to minimize the worst symptoms is effective. Take comfort in the fact that babies are far more resilient than we imagine, and – bad as you may feel – neither you nor your baby is likely to suffer any side effects.

Acupressure and other complementary therapies rely on the application of pressure to specific pressure points to stimulate or redirect energy flow through the body. Seabands are designed with an integral ball that applies pressure to the wrist when worn. Some people have found that this reduces nausea.

Food cravings

Cravings for certain foods during pregnancy, sometimes unusual combinations of foods, are part of the colourful folklore of childbearing. Nearly everyone has a tale of an odd craving that appeared during pregnancy.

A craving can be an overwhelming need for a specific taste or, sometimes, a smell. Quite often, the desired taste is strong: piquant, very cold, or hot and spicy. A favourite without flavour is ice, probably because of the impact of the cold on the taste buds.

Most cravings are harmless. They may be caused by the hormonal changes of pregnancy. Or they may indicate a nutritional deficiency; perhaps certain minerals or vitamins are missing from your diet, and the longed-for food supplies them.

On rare occasions, a pregnant woman develops a bizarre craving for non-food substances, such as sand, coal, or clay. Should you experience these cravings, known as pica, consult your doctor.

No treatment exists for these cravings (or for aversions to particular foods, which are also common), and it's probably best to regard them as harmless inconveniences that will pass shortly. Try to make sure that even if you lose your appetite for some foods, you continue to ingest those that you like and maintain a varied diet.

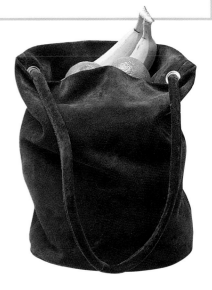

Eat little and often. When your stomach is empty, the excess acid has nothing to digest, which may make you feel nauseous. Eating between bouts of queasiness – even if you are not hungry – may prevent an attack and help to ensure that you are getting at least some of the nutrients you need. Carry healthy snacks in your bag when away from home.

COMMON PROBLEMS

The minor upsets of early pregnancy may make you feel "not yourself", but try to relax; get plenty of rest and wait for the improvement of the next few months.

As with pregnancy sickness (see pp. 84–85), the other problems that sometimes arise in early pregnancy differ from woman to woman; they also vary in degree of severity. More often than not, they are a nuisance rather than a serious problem.

CONSTIPATION

Very common in pregnancy, constipation may occur among women who have never suffered from it before. The pregnancy hormones (see pp. 66–67) relax the muscles of the digestive system, and the enlarging uterus may exert pressure on the bowel.

Dietary measures may help reduce this problem. Increase your fluid intake by having an extra glass of water with each meal. Take more fibre by including plenty of fresh fruit and vegetables in your diet. In addition, switch to whole wheat or bran breads and cereals. You may find that it helps to eat smaller meals and to add a meal or two so that your digestive system has less to work on after each meal, leaving you more comfortable.

Moderate exercise, such as walking or aerobics, helps alleviate constipation, as well as generally doing you good.

If you take iron tablets, they may contribute to your constipation. Talk to your midwife about trying a different kind or doing without them.

BREAST PROBLEMS

Tender breasts are typical in early pregnancy, and, in some cases, they can be uncomfortable. The tenderness should disappear, however, by the middle months.

Your breasts will begin to enlarge as a result of hormonal activity (see p. 67). Finding the right size bra is important for comfort and support (see p. 117).

HEARTBURN

The relaxing effect of pregnancy hormones on the muscles of the digestive system may cause heartburn. For information on how to treat this problem, see page 143.

FAINTING

You may feel lightheaded, even faint, because your blood supply is not yet adequate to deal with the demands of pregnancy. In addition, your blood pressure will typically fall slightly in early pregnancy (see p. 79). If you feel dizzy, take a few slow, deep breaths and find somewhere quiet to sit for half an hour or so. When you get up from a chair or from lying down, do so slowly. Tell your doctor if you faint or if you have any other symptoms.

VAGINAL DISCHARGE

Although an uncomfortable nuisance, increased vaginal discharge is common, again

Walking or jogging (if you jogged before pregnancy) can help relieve many minor discomforts of the first three months. Boosting your metabolism in this way helps combat the slowing of the digestive process and increases muscle tone, alleviating constipation and reducing heartburn.

because of hormonal changes. Most women stay fresh by using a panty liner, although some find that this causes thrush. If you find that you can't use liners, if the discharge becomes odiferous, or if you experience itching or soreness, see your doctor for treatment. The doctor will probably suggest vaginal pessaries or creams, neither of which will harm your baby.

MOOD SWINGS

A combination of factors may cause mood swings. The extra hormones circulating through your body may contribute to the highs and lows. So, too, may the psychological impact of knowing you're pregnant and beginning a whole new chapter in your life, which can be unsettling. Don't dwell on negative feelings. A good diet (see pp. 36–39) and exercise (see pp. 42–49) will help, as will keeping busy, seeing friends, and not spending too much time alone.

MEDICAL REMEDIES

It's natural to want to take something to relieve discomfort. Doctors base their knowledge of what is safe during pregnancy on experience or on theoretical assumptions founded on the active ingredients of the drug. Sometimes – as with the thalidomide tragedy of the 1960s – hindsight proves that a drug thought safe (to combat morning sickness) was not. Thalidomide had devastating effects on the limb development of the foetus.

We do know that some drugs (the acne preparation Accutane, for example) should not be taken at all, because they interfere with foetal development. Regarding others, we can only say, "as far as we know, they are safe". The best course of action is to take nothing without first consulting your doctor.

If you feel anxious because of medication you took before you knew you were pregnant, talk it over with your doctor.

Many homeopathic remedies are safe to use during pregnancy, but consult a doctor before taking a treatment. Yoga and other complementary techniques may alleviate problems for which medication would normally be prescribed (see pp. 52–55).

Many drugs, including some common painkillers and cough medicines, are not recommended for use in pregnancy. Certain herbs and aromatherapy oils, such as juniper and eucalyptus, should also be avoided. If you are in any doubt about the preparation you use, ask your midwife, complementary therapist, doctor or pharmacist for advice.

'I don't have a thing to wear...'

Feeling comfortable and looking good can require some thought in early pregnancy. You're too small for "maternity clothes", but your ordinary clothes may not fit you anymore, particularly if they have a tight waist.

Make a loop of elastic and thread it through the buttonhole in the waistband of your trousers. Slip one end over the other and pull. When you're ready to wear the pants, stretch the free end of the loop over the button on the other side. Wear large, loose T-shirts or tops to cover the gap that results.

Elasticated-waist skirts cut to flare over the hips will be most comfortable. A fitted skirt, even with its zip open at the top, will tend to ride up over your stomach.

If you can afford it, buy some clothes that are comfortable at your present size – one or two dresses or shirts that billow out may fit well into your pregnancy and be useful after the birth, while you're regaining your pre-pregnancy shape. Front openings are handy if you plan to breast-feed. (See also pp. 116–17.)

For comfort around the armholes and chest, borrow some shirts or sweaters from your partner. These may fit throughout your pregnancy.

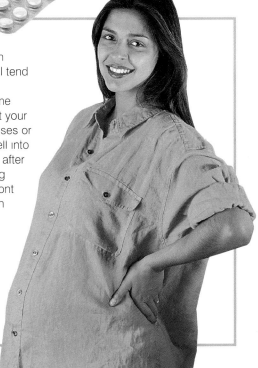

CHOOSING ANTENATAL CLASSES

Antenatal classes offer you and your partner advice on all aspects of pregnancy and childbirth. They also provide a good place to make new friends.

Q *What's the difference between childbirth classes, antenatal classes and parenting classes?*

A Sometimes, there's little difference. The name may reflect tradition more than the content of the class. When you are choosing classes, ask the course leader or teacher questions about the curriculum, how big the classes are, and when and where the class will meet. You should expect all of the classes to offer some element of preparation for childbirth. They should explain the physical process, teach how to recognize the start of labour and its different stages, and demonstrate the different positions you can adopt in labour and delivery.

Early parenthood should also be touched on and include such subjects as feeding your baby and returning to work. Some classes teach such elements of basic parenting as how to bathe a baby, change a nappy, and cope with fussiness in infants. Most also give advice on getting started with breast-feeding.

Q *What's the point of going to a class? Can't I get most of the information I need from my doctor or a good book?*

A The main advantage of classes is that they give you as an individual the opportunity for ongoing give-and-take with a professional who has the time to work through a wide range of questions with you. They help you set the agenda for your childbirth; give you information about the local hospital or unit you intend to have your baby in; allow you to express your own needs and concerns; and often teach you helpful techniques for coping with labour. You will also have a good source of new friends for you and your coming baby. There are stories about classmates who continue to meet once a month, even 10 years later, just for the fun and social support.

If you commute to work, you may want to choose classes nearer to home to make continued contact after the birth easier.

Q *I have just found out that I am pregnant. When should I think about starting classes?*

A Early antenatal classes usually meet once or twice. Classes usually begin in earnest about the sixth month and last around eight or nine weeks. Ideally, you should finish a few weeks before you expect to deliver.

Popular classes may be booked up early, so if you have heard that a particular set of classes is good, you may need to reserve your place well in advance.

Remember that you can go to more than one set of classes if you become unsure about the quality of the ones you have chosen or if they do not meet your needs.

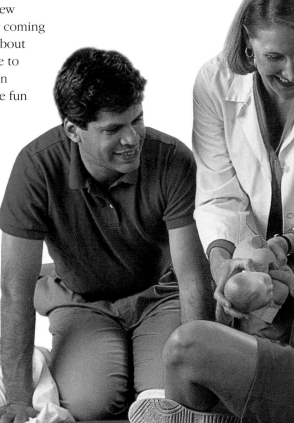

The best antenatal classes welcome partners who want to be involved. They also encourage plenty of personal contact between you and the instructor. You can ask any questions, confident that your concerns will be addressed fully.

Q *What should I know about those classes that teach pain-free birth?*

A The fad for describing childbirth as painless has disappeared. Good antenatal teachers speak honestly about labour. The truth is that for most women, childbirth involves some degree of pain, no matter what techniques are used.

In a good class, you will learn breathing or relaxation techniques that help you to cope with the pain, so you either won't need drugs or you'll need them later or in smaller quantities. These techniques also help you view birth as an enjoyable experience.

Fear and ignorance make labour more daunting than it needs to be. Good classes will inform you of all your options.

Where are the classes held? Do the times fit my schedule?

How much do the classes cost? Can I pay by session, or is there a discount for a group of classes?

How many participants are likely to be in the class?

Are the classes for couples only, singles only?

Are the classes for first-timers only?

Do they teach a specific method for labour and childbirth, or do they present me with options?

Jot down any questions you may have regarding classes before you sign up. You do not want to waste time attending classes that don't meet your needs.

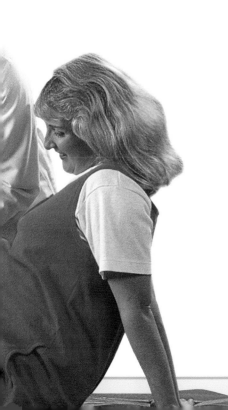

Q *What about fathers? Are they expected to attend?*

A Most classes these days are for couples, but a mother who doesn't have a partner, or whose partner can't or won't come, is welcome, too. Classes provide fathers with a unique insight into the experience of pregnancy and allow for discussion as well as information. Fathers, too, can find support in classes and learn ways to be a real help to their partners during labour and childbirth. They can practise massage techniques (for example, to relieve backache) and develop skills in offering encouragement and support to their partner in an acceptable way. Any fears and worries they have should be addressed, too.

Q *What if my partner doesn't want to come?*

A It would be a shame for him to miss out on what should be a shared experience. Encourage him to express his reasons for staying away. If need be, go to the first class by yourself, then tell him about it and how much you could learn together. He may fear that he'll be the only man, and it may reassure him to know that other fathers-to-be are attending the class. If he's adamant, don't pressure him. If he doesn't want to attend the birth either, you have the option of finding another birthing partner – your mother, sister or a friend. They will be welcome at your classes, too. Once the baby is born, the chances are that your partner will be more involved.

MISCARRIAGE

Estimates of miscarriage rates vary, but now that we can confirm pregnancy early, it's clear that more fertilized eggs fail to implant than was once believed.

Researchers now speculate that as many as one in four conceptions ends in miscarriage, but the usual figure given is one in six. Miscarriage is defined as the loss of a pregnancy before the 20th week. Most miscarriages occur in the first three months.

WHY WOMEN MISCARRY

Nature does a very good job of supporting strong, healthy pregnancies – and of abandoning those fertilized eggs that don't come up to scratch. Most early miscarriages are the result of a less than perfect conception: the fertilized egg may fail to implant in the uterine lining or fail to undergo cell division, or the cell division may result in some sort of error. Nature's solution is not to proceed with the pregnancy. Scientists don't understand why some eggs manage the complex process of fertilization only to fail at the next hurdle or two; one theory is that a normal egg may have been fertilized by an abnormal sperm or vice versa. When this happens, the resultant pregnancy used to be called a "blighted ovum" but is now more correctly referred to as an anembryonic pregnancy.

Between 1 and 2 percent of miscarriages occur at about the 20th week as a result of cervical incompetence. The cervix doesn't stay closed, but starts to dilate as the growing baby puts pressure on it. If your doctor

Pregnancy failure

A miscarriage is the most common form of pregnancy loss, and its causes are often unclear. A variety of conditions may result in the loss of a pregnancy. In other cases – despite test results – the woman may not be pregnant at all.

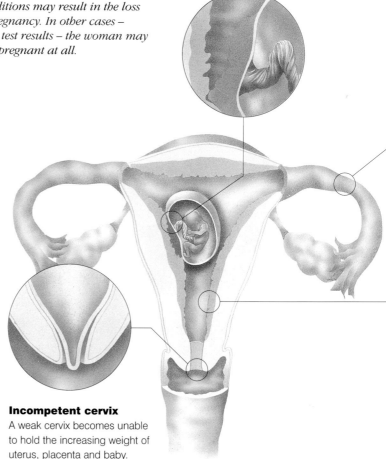

Separation of the placenta
Occasionally, the placenta does not form as it should. If the uterus is misshapen, the placenta may not attach itself firmly to the uterine wall. Or it may fail to produce enough hormones to sustain the pregnancy and will then spontaneously abort it.

Incompetent cervix
A weak cervix becomes unable to hold the increasing weight of uterus, placenta and baby.

suspects this condition, he or she can insert a stitch into the wall of the cervix to keep it closed. This so-called cervical cerclage can be removed just before you have your baby.

Miscarriages may also occur because the mother has kidney disease, hypertension, acute

emotional disturbances, anti-phospholipid antibodies, fibroid tumours or a misshapen uterus. They do not result from minor emotional disturbances, minor falls, normal lifting and other physical activities, moderate exercise, the occasional stressful day or sexual intercourse.

Ectopic pregnancy

The fertilized egg implants in the Fallopian tube, which can rupture as the embryo grows. Some parts of the tube are weaker than others, so the time at which the rupture occurs varies. An ectopic pregnancy must be removed (see p. 62).

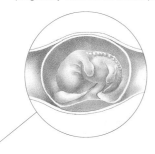

Hydatidiform mole

This is not a true pregnancy but a collection of fluid-filled sacs that grow from the chorionic villi. Pregnancy hormones are produced, which is why pregnancy tests show positive results. The mole grows faster than a baby would, which raises suspicions. A D & C (right) is usually performed to remove the mole.

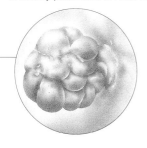

Dilatation and curettage

Left to itself, your body will usually take care of the physical after-effects of miscarriage, and you can assume that the pregnancy tissue has fallen away. But if you experience unexplained or prolonged bleeding, a D & C (dilatation and curettage) may be recommended. Doctors also use this procedure after a missed abortion – when the foetus has died but remains in the uterus. Your body would eventually expel the remains of the pregnancy naturally, but over a period of a few weeks; the tissue is usually removed surgically instead to reduce the possibility of its becoming infected.

This surgical operation to remove tissue from the uterus involves opening – dilating – the cervix by stretching the os, or small exit point. This allows the surgeon to introduce an instrument, the curette, which can suction or scrape over the inside of the uterus to remove any remnants of the pregnancy tissue.

A D & C is usually performed under general anaesthetic (although sometimes under a local), and it poses a small risk of damage to the cervix and uterus – and to any previously unknown twin that remains in the uterus (a rare occurrence).

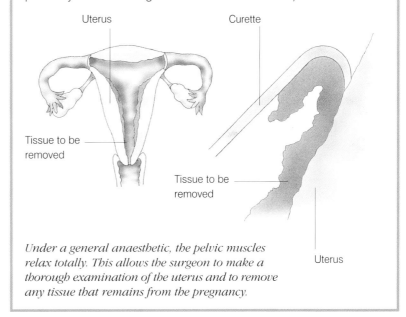

Uterus

Curette

Tissue to be removed

Tissue to be removed

Uterus

Under a general anaesthetic, the pelvic muscles relax totally. This allows the surgeon to make a thorough examination of the uterus and to remove any tissue that remains from the pregnancy.

BLEEDING IN PREGNANCY

Pregnant women may bleed lightly in the early months. Some women lose small amounts of blood throughout pregnancy. If you notice bleeding that's heavier than light spotting, or if spotting continues for more than a couple of days, seek medical advice.

The blood you see will always be your own blood, not the baby's. Bleeding that doesn't result in a miscarriage – the majority of cases – will not adversely affect either your health or the health of your baby.

THE WARNING SIGNS

These symptoms may indicate that you are about to miscarry. See your doctor or go to the hospital if you suffer from: **period-like pain** in your lower abdomen with vaginal bleeding; **severe or constant pain** without any bleeding; or **painless bleeding** that is as heavy as a normal period.

If there are any clots in the blood, or if you pass any tissue (usually grey or pink), you may already have started to miscarry. Try to save anything you pass in a clean container. This may allow your doctor to tell whether the miscarriage is only threatening, is partial, or is complete. Note any other symptoms, such as nausea or a raised temperature.

AFTER A MISCARRIAGE

Having a miscarriage is physically and emotionally traumatic. But the overwhelming majority of couples go on to have a healthy baby.

A miscarriage is a distressing, even devastating, life event. Not everyone will respond to it with the same degree of sadness, of course. But for many couples, there have already been some weeks or months of planning, of anticipation and, in the case of a late miscarriage, an attachment to the baby whose movement they may have felt in the womb.

THE PHYSICAL IMPACT

In all but the very earliest miscarriages, uterine contractions and the dilatation of the cervix will cause physical pain. If your doctor thinks there may be some pregnancy tissue left, you may have to have a D & C to avoid any possibility of infection (see p. 91). You may continue to notice blood spots intermittently for some weeks as your uterus returns to its pre-pregnancy state.

Your body has to adjust to the fact that it is not nourishing a baby. The extra hormone levels,

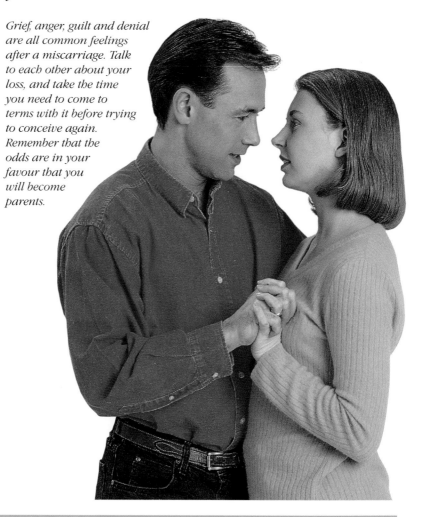

Grief, anger, guilt and denial are all common feelings after a miscarriage. Talk to each other about your loss, and take the time you need to come to terms with it before trying to conceive again. Remember that the odds are in your favour that you will become parents.

For partners

It's usually the woman who is the focus of care and concern after a miscarriage. You may be asked "How's your wife?" rather than "How are you?" or "How are the two of you?"

You need support too, however. While dealing with your own emotions, you may be acting as a buffer between your partner and the medical profession, asking questions about what has happened and what care she will need, while also supporting her during a physically and emotionally draining time.

Because you haven't experienced the physical sense of loss that your partner has gone through, you may be more upset than anyone realizes. But, especially in a later miscarriage, you will have focused on the pregnancy, and you may have felt the baby's movements. You, too, have made plans for the future and imagined yourself as a father and part of a family.

Acknowledging the difficulty and tension of the situation is important. Couples need to share their feelings and support one another. They should talk about what both have missed and admit how sad they feel. Then they can face the future, and the next pregnancy, with hope.

the increased blood supply, your weight and your enlarged breasts will all take time to return to normal. If the miscarriage occurs late in pregnancy, your breasts may even produce milk. This will dry up after a few days.

THE EMOTIONAL IMPACT

The weeks after a miscarriage can be a difficult, demanding time for the body, but the emotional effects can be hard to bear, too.

Allow yourself to grieve. In the case of late miscarriage, some couples choose to see their baby. Experts say that this can help you to accept what has happened. If you have started preparing the baby's room at home, don't let a well-meaning friend or family member clear everything away. Do it yourself when you feel able. If you plan another pregnancy, you may want to leave your preparations intact.

If you need time away from work to recover, take it. Or, if getting back to normal as quickly as possible helps, do this instead. Some women worry that something they drank, ate or did before they were aware of their pregnancy may have been to blame. But miscarriages are rarely caused by anything as clear-cut as something you did or didn't do. Focus on your own needs, rather than on any misplaced guilt.

People may find it hard to hit the right note of sympathy or understanding when you meet them. They may even avoid the topic because they don't know what to say. Accept this, and don't brood on their apparent lack of concern.

Talking to other women who have gone through miscarriages

A Case in Point
A Family's Loss

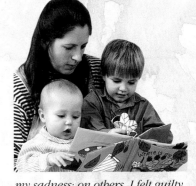

JESSICA, 35, AND HER HUSBAND WANTED A LARGE FAMILY.

"We conceived our first child easily and I had a marvellous pregnancy and birth. When Sam was a year old I was delighted to be pregnant again. We didn't tell anyone until I was 14 weeks pregnant, then broke the news. Only a week later, I miscarried.

"I felt that somehow having a beautiful, healthy child already should have made it easier to bear this loss, but it didn't. Watching Sam unfold into a little person seemed to make me more acutely aware of what this baby would have brought to us, and – young as he was – I felt the loss for Sam of a sibling who would have been close in age.

"Some days I threw myself into doing things with Sam to blot out my sadness; on others, I felt guilty that I should have mourned the baby for longer.

"Six months later I conceived again and spent an anxious few months, convinced I would lose this baby too. He's a year old now, strong and healthy. I know I'm lucky but I still catch myself sometimes, looking at the two of them and seeing the brother or sister who should be there between them. The pain has gone, but I can't forget my lost baby."

can be a support at this time. Some women also find that counselling or self-help organizations offering group sessions provide a release for their emotions. It can be a relief not to have to pretend everything's fine.

PLANNING FOR THE FUTURE

For most women, the best way to get over a miscarriage is to try again. Having a miscarriage does not mean that you won't be able to have a baby in the future. Most subsequent pregnancies are problem-free. If your doctor identifies a problem such as cervical incompetence (see pp. 90–91), he or she will advise you of treatment options.

Once you feel physically well and any vaginal discharge or bleeding has ceased, wait until you have at least one menstrual period before trying again. This allows you to date a pregnancy accurately and be sure that your body has recovered from the loss. Your period is likely to come about five weeks after your miscarriage, although it may take longer.

It is inevitable that, despite all the reassuring statistics, you will be worried about embarking on another pregnancy. Remember that having had a miscarriage has no effect on a future pregnancy. And your doctor will monitor your progress carefully if you have a history of miscarriage.

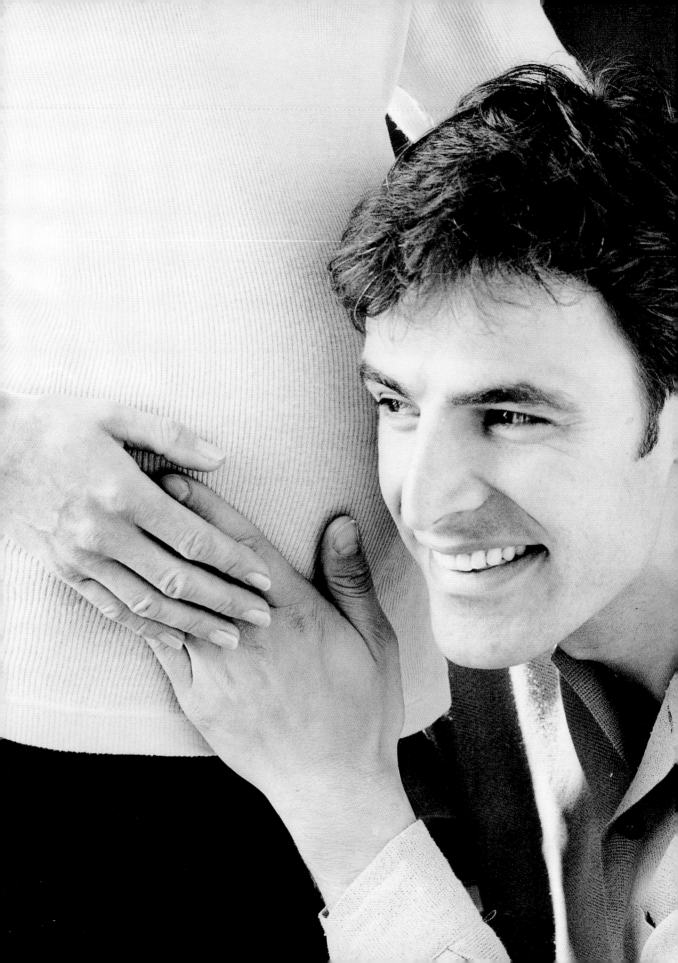

The second trimester

AS THE NEW LIFE *inside you becomes obvious to all, the second three months are likely to be those when you feel and look your best. In this period, you will probably:*

- Experience the bloom of pregnancy, when your hair shines and skin glows

- Have your first glimpse, through ultrasound, of this exciting new member of your family and tests to confirm his or her health

- Become increasingly conscious of your baby moving and growing

- Enter a period of deepening affection for your partner as the baby becomes a strong emotional bond between you

- Think about your future career plans and whether you'll need a carer to help you look after your baby.

The fourth month

FOR YOU

This month you are likely to experience renewed energy as the discomforts of the first trimester diminish. Your uterus rises out of the pelvis, forming a bulge that makes the waistbands of your clothes snug. The uterus will increase twenty-fold in size during pregnancy, and most of this growth occurs before the end of the fourth month.

Some women notice puffiness in their face during these weeks and beyond. This results most often from changes in your circulatory system that cause

As your abdomen rounds out this month, your pregnancy begins to be as noticeable to others as it is to you.

water retention. These changes also create the "bloom" that many women exhibit in these months.

Your blood volume increases as you produce more body fluids and more corpuscles. You may find that you are often thirsty and perspire more.

Your heart will increase slightly in size and pump more powerfully – but not faster – to move a greater volume of blood through your body.

During this time, you may be offered tests to check on the health of your baby (see pp. 100–101). Discuss all your options with the experts and your partner.

Changes to your skin

At about 16 or 17 weeks, you may start to notice a deepening of your skin colour, especially if you have an olive or light tan complexion. Fair- and red-haired women will notice this less. Heightened skin pigmentation is normal and can be attributed to the hormones circulating in your body during pregnancy. Moles, freckles and other areas of darker pigmentation become more pronounced; the most obvious change, however, is the "linea nigra", or dark line, that runs from your navel down the centre of your abdomen to the top of your pubic bone. Your nipples may be darker, and the areola (the coloured skin surrounding the nipple) may begin to spread farther across your breast. This heightened colouring will fade after the birth of your baby.

Sometimes facial colouring changes, too. In darker-skinned women, patches of light skin may develop on the forehead, nose and cheeks, forming a sort of "mask". (Pale-skinned women may develop darker patches.) This mask, or chloasma, disappears after the birth.

As the skin of your abdomen stretches, small lines or streaks may appear. These so-called stretch marks are pink or red in pale-skinned women and darker in women with black skin (see pp. 114–15). You may also find that your skin becomes drier.

FOR YOUR BABY

By this stage, your baby is moving vigorously and energetically, with his arms, legs, head and torso rolling and kicking (see pp. 102–103). You are unlikely to feel these movements, however, in part because they are buffered by the amniotic fluid (also known as "waters"). If this is your first baby, you may not realize that the fluttery feeling in your tummy is your baby moving. Once you have had one baby, the muscles of your abdomen tend to be more lax. This softening may make any movement of successive babies more apparent.

Hair
Your baby's hair begins to grow at about 16 weeks. Soft, fine hair known as lanugo has also grown all over his body. Its function is not fully understood, but it may have some role in protecting the baby's skin and helping to maintain a regular body temperature.

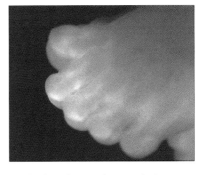

By the fourth month, your baby's fingernails and toenails have started to grow.

Major organs
All your baby's major organs are working, and the heart is beating at 120 to 160 beats per minute.

Around the eyes
Eyebrows and eyelashes start to grow at this time.

Genitals
The sex organs are more clearly defined, and the sex of your baby may be discernible on an ultrasound scan (see pp. 98–99).

The eyes and ears
Although not yet fully mature, the baby's eyes and ears function. He is aware of sound and light, which is perceived in the uterus as a faint, reddish glow. Among other sounds that he can hear is your heartbeat (see pp. 104–105).

Size
The baby is now about 17 cm (6½ in) long and weighs about 140 g (5 oz).

SEEING YOUR BABY

Ultrasound scanning gives you – and the professionals involved in your care – the opportunity to see your unborn baby in the uterus.

Ultrasound is one of the most useful tools in modern obstetric care, and when performed in the first half of pregnancy is able to tell accurately how far pregnant you are. It allows your doctor or midwife to gauge whether your baby is growing normally, especially if the baby is not the usual size for your stage of pregnancy. Ultrasound permits doctors to monitor the structure and size of the baby's major organs and bones, including the spine. It is used to check for signs of abnormality, such as the incomplete formation of the spine's vertebrae in spina bifida. It also shows how many babies you are carrying.

The position and condition of the placenta can be ascertained through ultrasound. In early pregnancy, it's necessary to know the location of the placenta – and the baby – if amniocentesis is being carried out (see pp. 100–101). In later pregnancy, ultrasound can be used to detect possible causes of unexplained bleeding. This happens most commonly when the placenta is starting to separate prematurely (a condition known as abruptio placentae) or is low in the uterus, and might interfere with the baby's safe exit.

In later pregnancy, scanning may be used to monitor the position of the baby in the uterus, which can affect the delivery. In certain cases, it may help to determine whether a caesarean is needed (see pp. 176–77).

You are likely to be offered a scan at around 18–20 weeks to confirm your dates and how many foetuses you are carrying, and to check for abnormalities. You may be offered another scan towards the end if any complications are suspected, or to check on your baby's growth if you develop a condition such as diabetes or hypertension.

HOW ULTRASOUND WORKS

Ultrasound scanning is painless, although you will be asked to fill your bladder by drinking lots of water, which may feel uncomfortable. (A full bladder pushes your uterus up so that the technician gets a better picture.)

Some lubricating gel – this will feel cold – is spread on your

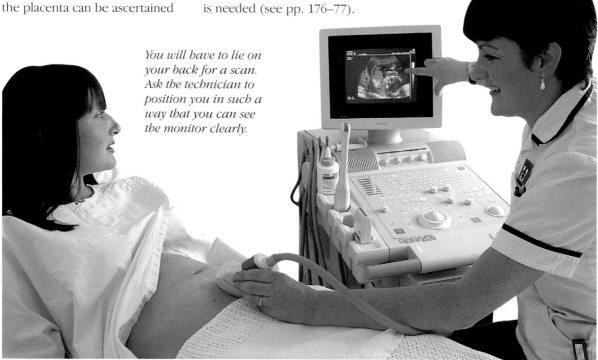

You will have to lie on your back for a scan. Ask the technician to position you in such a way that you can see the monitor clearly.

abdomen. The technician then passes a transducer over your abdomen. The transducer emits sound waves, which echo off the baby and are then interpreted by a computer, translated into picture form and transmitted to a screen. (Some machines use sound to track blood flow. This can supply additional information about the baby's health.)

INTERPRETING THE RESULTS

You may not recognize the baby's form when you see the image on the screen, but the technician can explain what appears. Ask him or her to trace the outline of your baby's body, to show you where the placenta is, and to point out the major body organs. You will probably be able to see your baby's heart beating and to discern quite clearly which way she is lying.

If you want to know, ask the technician if it is possible to determine your baby's sex. It's not always easy to do so – the way the baby is lying may obscure the genitals – and even when the baby is positioned so that the genitals are visible, it is possible to misinterpret the image. You will be warned of this and told that the sex information may not be correct. If you don't want to know the sex of your baby, tell the technician beforehand.

Try to arrange a time when your partner can go with you for your first ultrasound scan so that you can share the wonderful moment of seeing your baby for the first time. Some hospitals provide a print of the scan. If you would like one, ask.

Are there risks?

Ultrasound scanning has been in widespread use for 30 years, and today the majority of pregnant women in industrialized countries undergo routine scanning. Mainstream medical opinion holds that ultrasound causes no harmful side effects and that its many benefits outweigh any theoretical risks. Not only can problems be picked up sooner, but parents-to-be find this one of the most enjoyable aspects of their pregnancy care. Most say that their scans help them to feel more closely connected to their baby.

The theoretical risks of scanning centre on the effect of sound waves on foetal tissue. Some experts say that the waves simply bounce off, causing no harm. Others maintain that they cause hot spots or gas bubbles to form in the cells, which could result in cell damage. These risks exist in theory only. The many studies done to test the safety of ultrasound have found no evidence of harmful effects. Detractors argue that these were not random controlled trials*. Follow-up studies over 12 and 20 years have shown no conclusive deleterious effects.

The overwhelming evidence is that ultrasound is safe, so relax and enjoy the sight of your baby.

In random controlled trials, thousands of women are matched with an equal number of controls and they and their babies followed up for decades, until the next generation of babies is born.

Head
The head will seem large compared to the body.

Arm
The hands and fingers may be visible.

Ultrasound can detect an embryo from as early as the seventh week of pregnancy, but the larger the baby grows, the easier it is to identify the various parts of her body.

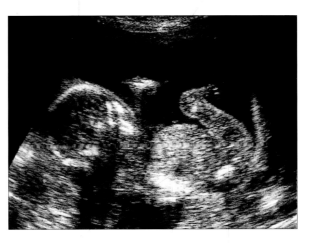

Heart
You should be able to see the heart beating.

Spine
The spine is curved: it becomes more bony as pregnancy progresses.

Leg
The baby's legs are tucked against the body.

ANTENATAL TESTING

When you are between 9 and 18 weeks pregnant, a number of tests can be carried out to confirm that your baby is healthy and developing as expected.

Q *What sort of tests are used to detect disabilities? Are they offered to everyone?*

A There are two types of test: one aims to establish a degree of risk to an individual mother of having a baby with disabilities; the other is more clear-cut and carried out to diagnose specific abnormalities.

Doctors typically offer certain tests only to women at higher risk of having a baby with a problem. For example, an older mother (above the age of 35), who is more likely to have a baby with Down's syndrome, may be offered chorionic villus sampling (CVS) or amniocentesis. Both tests increase the risk of miscarriage slightly, so doctors tend to be conservative about their use.

Tests may also be suggested after ultrasound has highlighted a possible problem. Thickened folds of skin on the nape of the baby's neck, for example, may indicate Down's syndrome. Amniocentesis can disprove (or confirm) the diagnosis. And mothers who have had a baby with an abnormality, or who are carriers of a genetic disorder, will be offered chromosomal testing.

Ask your doctor the reason for any tests you are offered, discuss their implications, and make sure that you will be shown the results.

Q *What are the differences between amniocentesis and CVS? When are they done?*

A Chorionic villus sampling (CVS) is available in only a few large hospitals, and is done when you are between 9 and 12 weeks pregnant. Either a fine catheter is inserted through your cervix or a fine needle through the abdomen into the uterus to remove a small sample of the chorionic villus. This is the tissue that burrows into the wall of the uterus and eventually becomes the placenta. A sample contains the genetic information needed to find out whether the foetus has a chromosomal disorder, such as Down's syndrome, or a genetic one, such as sickle-cell trait.

The results are available in 10 to 14 days. CVS increases the risk of miscarriage by 0.6 percent.

Amniocentesis is normally carried out between 14 and 16 weeks of pregnancy. The doctor will withdraw a sample of the amniotic fluid in which your baby floats with a needle inserted through the abdomen into the uterus and then into the amniotic sac. The cells contained in the fluid are tested for the presence of chromosomal abnormalities; the results are available in three weeks. The test increases the normal risk of miscarriage by an estimated 0.5 percent.

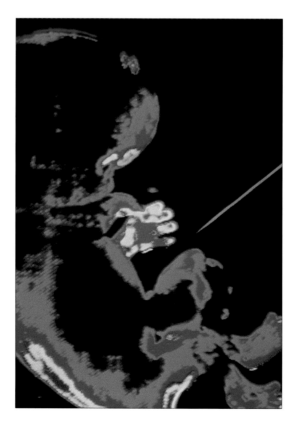

Before both amniocentesis and CVS, you will have an ultrasound scan to establish the safest place to insert the needle. In amniocentesis (shown at left), a small amount of amniotic fluid is taken for testing. In CVS, a sample of the tissue that will become the placenta is removed.

Q *Are there alternatives to these two tests?*

A Yes. CVS and amniocentesis are invasive – that is, they penetrate the womb. For some women, the triple test is more appropriate. In this test, a blood sample is taken at 16 weeks and tested for three hormones or hormone-like substances – alpha-fetoprotein (AFP), human chorionic gonadotropin (HCG) and unconjugated oestriols. A higher or lower level than normal of one or more can mean an increased risk of chromosomal problems or neural-tube defects (NTDs), such as spina bifida.

The results, available within about 10 days, will read as a "one in something" chance. "One in 380" or "one to 380" means that for every 380 pregnancies with the same result, 379 are likely to be normal.

If you feel the results indicate a higher than acceptable risk, you may choose to undergo amniocentesis or ultrasound to get more specific information.

Q *My sister lost a baby with spina bifida a few days after birth. Can my baby be tested for NTDs?*

A The alpha-fetoprotein test used to be used to indicate women at increased risk of having babies with NTDs. In expert hands, ultrasound is now better at detecting these structural abnormalities. Since most women have an ultrasound examination at 18 to 22 weeks, your doctor can ensure that your baby is carefully assessed.

Q *What other tests are available?*

A This area continues to develop, and many tests, most of them invasive, are still being assessed. In some hospitals, a blood sample taken from the umbilical cord is analyzed for a range of infections, abnormalities and such conditions as haemophilia. This test is not widely available.

The amniotic fluid can also be tested to determine the baby's lung maturity. This is crucial information if a decision has to be made about whether the baby can safely be delivered early and, if so, whether the newborn will need immediate special care.

Q *Do antenatal tests that show an abnormality always lead to a termination?*

A No. To begin with, most test results come back normal. However, you do need to think carefully before you have any test. How will you feel if the test shows that your baby has an abnormality? Will you consider a termination? If not, will you feel that the test has allowed you to find out as much as possible about your baby's condition, optimize delivery time and place, and prepare for his or her arrival?

Some couples prefer not to have any tests for abnormality because the anxiety engendered by the test, and then the wait for the results, can be emotionally draining. Others would not consider a termination under any circumstances, so they consider the tests to be pointless. Many people feel confident that they can accept and love their baby whatever his or her physical or mental health.

Your doctor will have his or her own views, but should give you only facts, not opinions. The final decision is yours.

Q *What is the procedure if we opt for a termination?*

A In early pregnancy, a D & C can be performed (see p. 91). Between 14 and 20 weeks, there are two alternatives. One is to go into "labour", which is induced by hormones and results in the vaginal delivery of your foetus and placenta. The other is to have a dilatation and evacuation, or D & E. In this, a hormone in tablet form is placed in the vagina, causing the cervix to become softer and more elastic. Some hours later, under general anaesthesia, your cervix is surgically dilated and the uterus evacuated of the foetus and placenta. Think about whether you want to see or hold the baby, or if you want hospital staff to take a photograph.

It is normal to mourn the loss of your baby, no matter when it occurs. The whole experience of being pregnant, having tests, making the decision to terminate, and losing a baby is enormously distressing. Even if you feel you made the right decision, it can be a period of grief for you, your partner and others who would have loved your baby.

Share your feelings with people close to you. You may also like to contact one of the support groups listed on pages 218–19.

The fifth month

FOR YOU

By the end of this month, you will look obviously pregnant. You may feel energetic and healthy, and your skin will be clear (see p. 114). Because the normal hair loss everyone experiences throughout life slows down in a pregnant woman and extra hormonal activity can make your hair richer in oils (see p. 115), your hair may be thicker and glossier.

Your uterus has risen farther out of your pelvis, and you now have a smooth, rounded bulge that makes the switch to clothes with an elasticated waistband necessary.

One of the most exciting moments of pregnancy occurs when you feel your baby move for the first time. You can expect this to happen at any time between 17 and 21 weeks. Movements feel fluttery at first – as if you had butterflies or fish inside you – but they become stronger and more frequent as the days and weeks go by. You will soon find them unmistakable. These sensations are called "quickening". Your midwife may want to record the date at which you first become aware of them.

Feeling your baby's movements

Your baby begins to move in about the 10th week, when he makes stretching motions that help to develop his muscles. These movements increase in frequency and intensity over the next few weeks and are essential to the formation of healthy limbs and muscle tissue.

You won't feel these movements until the fourth month at the earliest, when the inner wall of your abdomen is close to the outer wall of the uterus. You will feel a kick only when the baby is facing outwards: you won't feel when he kicks into the uterus. Later, as the uterus enlarges and the baby grows, you will notice movements frequently and clearly.

As your pregnancy nears its end, your baby may change position less often simply because there is less room for active kicking and punching. One of the best times to feel movement is a couple of hours after a meal. Lie down and put your hand on your abdomen. Encourage your partner to do the same. Count the movements: 10 in 10 minutes is an indicator of foetal good health. Remember that natural lulls in movement occur when your baby is asleep. However, if you haven't felt your baby move at all for more than half a day, drink some juice and lie on your left side. If you still feel nothing, ask your doctor to listen for the baby's heartbeat to reassure you that all is well.

Although vigorous kicks and punches may take your breath away, enjoy them as a sign that your baby is active and strong.

FOR YOUR BABY

During these weeks, your baby's movements become more energetic, more vigorous and more complex.

From now until the end of your pregnancy, your baby recycles the amniotic fluid in your womb, swallowing it and excreting it via his bladder and urethra. This is the baby's way of exercising his immature swallowing and digestive mechanisms.

Beginning at around 20 weeks, your baby's skin develops an all-over coating of vernix, a greasy, whitish substance. This remains on your baby's body until birth, although it diminishes on babies born after about 37 or 38 weeks. Very premature babies may have more.

Bones and muscles
The muscle tissue is growing stronger, and the skeleton is becoming bonier.

Hearing
Babies at this stage seem able to hear more clearly than once thought. Your baby may jump in response to a loud noise.

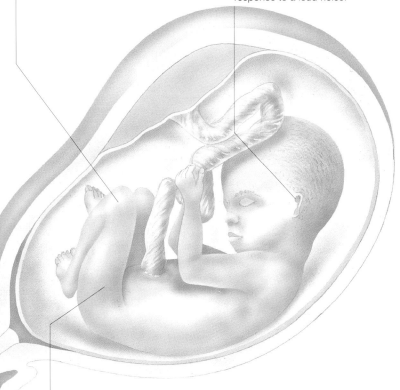

Size
At the end of the 21st week, your baby will measure approximately 28 cm (11 in) in length and weigh 450 g (16 oz).

Skin
The baby's skin is covered by vernix, which acts as a sort of waterproofing and helps to maintain the skin's texture and temperature.

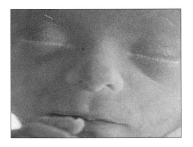

The teeth are present in the jaw from about the fifth month. Most babies have no teeth at birth, but occasionally a baby is born with one.

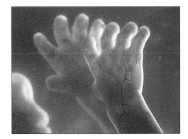

By the fifth month, the baby's hands and feet are developed enough for him to flex and suck his fingers and flex his toes.

IN TOUCH WITH YOUR BABY

*Babies' senses develop while they are in the uterus.
You can start to establish a close bond with your
baby even before she is born.*

We now know that unborn babies are aware of much of their surroundings and are able to respond physically to a variety of stimuli. We also understand a great deal about the way a baby's body functions in the uterus and what she can hear and see. It can be a warm and rewarding experience for parents to capitalize on the baby's awareness by making contact as she grows.

Studies of unborn babies and their parents suggest that babies remember certain aspects of their life in the uterus. In one study, babies whose pregnant mothers regularly sat down each afternoon to relax and watch their favourite programme on TV were found to relax after the birth whenever the familiar sound of the show's signature tune was played to them.

Unborn babies have a sense of taste as well as likes and dislikes. Researchers added saccharin to the amniotic fluid and observed (via ultrasound) that the babies' swallowing rate doubled. When a foul-tasting oil was added, the babies grimaced, and their swallowing rate dropped sharply.

Your baby's ears are acutely sensitive from the 24th week on. Inside the uterus, the baby can hear your heartbeat and digestive noises, the sound of your voice and that of other people. The sound of a heartbeat-like noise always soothes a newborn, and tapes of womb noises, simulated or real, are available for use after the birth to calm the baby's crying.

A baby's eye muscles develop early in pregnancy, and from about week 16 the baby becomes sensitive to light. If a bright light is shone on your stomach, your baby may move away from the light. She will perceive the sunlight if you are sunbathing with your stomach uncovered.

The neural circuits of the brain are fully developed in a baby of 28 weeks' gestation. At week 32, brain-wave tests detect REM (rapid eye movement) sleep, which in adults indicates a dream state. It seems likely that the unborn baby is reliving, in dreams, some of the experiences she has already had of moving, hearing, seeing and feeling.

YOUR MOODS
Many mothers-to-be want to know whether their moods can affect their unborn babies. Such links are difficult to prove or disprove. Babies have been born to mothers whose financial circumstances and emotional outlook on their children were less than ideal and have grown up healthy and happy. Babies of women who seemed to have an abundance of love and material comforts have become emotionally disturbed.

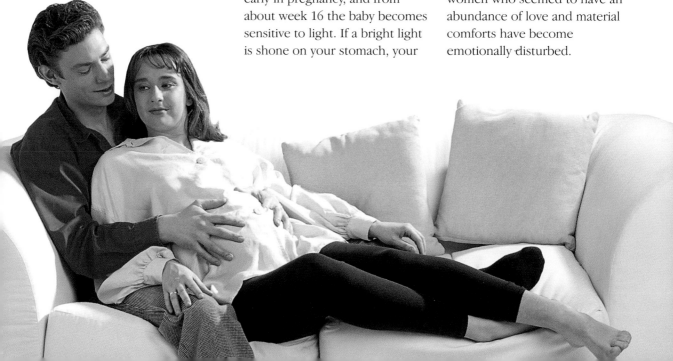

Still, when you are happy, you produce endorphins – hormones that enter your bloodstream and cross the placenta to your baby. When you are frightened or anxious, the adrenal hormones you produce are similarly transmitted to your baby. It seems likely, therefore, that your baby can react to your emotions – both positive ones, such as love, and negative ones, such as fear.

But even without these links, women who are positive about their pregnancy tend to be those who have more satisfying childbirth experiences. For this reason, if for no other, dwell on your positive feelings towards your baby and do your best to transmit your love and happiness to her.

NAMING THE BABY

Many couples share a pet name for their unborn baby, often one they would never dream of bestowing officially. This is a loving way of recognizing that they are a threesome and of feeling closer to their baby without voicing any expectations of gender, looks or personality.

You will probably want to choose your baby's "proper" names before the birth. You may have your own favourites or a family name that you want to pass on. Or perhaps you want to name your child after someone you admire or love.

Massaging your baby in the womb is a wonderful way to give her the experience of a loving touch. You can continue to massage the baby after the birth; you may see her visibly relax as you stroke and touch her.

What you can do ...

To stimulate your baby's listening response

Start playing music regularly to your baby beginning five or six months into your pregnancy: set aside about 10 minutes several times a week. Choose a time when the house is quiet, and sit or lie close to the speakers so that no extraneous noise interferes with the music. Research shows that unborn babies are more restful, as if actually listening, when simple melodies are played. Simple flute music elicits an especially good response; more complex sounds at this stage are apparently too difficult to decipher. Loud orchestral or rock music with the occasional boom or clang causes jumpier, more agitated movements.

To make the sound of your voice familiar

Talk to your baby when you are lying down and relaxing. She can hear your voice. Help her to know it better without the distractions of other everyday noises.

It doesn't matter what you say – read poetry if you're not sure where to start – but use a calm, regular tone of voice. Or sing soft, soothing melodies to her.

To communicate your touch

Babies are sensitive to touch from very early on. When you can feel your baby as she moves, and even see the shape of her kicking legs and punching arms, touch and massage your abdomen gently, smoothly and regularly. You can use baby oil, or a mild vegetable or nut oil such as almond oil, to enhance the experience for you. Your partner can share or even take over the massage as you continue gently communicating with your baby.

To avoid superbaby syndrome

One word of warning: stories abound of parents reading the classics or playing symphonies to their unborn babies with the intention of getting them into the best kindergartens by the age of three. No real evidence exists that such hot-housing works or – even if it did – that any initial advantage is sustained as a child grows up.

Let your baby know that she is loved and wanted, both before and after birth. Then allow her to develop at her own pace.

Playing music to your baby while she is in the uterus will help you to feel especially close to her. You may also reap rich rewards after the birth: music is often effective in soothing a crying baby.

The sixth month

FOR YOU

This is a time when your uterus grows rapidly and you gain weight quickly. Your midwife may measure your stomach with a tape; this provides a relatively accurate guide to the size of the uterus and the baby inside it.

You will probably feel healthy and fit, and you may be tempted to maintain a high level of activity. But remember that your heart

The uterus rises above your navel at 24 to 25 weeks, and you will notice your navel flattening, or even popping outwards under the pressure.

and lungs are now working 50 percent harder than they were before you became pregnant (see pp. 56–57 and 96). Be careful not to exhaust yourself.

You may notice that you have started to produce colostrum, or early milk; in some women a little of this leaks from their nipples.

At this stage it is fairly easy to hear your baby's heartbeat. Borrow a stethoscope for yourself; your partner should be able to hear the heartbeat by putting his ear to your abdomen.

How your breasts change

Your breasts are composed of glandular tissue made up of 15 to 20 lobes, each divided into smaller lobules. The lobules contain sacs (alveoli) that consist of clusters of cells. Each lobe is drained by a duct. The ducts converge beneath the nipple. There they widen into milk reservoirs before narrowing again to emerge as openings on the nipple's surface.

Influenced by oestrogen and progesterone, the milk-duct system expands in the first five or six months of pregnancy, and more lobules are formed. As the

lobules enlarge, protein and fat accumulate in the cells lining the alveoli. In later pregnancy and in the first days after your baby's birth, your breasts release colostrum, a yellowish, watery substance that contains protein, sugar and antibodies.

You will not produce milk until after the birth, but the breasts are capable of producing milk after about six months of pregnancy. As a result, women whose babies are premature make milk to feed them within days of the birth, just as women whose babies are born "on time" do.

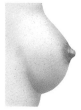

Non-pregnant

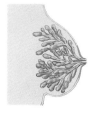

After 6 months

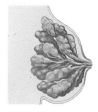

While breast-feeding

FOR YOUR BABY

Your baby is continuing to grow but has so little body fat that he still looks very thin. During these weeks the baby will fill out, becoming bigger and stronger. The skin still has a thick covering of vernix, and vernix production continues to increase during these weeks.

If your baby is born at any time from now on, he has the capacity to survive. The lungs are not mature enough to function alone, however, and many babies born as early as this need a great deal of neonatal intensive care.

Size
At 25 weeks, the baby is about 34 cm (13½ in) long and weighs about 600 g (21 oz).

Hands
A unique set of fingerprints starts to appear on the fingertips.

Eyes
The eyes are open by week 25, and the baby responds to light (see pp. 104–105).

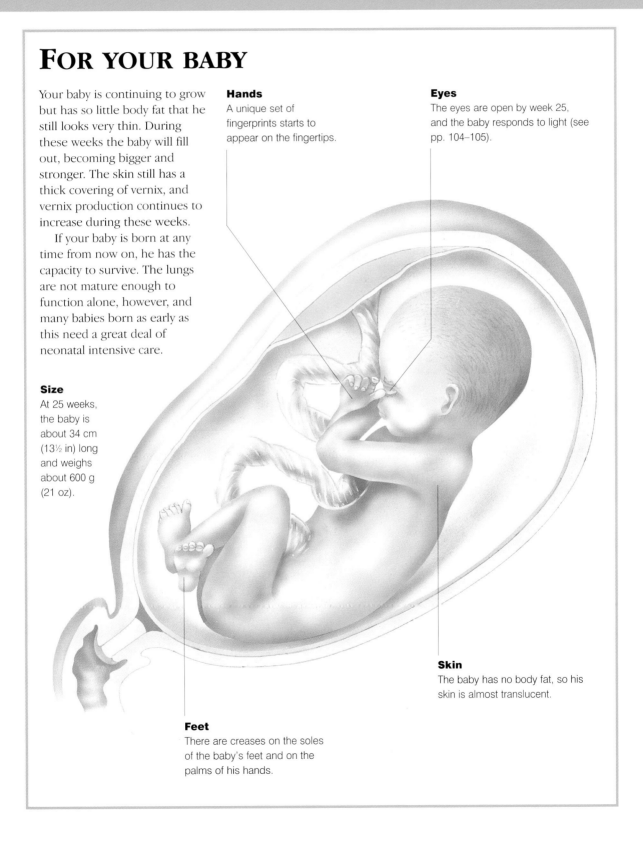

Skin
The baby has no body fat, so his skin is almost translucent.

Feet
There are creases on the soles of the baby's feet and on the palms of his hands.

THE EMOTIONAL IMPACT AFTER SIX MONTHS

Once the euphoria of learning you are pregnant has worn off, and the birth itself draws closer, you and your partner may experience mixed emotions.

Pregnancy is a time for sharing and for feeling close to your partner. You are embarking on one of life's greatest adventures together, one that began with your love for each other. Whether your pregnancy was planned or a surprise, happened quickly or was eagerly awaited for years, it will naturally cause some anxieties and concerns about the future. You may be able to imagine the first few days of parenthood after childbirth, but it's always difficult to look beyond them. You know you are facing a test of character. Are you ready and able to meet the demands of parenthood?

Your feelings about your own childhood may surface now. If you had parents you love and respect, you have a hard act to follow (see p. 68). If your background was less happy, you may be concerned about the lack of role models to guide you. If your parents are no longer living, you may find you miss them acutely.

Many antenatal classes begin around now. These provide a forum for airing your feelings and give you the chance to raise topics that concern you with a wider audience. Many of your anxieties may be addressed: you will learn, for example, what happens during the birth and discover ways of supporting each other.

YOUR CONCERNS

Your major concern is likely to be your baby. The first question most new mothers ask – even those who have had antenatal tests to confirm their baby's health – is not "Is it a boy or a girl?" but "Is it okay?" You may then start to wonder what you will do if all is not "okay".

It is worth putting children's special needs in perspective: one in six children has some form of special need. The overwhelming majority are minor physical problems or slight, often temporary, learning difficulties. This statistic does not lessen the impact of your child's needs, but it may help you to realize that many other parents have faced a similar challenge. Severe, life-threatening

---

A Case in Point
Hidden Anxieties

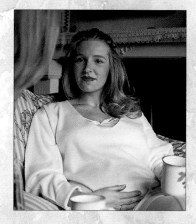

CLARE, 30, HAD AN EASY PREGNANCY FOR THE FIRST SIX MONTHS.

"*My pregnancy came as a surprise, although we'd talked about starting a family some time in the future. Luckily, I escaped all the worst early symptoms. Then, at around six months, I started having the most terrible dreams. In the worst one, which recurred and seemed more real every time, labour went on for days and was very painful. And when the baby was finally born, they wouldn't let me see it. I knew I must have given birth to a monster. The other dreams weren't as bad, but in all of them I was frightened or in pain.*

"*After about a month of having the dreams, I started going to antenatal classes. To my relief one of the other mothers-to-be asked if frightening dreams were normal because she was having ones similar to mine. We discussed them a lot. Gradually, I realized that they stemmed from my fears about how I would cope with the birth, anxiety that I wouldn't be a good mother, and also a sense of guilt that I hadn't really wanted a child yet.*

"*Once I talked those feelings through and came to terms with them, the dreams stopped. I handled Sophie's birth better than I could have hoped, and, of course, she's perfect.*"

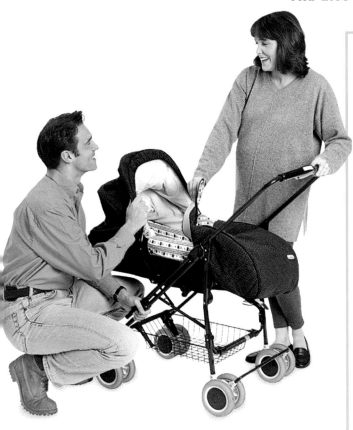

A second baby

If this is not your first baby, your feelings may be even more complex as the birth of the new baby draws near. You know what to expect of childbirth and of the first few weeks with a newborn, and you probably feel more secure in your parenting skills. But you may wonder about the impact of the new baby on your first child and feel overwhelmingly protective towards her.

Mixed reactions to a sibling are normal. Your child has had your sole attention up to now and will have to learn to share you. New babies take a lot of time, and their needs cannot be put on hold for long.

You cannot resolve in advance all your child's feelings about the newborn. (If your first child is still a baby, she won't even be able to articulate them.) But in these few months, spend as much time as you can with your child, making her feel secure in the knowledge that you love her and enjoy being with her. If she is old enough, take her on a couple of "grown-up" outings that she will treasure. When the baby is born, these efforts will help her to understand her own special place in your family.

Talking of the baby as a playmate can be misleading, since a young child may then expect the baby to be able to play immediately. But talking about what the baby will bring to your family – someone to look after, another person to love – can give an older sibling a greater sense of involvement. Emphasize your child's role as the older sibling whom the baby will love and need.

Try also to make sure that your partner spends plenty of time with your child so that when you are wholly involved in baby care, their strong relationship can bridge the gap.

disabilities are relatively rare. Whatever the need, support groups abound and provide information and friendship.

As the birth draws closer, acknowledge your questions and fears about the birth process itself. Talk to your partner and other new parents so that you are as well prepared as possible.

PARTNERS: YOUR CONCERNS

You will share many of your partner's feelings – elation at the prospect of being a parent and anxiety about the new person who is about to join your lives. If you have no previous experience of childbirth, you may wonder if you will be able to offer the support your partner needs. You may be concerned about your involvement with the baby or fear the changes that the baby's arrival will inevitably cause to your relationship. Talk about your concerns with your partner.

One way many couples prepare to become a threesome is to pursue activities that make the baby seem more real. Shopping together for baby paraphernalia helps to bring the baby closer to you even before the birth.

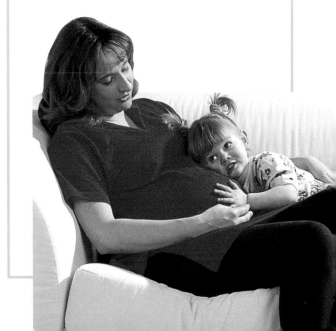

SEX DURING PREGNANCY

Whether you are highly aroused during pregnancy, or too tired or anxious to relax and enjoy sex, loving communication with your partner is important.

Your feelings about sex may change during pregnancy. You may want more sex, or you may want less. Your attitude towards lovemaking may change from week to week; you and your partner may suddenly find that you have different needs, even if you were well matched before.

During the first three months, you may be too tired and too nauseous to enjoy sex. But later, it's normal to have a heightened libido. By the fourth month, the increased blood supply to the tissues of the vagina causes many women to experience a state of more or less permanent arousal. You may find that your increased breast size makes you feel sexier. And many men find the sight of their partner's newly rounded body exciting. There is, after all, no more womanly shape than the pregnant abdomen.

On the other hand, the downside of a society that places so much emphasis on being slender is that many women feel they become unattractive once their contours start to round out. Remember, first, that you are gaining weight to support the life inside you, not because you are weak-willed or have let yourself go. Weight gained eating healthy food that is good for you and the baby will disappear after the birth. Your partner has his own unique viewpoint: your curvaceous torso is the final proof of his (and your) fertility. If weight is in danger of becoming an issue between you, talk about it.

IS IT SAFE?

Sexual intercourse while you are pregnant will not harm your baby in any way: he is cushioned by fluid in the amniotic sac, even at the end of pregnancy when his head is well down in your pelvis. At this later stage, the baby may be dimly aware of your partner's movements during intercourse, especially if they are vigorous, but this is in no way harmful.

Your doctor may advise against sexual intercourse if you have had one or more miscarriages. In this case, you may be asked to abstain around the time when a period would have been due, usually until after the first three months have elapsed. Then most doctors give the all clear.

Your doctor may also advise against sex if placenta praevia has been diagnosed (see pp. 176–77) or if you are considered at risk of premature labour. Ask your doctor or midwife about non-penetrative sex, and talk together as a couple about activities that enhance your enjoyment of intimacy.

Anxiety about miscarriage can be a cause of stress. Some couples become unwilling to cuddle or touch in case they become too aroused to stop. You can't cause miscarriage or premature labour (if it's not about to start anyway) by anything you do sexually, so follow your feelings. Spotting is common around the time of a missed period and almost always nothing to worry about – it's not caused by having intercourse.

Sex and labour

Sexual activity of any kind releases oxytocin, a hormone that causes the uterus to contract. For this reason, couples are sometimes advised to have sex if their labour is overdue and they are tired of waiting for something to happen.

While you may not feel up to sexual intercourse itself, you can use nipple stimulation, masturbation or manual stimulation. Make sure you have adequate privacy, or you won't be able to relax.

If you are not too tired or uncomfortable for penetrative sex, remember that seminal fluid contains prostaglandins, which can sometimes speed the "ripening" of the cervix when labour is about to begin anyway.

You should certainly avoid penetrative sex once your waters have broken, since there is a risk that you might introduce infection. Some doctors advise that you avoid penetrative sex as soon as the cervix has begun to dilate, even if the membranes haven't ruptured. Again, there is a slight risk of infection.

Remember: sex can't precipitate labour if it's not about to start anyway, so there is no risk of premature labour beginning or of your going into labour before you and your baby are ready.

COMFORTABLE POSITIONS

In the first three months of pregnancy, especially if there is little outward change in your body, there may be no need to change the positions you normally adopt for lovemaking. You may, however, find it more comfortable to avoid deep penetration.

Almost from the start, however, the changes in your breasts that prepare them for feeding your baby (see p. 106) can make some positions uncomfortable: in the missionary position, for example, your breasts are constantly stimulated, which can make them sore. Many women say that their breasts become so tender they feel almost bruised. During sexual arousal, blood rushes into the veins, making the tissue further engorged – the average breast is 25 percent bigger when you are aroused. Breast and nipple stimulation during pregnancy

should be very gentle, whatever your prior preferences.

In later pregnancy, some change is almost inevitable. Some couples find man-on-top positions awkward or uncomfortable unless he supports himself on his elbows to avoid placing all his weight on his partner's abdomen. If you find that you get dizzy when you lie on your back, you may prefer to lie side by side, with your partner entering you from behind. This reduces pressure on your abdomen and limits the depth of penetration, but, obviously, you are not face to face.

Woman-on-top positions offer the advantage of face-to-face contact. They also allow you to control the depth of penetration and set a pace that feels comfortable.

During the last trimester, backache can be a problem. Once the baby's head engages into the pelvis, you may also feel that the baby is taking up all available space. In addition, your partner may worry that he will somehow hurt the baby (he won't). You may be more comfortable kneeling with your forearms on the bed so that the baby's weight is taken off your cervix and have your partner enter you from behind.

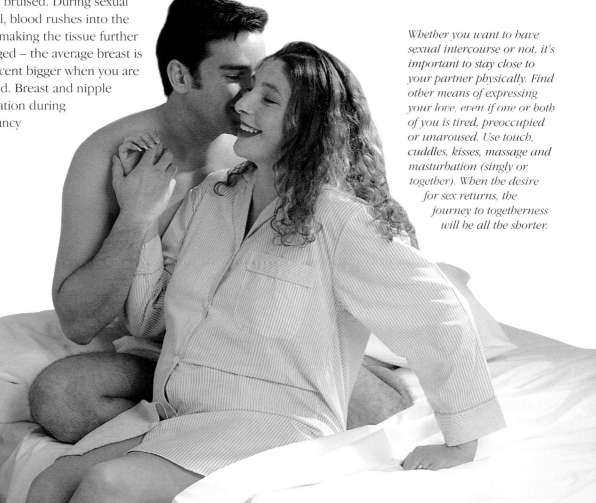

Whether you want to have sexual intercourse or not, it's important to stay close to your partner physically. Find other means of expressing your love, even if one or both of you is tired, preoccupied or unaroused. Use touch, cuddles, kisses, massage and masturbation (singly or together). When the desire for sex returns, the journey to togetherness will be all the shorter.

COMMON DISCOMFORTS

The minor problems of the second trimester are easy to deal with, and many can be avoided completely by paying attention to diet and overall fitness.

Some of the minor irritations of the first trimester may continue. The pressure of the uterus makes the bladder feel full even if it is not, and pregnancy hormones relax the bladder, making you want to urinate more often. Other, mostly minor, problems may arise as your baby grows.

THRUSH

As levels of acidity and sugar in the vagina alter during pregnancy, the fungus *Candida albicans* may multiply rapidly, which in some women results in thrush. Symptoms include itchy skin around the vagina and anus and a milky-white, flaky vaginal discharge. Your doctor may prescribe pessaries or a cream that will be safe to use in pregnancy.

About 25 percent of women have a *Candida* infection at term. This is normally treated only if the discharge is irritating.

CYSTITIS

This bacterial infection is common during pregnancy due to the pressure of the uterus on the ureters and the effect of hormonal changes on muscle tone. The bladder cannot empty completely, and bacteria multiply.

Symptoms include a constant desire to urinate and irritation, pain or burning during urination. Drinking lots of water can help to flush out the infection.

To prevent cystitis, drink cranberry juice, which can inhibit

How pregnancy affects your organs

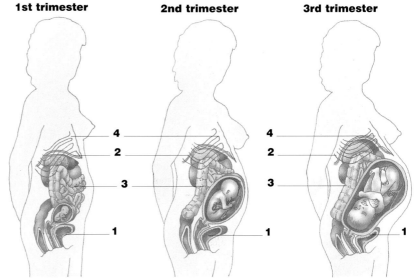

1st trimester

2nd trimester

3rd trimester

1 Bladder
The growing uterus presses on the base of the bladder until the uterus rises out of the pelvis (about week 12); as the baby's head moves down to engage, pressure returns.

2 Diaphragm
In the later months, the expanding uterus presses on the diaphragm, pushing it into the chest cavity, thus decreasing the lungs' ability to expand.

3 Intestines
As the uterus expands, space for the intestines becomes limited, and they are pressed up against the diaphragm into the chest cavity.

4 Rib cage
The increase in blood circulation demands more oxygen from the lungs. The lungs expand to cope, which may cause your ribs to flare out to the sides and front.

bacterial growth. Urinate before and after having sex, and try to empty your bladder completely. Continue to drink lots of water. Your doctor may want to do a urine culture every month, or prescribe antibiotics if cystitis is a recurrent problem or you have had a kidney infection.

VARICOSE VEINS

Swollen veins in the legs often result from poor circulation, although a hereditary factor also

exists. Varicose veins occur during pregnancy because the extra weight you are carrying puts stress on the veins of the lower body. As the volume of blood in the veins increases, the walls stretch, causing blood to pool in the veins.

Try to avoid standing for long periods, which puts more strain on your lower body. Sit with your feet raised as often as you can, and raise the foot of your mattress by about 15 cm (6 in). If you must be on your feet or sit for long periods of time, wear support tights and walk for at least 2 to 3 minutes every 30 to 45 minutes.

HAEMORRHOIDS

Varicose veins of the anus, or haemorrhoids, are common in pregnancy, again because of pressure from the uterus. They usually become a problem only when they are exacerbated by constipation. Then they can become painful and may bleed or itch. To avoid constipation, eat plenty of fibre-rich foods and drink lots of fluids. Pelvic-floor exercises (see pp. 44–45) may also help to improve the blood flow to the veins and relieve pressure.

Varicose veins of the vulva are also common; wearing a sanitary pad may relieve pressure on them.

GESTATIONAL DIABETES

Diabetes related solely to pregnancy may occur in the second half of pregnancy. This is discussed on page 143.

Sitting with your feet up helps to prevent blood (and other fluid) from pooling in your lower limbs, a cause of swelling, pain and varicose veins. Do foot-circling exercises (see p. 48) to improve circulation in your lower legs.

How can I avoid stretch marks?

The chances are that you can't. Almost all women develop the pinkish streaks known as stretch marks to some extent. They usually appear on the breasts early in pregnancy, then on the abdomen, hips, thighs and elsewhere later.

Women who manage to avoid them are usually those who inherited supple skin or maintained a healthy diet and got plenty of exercise before they were pregnant (one more reason to get yourself in shape before you conceive). Stretch marks are more common in women who have delicate skin. They can be minimized by keeping your weight gain gradual and moderate.

Creams can prevent your skin from feeling too dry. They can be pleasant to use, but they cannot stop the collagen, well below the surface of the skin, from stretching and tearing as the baby grows and you gain weight.

Stretch marks do shrink and become silvery and less noticeable over time, but they rarely disappear.

BACKACHE

Backache is avoidable during pregnancy. If you were fit before you conceived, you stand a good chance of escaping it. Strong back and abdominal muscles help you to maintain good posture even as your abdomen grows.

Several factors contribute to backache during this time: the effects of the hormone relaxin on the ligaments; the loosening of the joints of the pelvic bones; and a shift in your centre of gravity as your abdomen grows. Spending long periods of time on your feet may also give you backache.

Wear shoes with a low heel, and sit and stand with your back straight and shoulders back. Lift objects carefully, bending your knees. Avoid carrying a heavy bag over one shoulder only – doing so throws your spine out of line, which may cause back stress.

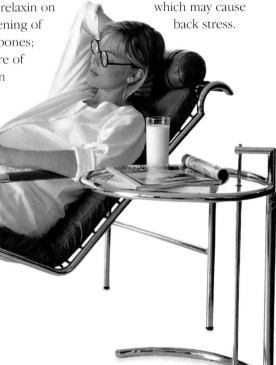

LOOKING THE PART

Although pregnancy hormones are likely to affect your hair, skin, nails and teeth, more often than not the changes are for the better.

You may find that you look healthy and radiant all through your pregnancy. Or there may be times when your skin, hair and general appearance seem dull

Hair
Choose an easy-to-manage style and have your hair trimmed regularly to keep it in good condition. A visit to the hairdresser in the last month is a good morale booster – you may not get the chance again for a while!

and fatigue shows in your face. Still, the phenomenon known as the "bloom of pregnancy" is experienced at some stage by most women. You are likely to notice it after about three months, and it will continue until the last few weeks of your pregnancy. In the interim, any sickness you've had is probably gone, or less severe. Also, you may not feel as anxious or tired as you did at the

beginning or may at the end of the nine months. You may be eating better than you did before you became pregnant, and this will have a positive effect on your skin and hair. But the main causes of the bloom of pregnancy are your increased metabolism, which now filters out toxins more quickly, and increased oestrogen production, which offsets any tendency towards skin blemishes and widens the arteries supplying blood to the skin.

YOUR SKIN
Some women notice a darkening of skin pigmentation during pregnancy (see p. 96). More common, however, is an unpredictable reaction to cosmetics. Products you've used in the past may no longer suit you. Dry skin may become drier, and red, itchy palms may develop, again because of an increase in hormone production. If you have oily skin, you may notice that it becomes even oilier.

You may sweat more; some women develop a visible rash where perspiration hasn't evaporated. This increase, too, occurs because of your raised metabolism. Wearing loose cotton clothing helps, as does using cornflour after a bath or shower.

Sunlight benefits the skin because it helps the body to produce vitamin D (which your body needs in order to metabolize calcium effectively). You may find that you burn more easily during pregnancy, however, so remain in direct sunlight for

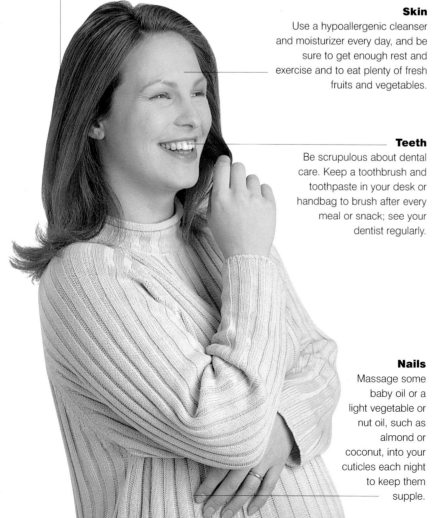

Skin
Use a hypoallergenic cleanser and moisturizer every day, and be sure to get enough rest and exercise and to eat plenty of fresh fruits and vegetables.

Teeth
Be scrupulous about dental care. Keep a toothbrush and toothpaste in your desk or handbag to brush after every meal or snack; see your dentist regularly.

Nails
Massage some baby oil or a light vegetable or nut oil, such as almond or coconut, into your cuticles each night to keep them supple.

only short periods, and avoid the "peak hours" – 10 AM to 2 PM. Wear a hat, and use a sunscreen with a high sun protection factor (SPF), especially on your face, whenever you're out in the sun. Using tanning machines isn't recommended because of the risk of burning.

YOUR TEETH

There's a widespread idea that your teeth suffer during pregnancy. This isn't inevitably the case, of course, but it's true that your gums are more susceptible to infection while you are pregnant. The pregnancy hormones make them softer; as a result the gums are more likely to become swollen, inflamed or broken, and they may bleed.

Broken skin can lead to infection, which causes the gums to recede and to expose the more sensitive part of the teeth. This, in turn, creates a greater risk of decay. Use only a medium or soft-bristle toothbrush to avoid damaging the gums.

You can make a difference by practising good teeth care while you are pregnant. Pay attention to cleaning and flossing. (Keep a toothbrush at work.) See your dentist for regular check-ups. Have your teeth cleaned to remove plaque – build-up may exacerbate gum problems. Bleeding gums are common and rarely indicate an infection, but see your dentist to make sure that all is well.

A healthy diet pays dividends for your teeth. Avoid refined sugars and eat plenty of foods rich in vitamin C (to strengthen gums) and calcium (important for your teeth and bones, as well as those of your baby).

Your hair during pregnancy

You may find that your hair feels thicker than before you were pregnant because the normal level of hair loss slows down during pregnancy. You actually keep more of the hair you grow. This is reversed after you give birth, when the decline in hormone levels may make your hair fall out more quickly than usual. Don't worry – new hair is already growing, and you will be back to normal in a few months: no treatment is necessary.

Most women find that their hair is more lustrous during pregnancy because the pregnancy hormones often stimulate oil production in the scalp. If you had a tendency to oiliness before pregnancy, it may become more pronounced. In a few women, the reverse happens – hair that is usually dry becomes drier.

It is usually best to avoid perms and colorants. The hair often changes during pregnancy, which means that your hairdresser will not be able to predict your hair's reaction to the chemicals in these products. A perm may not take at all, and colour may be patchy. (Some hairdressers will not use chemicals on pregnant women for this reason.)

More important, the chemicals contained in these products are absorbed by the hair shaft and pass through the scalp into the bloodstream and, perhaps, across the placenta. Studies so far have cleared such products of causing foetal damage (so don't worry about past treatments), but a theoretical risk exists. Some colour products contain lead.

If you really want to change your hair colour or simply give yourself a boost, try rinse colours – either natural ones, such as henna or lemon rinse, or chemical ones that only coat the hair rather than penetrating the hair shaft. If you don't like the result, you can fix it more easily.

YOUR NAILS

The increased metabolism typical of pregnancy may make your nails grow faster, but they may also become brittle and develop grooves. A professional manicure can help to improve your nails' appearance (and is a wonderfully self-indulgent experience).

Not only are your feet carrying your extra weight, but they may also be swollen by fluid retention. The hormone relaxin softens the ligaments between the joints, which may make your feet spread, so that your shoes feel tight. Pamper your feet – or get your partner to do so for you. A foot massage at the end of the day is a relaxing way to wind down.

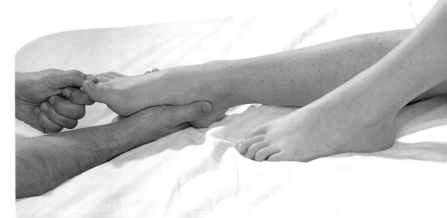

DRESSING THE PART

Looking good during pregnancy makes you feel good, too; you can choose from a wide range of clothes without compromising your own style.

Some of your clothes may start to feel tight from as early as 10 or 12 weeks, but you probably won't need to buy anything special until the fourth or fifth month. Men's sweaters and shirts (borrow your partner's) are often cut big and baggy and can work for casual wear right until the end.

You needn't worry about the baby if your clothing is tight – he is totally protected from any pinching or squeezing. However, clothing that constricts at the waist (or where your waist used to be) will be uncomfortable. Traditional-style flowing dresses are no longer the only option: stretchy fabrics, such as Lycra, allow for comfortable, figure-hugging styles if you want to show off your beautiful new shape.

Trousers or leggings (cut for pregnancy, with extra room in the front) worn with sweaters or T-shirts are great for weekends. For work, look for well-cut trousers and team them with a long blouse or shirt over the top (again, your partner's shirts may fit the bill – and you can even add a tie occasionally, just for fun). A maternity jacket can be expensive, but you may feel this is justified if you wear it almost daily for three or four months.

Layered clothing is ideal. If you get too hot – as you may, if you are pregnant during the summer – blood flows away from the uterus (and your baby) to the skin in order to cool you down. Being able to add or shed a layer will enable you to regulate your body temperature more easily.

If you buy clothing that can be worn while you are breast-feeding, you will get several more months' wear out of it while you are getting back to your pre-pregnancy contours.

YOUR SHOES

Have your shoe size checked after the fifth or sixth month. As the ligaments in your feet soften (see p. 115), you may find that your feet are half a size bigger, making previously well-fitting shoes tight.

A slight heel is better for your posture and your back than either a high heel or a totally flat one. Very high heels and slingbacks may make you totter dangerously. Choose leather or canvas so that your feet can

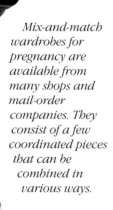

Mix-and-match wardrobes for pregnancy are available from many shops and mail-order companies. They consist of a few coordinated pieces that can be combined in various ways.

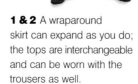

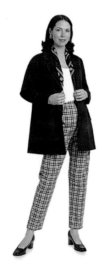

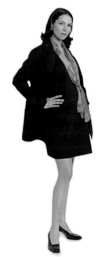

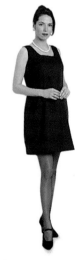

1 & 2 A wraparound skirt can expand as you do; the tops are interchangeable and can be worn with the trousers as well.

3 Elasticated trousers are comfortable and can be dressed up with a jacket.

4 A simple dress and jacket combine for a smart office look.

5 The same dress, set off with jewellery, becomes an elegant formal evening dress.

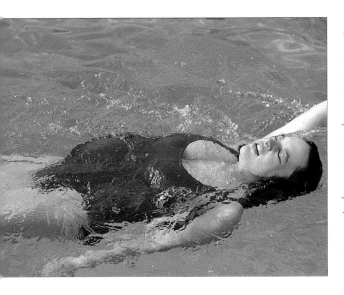

A regular swimsuit won't work for long because over-stretching weakens the fibres. If you swim often, you may find the expense of a maternity suit justified. Or ask your friends if anyone has a maternity suit that she is no longer using.

Your personal style

Every woman is different and every pregnancy unique. You don't need to sacrifice your personal style simply because you are pregnant. In fact, some women are so proud of their enlarged breasts and rounded stomachs that they want to show them off.

Find the elements of your style that can be maintained through nine months of body changes (and beyond). Concentrate on colour, the cut of necklines and sleeves, skirt lengths, trouser styles and accessories.

Clothes such as dungarees, stretchy skirts and leggings that are simply one or two sizes bigger than normal may fit until well into your pregnancy. A flowing skirt may fit for longer if you replace the waistband with a drawstring. A collection of scarves or jewellery can be augmented all through your pregnancy, especially as your choice of clothes becomes more limited.

The point is, pregnancy may make you feel unfamiliar with your own body, but you needn't feel frumpy.

breathe. Sneakers with good support for your arches and heels are excellent footwear for both home and leisure.

CHOOSING UNDERWEAR

Some women find that their normal size and style of bra fits until they are about six months pregnant; others need a larger size well before then. Your rib cage may expand, making a larger size necessary, and you will probably increase by two or three cup sizes in a first pregnancy (in subsequent pregnancies, the breasts may need less preparation for breast-feeding). If your breasts become very large, you may be more comfortable wearing a lightweight cotton bra when you sleep as well.

It is worth being measured for a bra that will give you support in the last few months of pregnancy and beyond. It should have some form of front opening for easy breast-feeding. Choose a style with a wide, long fastening at the back; this allows you to increase the size in the first few days after the birth, when you may need extra room. Wide shoulder straps

are more comfortable and supportive than thin ones. Cotton or cotton blends feel coolest and stand up to frequent washing (it's not uncommon to leak colostrum before the birth and milk afterwards – you will need to launder your bras frequently).

Buy pants that you can wear under your tummy, bikini-style, or choose a large, stretchy style that you can pull right up over it. Anything you wear halfway up may irritate the skin on your abdomen where it is stretched most thinly. Waist-high pants will have a tendency to roll down at the top, causing uncomfortable and unattractive bulges. Cotton and cotton blends are the best fabric options, especially for women who are prone to thrush (see p. 112) – the fungus that causes this is more likely to thrive under hot synthetic fibres.

If you wear tights, you don't need to buy the more expensive maternity tights when you get too big for non-maternity styles. Extra-large regular tights should fit if you wear them back to front,

so that the largest part is over your stomach.

Support tights can help ease aching legs, especially if you need to be on your feet a lot. If you have varicose veins, support tights are most effective when you put them on before you get out of bed in the morning. Avoid elastic-topped socks and stockings, which can restrict your circulation. Your doctor may prescribe custom-made anti-embolism stockings if varicose veins are very pronounced.

YOUR RIGHTS AT WORK

Pregnancy brings some entitlements at work, which are intended to safeguard your health and well-being and that of your baby.

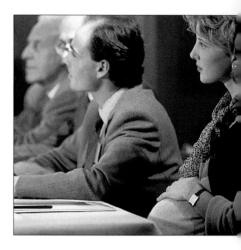

Q *I am pregnant. What are my rights to maternity leave?*

A In both Australia and New Zealand, employees who have worked for a period are entitled to parental leave, which includes maternity leave and generally allows for 52 weeks' unpaid leave. In the public sector in Australia, there is also provision for paid maternity leave; this is becoming increasingly available in the private sector as well. You should check with your union, your employer or your local Department of Labour.

Q *I've read so much about safety at work during pregnancy. How can I make sure my workplace is safe?*

A Most jobs and most workplaces are absolutely safe while you are pregnant. The main exceptions are jobs that involve chemicals or radiation; health-care work; work with animals (although you can take steps here to prevent infection); and jobs that involve heavy lifting and long periods on your feet.

You have a right to know the risks to which you are exposed in the workplace, and your employers have a duty to tell you. If you are in any doubt about workplace safety, contact your local Department of Occupational Health and Safety.

If your job is sedentary, you may feel able to work almost to the end of your pregnancy. Be sure to take a lunch break – spend the time with your feet up, if you can – and try to travel outside peak hours.

Q *My employers want me to take part of my annual holidays to cover my antenatal appointments. Am I obliged to?*

A No. These appointments are part of your medical care, and you should therefore be able to take time off without losing any part of your holiday entitlements or regular pay. Make sure you make the proper arrangements with your supervisor for the necessary time off.

Q *My job sometimes involves heavy lifting. I'm worried about the safety of this while I am pregnant. Can I be excused from this part of the job?*

A You can request a transfer to another job or ask to be excused from unsuitable parts of your job. Your doctor can assess the risks involved and provide an appropriate certificate or letter for your employer. If you have any doubts, it is worth getting advice from your union representative, your company's personnel director or your local Department of Labour or Industrial Relations.

Q *I suffered badly with morning sickness in early pregnancy and took quite a lot of time off work. Will this count as part of my maternity leave?*

A No. You were off work because of sickness, as you might have been if you were not pregnant, and this time counts as sick leave. It does not affect your rights to maternity leave and pay.

Q *I had only been back at work a couple of months after having a baby when I found out I was pregnant again. Will I get maternity leave again?*

A Yes. You have the same rights to maternity leave for each pregnancy.

Q *Do I get my old job back when I return to work?*

A Yes. You are entitled to return to your old job if it still exists, or else to a position as close as possible in salary and status to your former job.

Q *I'm on my feet for five or six hours a day at work and am beginning to find it tiring. What should I do?*

A Long periods of time on your feet can give you backache, may lead to swollen ankles, and will aggravate varicose veins and haemorrhoids, if you are suffering from them. Think first about whether it is necessary for you to be on your feet so much. Many jobs can be done just as well sitting. If you work in a shop, for example, could you sit for part of the day; if you are a waitress or a hairdresser, could you take a break between customers; if you are a police officer, could you spend more time at your desk?

If you must remain standing for long periods, make sure you get enough rest with your feet up at other times. Make a point of eating well, so that you have plenty of energy. Wear support tights to minimize discomfort from varicose veins.

All these measures may go some way to easing aches and pains, but you may still find that you will have to consider starting your maternity leave earlier than you planned.

If you work with young children, you may find your job tiring, so make sure that you get plenty of rest. You will also be exposed to more childhood infections. Take the same precautions other pregnant women do: eat well; avoid being on your feet for long periods; avoid heavy lifting; and avoid bending from the waist – bend your knees if you want to get down to child level.

Q *Can my partner take some paid time off when the baby is born?*

A Parental leave, which is recognized in both Australia and New Zealand, provides for paternity leave under certain circumstances. Generally, this leave will be unpaid, but many public sector and some private sector awards or workplace agreements provide for paid leave.

Q *We are planning to adopt a child. Can I take time off to help the baby settle down?*

A Yes. Adoption leave is provided for under the parental leave provisions, and generally applies to the adoption of a child under five years of age.

Q *What happens about parental leave if I have a miscarriage, my baby dies or the adoption does not proceed?*

A If the employee has not yet started parental leave, then the leave is automatically cancelled. If the employee is on leave, he or she must apply to return to work and should be allowed to do so within a reasonable time. In some cases, special maternity leave is available to allow the employee time to cope with the loss.

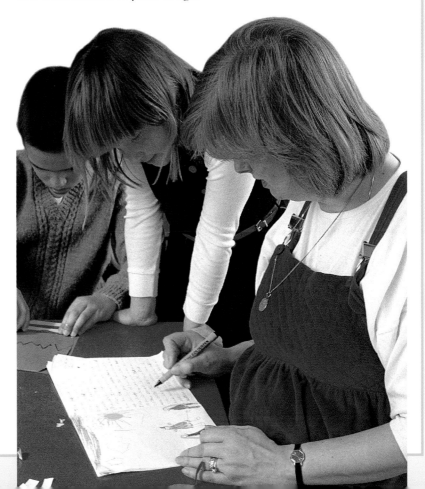

CHILD CARE: THE OPTIONS

Start thinking about your options for child care now, before you start finalizing your own career plans.

There are few rights and wrongs when it comes to child care – but there is a right way for your baby, you, and the other members of your family. Some full-time mothers have babies who thrive on being cared for at home; other at-home mums find themselves embroiled in household chores and less able to give a baby the care and attention he needs. Some babies benefit from the early socialization a nursery gives them; others seem to need more individual attention.

THINKING ABOUT YOURSELF

If you know that full-time motherhood is not for you, spend as much time as you can finding a carer for your baby (see pp. 122–23), but don't feel you have to get back to work right after the birth just because your child care is arranged. You need time to recover physically from the birth and to get used to all the changes, mental and emotional, that motherhood brings.

Making the most of the time you spend at home will help to build your relationship with your baby. You will have an opportunity to lay to rest any nagging doubts about whether you should stay at home or for how long. If you stay at home until breast-feeding is well established, you may be able to express milk for your baby to have during the day and maintain a couple of breast-feeds – perhaps early morning and bedtime – once you return to work (see pp. 206–207).

If you think that you would like to stay at home but worry that you will not be able to afford it, include in your calculations what you will save by not working – fares, lunches, business wardrobe, and, of course, the cost of child care. Work out exactly how much you need to pay for the essentials and consider changes that might help you manage. When they sit down to work it out, many couples are surprised by how little they *have* to earn.

Which type of care is right for you?

At-home care by a family member

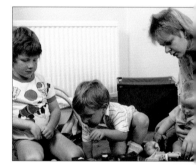

Today more and more fathers take an active role in raising their children, and for some couples, Dad's staying at home is a good option. As long as your baby has a stable environment – with a carer who loves him, is there for him, and makes him feel important – the gender of the carer really doesn't matter.

The other obvious family member to ask is one of the baby's grandparents.

Care in another's home

A childminder – often another mother – may care for your child, perhaps along with her own children, in her own home.

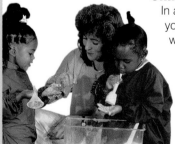

Child-care centres

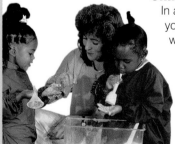

In a child-care centre, your baby is cared for with other children by trained staff. Many centres take children of all ages, from babies to school age.

At-home care by a nanny

A nanny is an employee paid to look after your child. Some live in, becoming part of the family; others come on a daily basis. "Nanny sharing", by which you and a friend employ a nanny to come into one of your homes and look after both babies, is also an option.

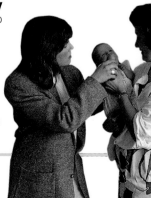

Advantages

- Your baby has all the advantages of home – the security of familiar surroundings, his own toys and equipment, and his own cot.
- He has the full, individual attention of the carer.
- You do not have to add travelling to a childminder or child-care centre to your already busy day.
- Since he is exposed to fewer other children and their germs, your baby is likely to get fewer coughs, colds, and childhood illnesses.
- Fathers who take such an active role in raising their children tend to have a stronger relationship with them in later life.
- Grandparents are often revitalized by this new role.

Disadvantages

- You may start to resent the close relationship building between your partner and your baby and feel you are somehow missing out.
- Despite the growing number of at-home fathers, dads are still in the minority at parent-and-toddler groups. If this makes your partner unwilling to frequent such gatherings, your baby may not get many opportunities to be with other children.
- If you ask your parent or parent-in-law to be the carer, you may find he or she has fixed ideas on child rearing that are different from yours. Do you have an honest enough relationship to be able to tell him or her that this is not the interaction you want with your child?

- This type of care usually costs less than a nanny, since the carer is not devoting herself to one child only.
- Her care is more personal than that of a nursery and she may be more flexible about hours.
- Your child will have plenty of opportunity to socialize with others – this can be especially important for only children, who need to learn respect for the feelings of other children.
- Childminders have to be registered and their homes must meet certain safety standards.

- Since she has more than one child to care for, a childminder may be unable to give your child the individual attention you might prefer.
- The childminder may be unwilling to have your child if he is sick.
- You have to add travelling time to your schedule.
- The childminder will have her own ideas on baby care and may be unwilling to listen to yours.
- There may be no back-up if a childminder is sick.

- Staff trained in baby and child development can provide plenty of opportunities for stimulating play geared to your baby's level of development.
- A centre offers social contact for your baby, although this is less important for infants than for older babies and toddlers.
- Since there are several carers, your baby is unlikely to be upset by a change of carer: someone familiar is always close by. Such continuity of care can be important.

- A child-care centre can be expensive, unless it is subsidized by your workplace.
- Because of the large number of children in such facilities, the rate of childhood illness tends to be higher than with other options.
- Your baby will not enjoy the same one-to-one relationship as with a nanny or family member.
- You have to add travelling time to your schedule (unless the centre is at your workplace).

- As with at-home care by a family member, your baby is in familiar surroundings and has all his toys around him.
- He is likely to be exposed to fewer germs than in other situations.
- He has the benefit of individual love and attention from an adult other than Mummy and Daddy.

- Exclusivity can be costly.
- You may resent having another person in your home, particularly one who, as you hope, is developing a close relationship with your baby. If the carer lives in, you may suffer a loss of privacy as a couple.
- Once the baby has formed a bond with the carer, he will suffer a loss if that person is not there, through sickness, family problems, or another job offer.
- Your baby may also not get much opportunity to mix with other children.

CHOOSING A CARER

If you are going to leave your baby in another's care, you must be absolutely sure that the person will be attentive, loving and responsive.

You need to start looking for a carer at least two months before you'll need one. But it is easier if you have done some preliminary work in advance.

If you are planning to return to work while your baby is young, do some investigating now, before finding care is a necessity. If you want to employ a nanny, either to live in or to come on a daily basis, contact agencies to find out their procedures for checking credentials and how much they charge. Visit child-care centres to get a feel for the range of services they offer. Similarly, visit a couple of childminders – even if they don't have vacancies – so that you know what to look for when the time comes.

VISITING CHILD-CARE CENTRES

A visit should allow you to learn the staff-to-children ratio (one to three is optimal for infants), the qualifications of the staff (what training they received), how they are licensed, and their attitudes (their philosophy of child care and their methods). Obviously, a staff member should respond to your questions, but she should always have her eyes and ears on the babies in her care.

Note whether the children are separated according to age (those under one year should not be with the boisterous toddlers), and observe the children. Are they happy and occupied? Even a small baby benefits from being

A Case in Point
When Dad Stays Home

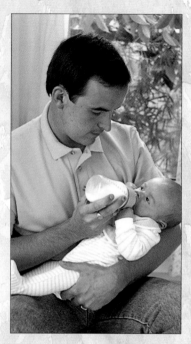

PETER AND SARAH, BOTH 35, WERE LIVING AND WORKING 500 KM (300 MILES) APART AND SAW EACH OTHER ONLY AT WEEKENDS WHEN SARAH BECAME PREGNANT.

"Although it came as a shock, Sarah's pregnancy put our shared life and logistics in perspective. We wanted this baby and had less than nine months to get organized.

"Sarah didn't want to give up her job as a special-needs teacher; I was less involved with my career. So I sold my house, left my job, and moved in with her. The decision to be a full-time dad came slowly. I could only get work that took me away from home for days on end, which wouldn't be an option once the baby was born. Sarah's house was too small for us to employ someone to live in, and neither of us could face another upheaval. The only childminder we liked didn't have a vacancy for a baby. With two weeks to go before Laura was due, I suggested I take a year off to look after the baby.

"Sarah went back to work when Laura was 10 weeks old. I don't know if I was just lucky, but she was a happy baby from the start. She was always pleased to see Sarah, but didn't fret when she left for work. She gained weight, slept well and rarely
cried. Every afternoon I took her to the park, and as soon as she could sit up, I put her in a baby swing and listened to her laugh. But the best thing was giving her a bath so that she was all clean and snuggled into her sleepsuit when Sarah came home, gave her a last bottle and put her to bed.

"As it turned out, I was home for 15 months, and I can honestly say that it was the best time of my life. I had a fulfilled wife and a thriving daughter, and I went to bed each night marvelling at whatever new accomplishment of Laura's I'd witnessed that day."

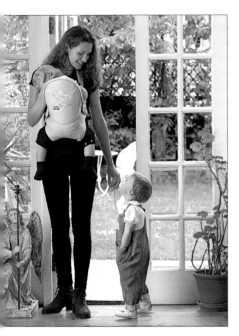

talked to or having a toy to play with. Is anyone crying – and how long does it take a carer to do something about it?

Are there plenty of toys appropriate to the ages of the babies and children? Ask whether children are encouraged to bring a special toy from home. Are there outdoor activities or trips?

Note whether the building is light, airy and a comfortable temperature. Look at areas where food is prepared and ask to see where bottles are stored. Is it all spotless? Do carers wash their hand frequently? Check on attitudes towards special dietary requirements.

CHILDMINDERS

Childminders' homes are inspected regularly to make sure that they comply with safety standards, and

When interviewing carers, decide in advance which issues are most important to you. These questions give you an idea of some of the subjects to cover – tailor them to suit your own needs.

Your baby or child is the best barometer of whether your child-care arrangement is working. If he seems happy, sleeps normally and continues to put on weight, all is probably well. If a happy baby suddenly becomes fretful or starts to cry more than usual, this may be a sign that the carer is not giving your baby what he needs.

approval from local council or government authorities is usually necessary. However, you should take a good look at the childminder's premises. It may be a busy family environment, but all food-preparation areas and bathrooms should be clean and tidy.

The number of children a childminder can care for at any one time is restricted by law, and the ages of the children will vary. Check that there are toys suitable for all the children to play with. If your baby takes some of her own, will they be taken care of? Equally important, are there signs that the minder spends time with the children in other activities – drawings stuck to the fridge, clay models on the table? This shows that the carer is interested in

stimulating the children, not simply watching them.

Check attitudes towards flexible hours, special dietary requirements and holiday arrangements. Ask if any back-up is provided if the minder gets sick. What happens if one of her own children is sick?

FINDING A NANNY

In some ways, a nanny can be the easiest type of carer to find because you are in the position of employer and in theory do not have to compromise. But in practice, if demand exceeds supply in your area, you may not get exactly who you are looking for. Decide in advance what your priorities are. For example, you may prefer someone who is open to your ideas on child care rather than wanting to do it all her own way.

Sift through applicants' CVs and make a shortlist of possibilities. Check all references and be prepared with questions for former employers. If you don't find someone the first time around, try again.

Previous employment
What age was the youngest child you have looked after?
How long were you with your last employer?
Why did you leave? Do you have references?

Familiarity with babies
How would you spend a day with my baby?
What do you think a baby this age needs most?
Have you studied child care or development?

Personal details
Why do you want this job?
How many days have you taken off sick in the last year?
Do you have children?
Do you smoke?

Fitting in
How would you react if I came home late? Would you consider sitting at night?

Personal skills
Are you certified in first aid?
Do you have a clean driver's licence?

TWINS: YOUR PREGNANCY

You will have twice the love and twice the joy with twins; but carrying two babies often augments the minor irritations of pregnancy.

Today multiple pregnancies are almost always diagnosed before delivery, usually at your first ultrasound scan. Your doctor will also check to see if your uterus is larger than typical for your stage of pregnancy. He or she may hear more than one heartbeat or feel more limbs than one baby could have, and, in later pregnancy, feel two distinct heads.

The uterus becomes crowded with two babies, two umbilical cords and two placentas (or one larger one for identical twins). You will look bigger earlier than someone expecting just one baby: as a guide, you can expect to look the same at 30 weeks as the mother of a single baby looks at full term.

MINIMIZING PROBLEMS

Carrying twins challenges your physical resources. Some problems are particular to – or more common in – twin pregnancies (see pp. 126–27). You may also suffer more acutely from such minor irritations of pregnancy as backache, fatigue, heartburn, nausea, constipation and haemorrhoids than a woman who is carrying a single baby.

Rest is vital – you need to rest more, earlier in pregnancy. This may mean giving up work sooner than you would wish. Rest is important to get you through both pregnancy and the first weeks after the birth. It can also help to alleviate other problems, such as nausea and backache, which are magnified when you are tired.

As your pregnancy advances, finding a comfortable position in which to rest (and a comfortable chair or bed) may be a challenge. You may find it helpful to support your abdomen in your lap by sitting more or less upright. Alternatively, a lounge chair whose head and foot you can raise may be a good choice. Take care – or have someone close by – when you are getting up or sitting down.

Backache not only strains your muscles but also saps your strength. Yoga can help give you more energy and tone your muscles (see pp. 52–53). So, too, can swimming, as the water supports all your extra weight. Pelvic-floor exercises (see pp. 44–45) are particularly important since these muscles are supporting so much extra weight in a twin pregnancy.

Upward pressure from your uterus as early as 20 to 24 weeks can cause heartburn and make you feel full at a time when good nutrition is vital. From the middle of your pregnancy onwards – and especially towards the end – you may find it easier to graze throughout the day than to eat three full meals. This approach may also help if constipation is becoming a problem. Be sure to drink plenty of water and fruit juice, too.

Total weight gain

You can expect to gain about 50 percent more weight than a woman who is carrying only one baby, or 16–20 kg (35–45 lb) in total. You will also get bigger faster and can expect your uterus to rise more quickly out of your pelvis. This means, of course, that you will need maternity clothes sooner than other women.

Twins are often born early, and the larger they are, the less your doctor will be concerned about their condition. In practical terms, this may mean that your babies spend less time in intensive care or less time in the hospital before you take them home.

Eat healthily, choosing fresh, unprocessed foods as often as you can (see pp. 36–39) to give your twins the best start possible.

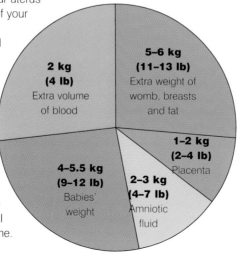

2 kg (4 lb) Extra volume of blood

5–6 kg (11–13 lb) Extra weight of womb, breasts and fat

1–2 kg (2–4 lb) Placenta

4–5.5 kg (9–12 lb) Babies' weight

2–3 kg (4–7 lb) Amniotic fluid

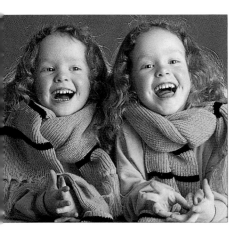

Identical twins share a great deal; in childhood, their names may be their main means of establishing their individuality. Try to avoid names that sound the same – in tone, initial letters or number of syllables – to help most people get the right name for the right child most of the time.

DRESSING FOR COMFORT

Finding clothes that fit and are comfortable can be tricky. Despite the increasing incidence of twins, few manufacturers of maternity clothes cater to women carrying more than one baby. Stretch fabrics may help, but the itchiness that many women experience as a minor discomfort may become intolerable if you wear anything constricting, simply because the skin of your abdomen is being stretched so thin.

Men's shirts and dungarees, or loose dresses from shops that cater for large women, may be the answer. In general, buy the largest, loosest-fitting clothes you can find in natural fabrics and assume that nothing will be too big. Accept any large-size hand-me-downs.

Buying for the babies

Equipping twins is considerably more expensive than having two children close in age. Twins require you to have two of everything at the same time; single siblings pass their outgrown clothes and equipment down the line.

Many parents are superstitious about getting everything ready for a baby, "just in case", but with twins you really don't have a choice: wait too long and they may arrive before you are ready (remember this if you are planning to paint their room). The extra weight may leave you too tired to look at nursery essentials after about six months; and you will be too busy with your babies after the birth.

Transportation

Twin prams and double strollers are less expensive than two singles, and there is usually a thriving secondhand market in these goods. Bear in mind that double strollers can be difficult to manoeuvre: if you are taking two tiny babies out, you may find it easier to carry one in a sling and

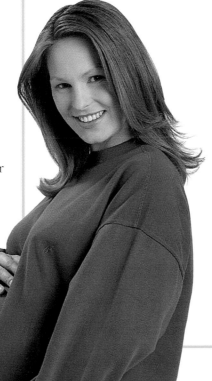

push the other – or take someone with you to carry the second baby. Two baby capsules are vital both for safety and to comply with the law.

Sleeping

You can put off buying two small cots for the first weeks but only until your babies become too big and mobile to fit into one without disturbing each other's sleep. Consider one full-size cot for them to share from the start; buy a second after a few months.

Clothes

It makes sense to accept as many hand-me-downs as you can, particularly of newborn size: most single babies under-use this size, so you may get almost new clothes that will be perfect for your smaller-than-average babies. Many parents of twins like to dress them alike, even from the start. It is more practical not to. Will you want to change both if one soils his or her outfit, for example? And remember that twins, inevitably, share a great deal. While for some this intimate relationship with what may be a mirror image is a delight, for others it causes problems over time. Experts suggest that you treat your babies as individuals from the beginning.

Other essentials

A double quantity of other baby essentials – bedding, nappies (see pp. 136–39) and bottles (if you are going to bottle-feed) – is unavoidable.

Practical arrangements

If twins are creating a serious financial burden for you, find out whether you are entitled to any government benefits; arrange for extra help at home for after the birth (see p. 127); and consider contacting a multiple-births support group (see p, 219).

TWINS: SPECIAL CONCERNS

The diagnosis of twins may make you feel special, or it may make you nervous. You will almost certainly benefit from extra care during your pregnancy.

If you are expecting twins, or more, you – and the babies – will be monitored closely throughout your pregnancy and during labour and birth. You will also be closely cared for after the birth. This is due to certain problems that occur more often in multiple pregnancies. These can almost always be treated, but spotting them early can be vital.

ANAEMIA

Beginning at about the 20th week of any pregnancy, your baby's growing blood supply draws on your iron stores to develop properly. If you started pregnancy deficient in iron, the concentration of red blood cells – which depend on iron for their formation – may not have kept pace with the increased volume of body fluids that is normal in pregnancy (see p. 96). The body's red blood cells contain haemoglobin, which carries oxygen from your lungs around the body. If the shortfall in blood cells becomes excessive, you become anaemic.

Women carrying twins are prone to anaemia because they have two babies drawing on their iron stores, and they have a greater increase in body fluids.

The major symptoms of anaemia are weakness, shortness of breath and, sometimes, dizzy

---

A Case in Point

Warming to Twins

SUE, 32, FELT TRAPPED WHEN SHE WAS TOLD SHE WAS EXPECTING TWINS.

"Even before I became pregnant, Joe accepted that I needed to work outside the home. But I earned far less than he, so I knew that we couldn't afford for him to stop work. Where would we find someone to take care of two babies? I wasn't sure I would be able to look after them myself. I'd never even changed a nappy.

"All my mental images had been of pushing one baby in a pram, holding one baby in my arms, a baby nestled between us in our bed ... I couldn't imagine two strollers or two cots. Where would we put them?

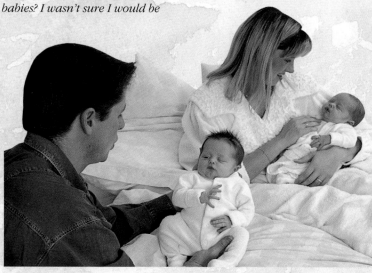

"Joe was great from the start. He didn't try to persuade me that it would all be okay but gradually started talking about 'the babies' and 'when we're a foursome', easing me into the idea of twins. He came to all my appointments and in unobtrusive ways made me take care of myself.

"Alex and Chloe were born at 37 weeks. For three months, Joe and his mother did all the housework – all I did was rest, eat, and bathe, change and breast-feed the babies. It brought me so close to them. I couldn't believe I hadn't wanted them.

"Then Joe's company's day-care centre had a couple of part-time vacancies, and he suggested that we take them. We've done a lot of juggling, and I've cut my work hours, but so far it's okay. Alex and Chloe know I'm their mum, and I love them, but I'm not the only person who looks after them. They have time apart from me."

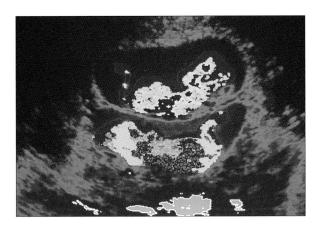

Usually, as shown here, each baby has a separate amniotic sac. Whether the twins resulted from one egg or two, each baby may have a placenta, or the placentas may become fused.

spells. In severe cases in which anaemia is neglected, your babies may receive less oxygen.

The best treatment for anaemia is prevention through eating plenty of iron-rich foods (see pp. 36–37). You may be advised to take supplements and, perhaps, extra folate. If you develop anaemia, additional supplements may be recommended. If you are diagnosed with anaemia, don't worry: babies of mothers whose anaemia is treated are rarely iron-deficient at birth.

HIGH BLOOD PRESSURE

Twin pregnancies are more likely to be complicated by high blood pressure. Because high blood pressure reduces the efficiency of the placenta, doctors monitor blood pressure carefully for signs of problems.

A good diet and moderate exercise are the best ways to prevent high blood pressure. Yoga often helps to lower raised blood pressure, too. You will be advised to rest – at home if your doctor is satisfied that you will get rest there, in the hospital if not. High blood pressure is also one of the symptoms of pre-eclampsia (see p. 143), which is more common in twin pregnancies.

BLEEDING

Light spotting around the time a period would be due is normal, whether you are carrying one or more babies. However, later in pregnancy, and especially in a multiple pregnancy, bleeding can be an indicator of premature labour or abruptio placentae (the placenta has started to come away from the wall of the uterus).

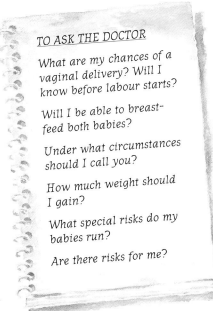

TO ASK THE DOCTOR

What are my chances of a vaginal delivery? Will I know before labour starts?

Will I be able to breast-feed both babies?

Under what circumstances should I call you?

How much weight should I gain?

What special risks do my babies run?

Are there risks for me?

You will have more antenatal checks than a woman carrying only one baby, and more questions to ask your doctor.

Extra care

Organizing help if you are expecting twins is a priority. Since you can't rely on your pregnancy lasting 40 weeks, start planning early (around six months). Studies show that parents of twins enjoy their babies more if they are not physically and emotionally drained by trying to do it all themselves.

Asking for help does not reflect poorly on your ability as a mother. It frees you to concentrate on being a mother: feeding, cuddling, changing, bathing your babies. Those tasks that are unrelated to motherhood, such as cooking, cleaning, and washing, can easily be done by someone else.

Try to choose helpers who will not require too much supervision from you. Allow a friend to stock your freezer with nutritious dishes once a week, or hire a house cleaner for a couple of hours.

In mild or even moderate cases of abruptio placentae, rest may be all that you need. You will, however, be closely monitored, and if there is any sign that your babies are in distress, a caesarean will be suggested.

Rest may also be advised, if your doctor thinks you are going into premature labour. If bedrest does not halt labour, you may be given medications to delay the birth. You may be monitored at home or in the hospital and may have to be prepared for a lengthy stay.

For information on giving birth to twins and caring for two newborn babies, see pp. 194–95.

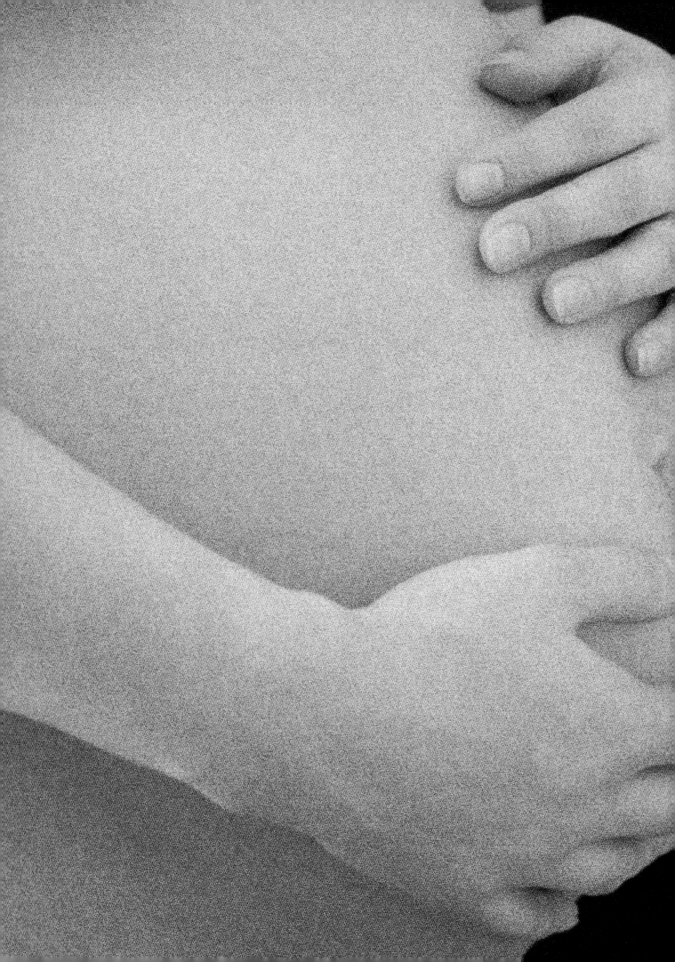

The third trimester

FOR SOME WOMEN *this trimester passes slowly. They become increasingly excited to see the baby they can feel moving, kicking and even hiccuping inside them. But there is still plenty to do at this time. You will probably:*

- *Think in detail about your hopes and plans for the delivery, now that it is close at hand*

- *Make some shopping trips to buy the clothes and equipment your baby will need for his or her first few months*

- *Experience some discomforts as your size makes you feel awkward and contributes to fatigue.*

The third trimester is a time of rapid growth and maturity for your baby. If the baby were born at the beginning of this period, he or she would need a lot of specialist care to survive. At its end, the baby will be strong and healthy.

FOR YOU

You will probably feel healthy and energetic most of the time. You may notice some swelling around your face, hands and ankles. If so, tell your doctor or midwife; you are probably retaining fluid. Your doctor will want to monitor you, because severe swelling, if accompanied by high blood pressure and protein in the urine, can signal pre-eclampsia (see p. 143).

You may feel the pressure on your diaphragm, as well as your bladder, as your baby begins to crowd your organs. The skin of your abdomen will feel thin and stretched.

Your breasts may leak a little colostrum (a thin yellowish liquid), if they haven't before. Some experts recommend preparing the nipples for breast-feeding by expressing colostrum and rolling the nipples between thumb and forefinger, but wait until week 36 before you try this.

Around this time you may have another blood test to check for Rhesus (Rh) antibodies, if there is a chance your baby could be at risk (see p. 24). You may also be checked for anaemia (see pp. 126–27).

What if my baby is premature?

Far more babies are born late than early, but many women worry that their baby will be premature – that is, born before the 37th week of pregnancy.

In some cases, the cause of premature labour is unknown, but there are many contributing factors. Cigarette smoking, alcohol abuse and drug use may induce premature labour, as may a poor diet and inadequate weight gain. Other, less avoidable factors include your health (having high blood pressure, diabetes or a heart problem increases the risk), exposure to the synthetic oestrogen drug DES, something wrong with the baby (in which case treatment may be attempted; see pp. 146–47), carrying more than one baby, or having a history of premature births.

In recent years, the survival rates of premature babies have increased dramatically – with no long-term side effects. Survival rates are affected by: how close to term you are; the baby's size; whether she has any birth defect or disability; and the availability of specialist care.

Babies rarely survive more than a few hours if born before 23 weeks. At 24 weeks, just under half survive. Thereafter, the statistics improve dramatically. A baby born at 25 weeks has a slightly better than 50 percent chance of survival. At 26 weeks, it's 75 percent; at 28 weeks, 85 percent of babies survive. By the time your pregnancy has reached the 35th week, the baby is almost certain to be fine.

See page 134 for information on recognizing premature labour.

FOR YOUR BABY

During these weeks, your baby starts to accumulate fat under her skin. This fat will provide her with energy during her first few days of life and help to regulate her body temperature. She still looks very small and skinny compared with a full-term baby, however.

Her lungs are beginning to mature, but if she were born now and had not had the benefit of in utero steroids (see p. 147), it would be several more weeks before she could breathe without the help of a respirator.

Skin
Her skin becomes less translucent and papery because of the fat beneath the outer layers.

Genitals
In a boy, the testes descend into the scrotum at about week 29.

Arms and legs
Fat under the skin makes the baby's thighs and arms chubbier. She is still able to freefall in the uterus, but space is getting more restricted.

Head
The baby's head is starting to look more in proportion to the rest of her body, and her face has filled out a little, especially in the cheeks.

Size
The baby measures about 40 cm (16 in) and weighs 1.3–1.8 kg (3–4 lb).

MAKING A BIRTH PLAN

Recording in advance your hopes and wishes for the birth of your baby helps everyone involved in your care to understand your expectations.

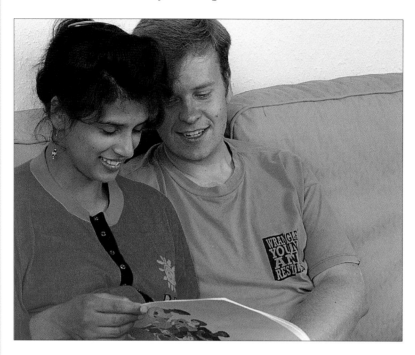

Q *My sister had a baby last year and didn't have a birth plan. Should I have one?*

A Yes. Many mothers-to-be (and their partners) find it useful to consider the options that will be available to them during labour and delivery. They discuss the options with someone whose opinion they trust and who can advise them on the medical aspects of their choice.

A birth plan is simply a means of giving this sort of discussion formality. It records your preferences so that they are clear to anyone who may be caring for you during labour. Then, if everything goes smoothly, you will be able to give birth to your baby in the way you have chosen.

Remember when compiling a plan that it is an ideal: obviously, the health and safety of you and your baby come first, and circumstances may necessitate changes.

Q *If I make a plan, will I have to stick to it?*

A No. Labour and birth can be unpredictable, as can your responses. You may change your mind about some aspects when it comes to the real thing. Or circumstances may change in such a way that you need to depart from what you thought you might want. But your plan should be respected, and departures from it should have your (or your partner's) permission and approval.

Q *What sort of issues should I be thinking about?*

A Consider different labour and birth positions. Is it important to you to be able to move freely? Do you want a variety of furniture available in the labour room?

Who do you want to be your labour companion? If not your partner, have you chosen someone else – sister, mother, friend – or do you want your midwife or doctor to help you find someone? (Student midwives are often happy to fill this role.)

Ask about the hospital's policy on video cameras (if that's important to you). Think about pain management (see pp. 170–73) and record your wishes. Will you want an epidural, for example, or at least the option of one? What other pain relief is available? What are your feelings about it? Would you like encouragement and support to manage without medication?

Your doctor may suggest inducing labour or accelerating it with drugs (see pp. 168–69). How do you feel about continuous foetal monitoring (see pp. 174–75)?

Make it known if you want to breast-feed so that your baby can be given to you to hold and feed as soon as possible after delivery. It is usual for babies to stay with their mothers day and night, but ask whether nursery care is available in case you need a break.

Finally, what are visiting policies, and how long, typically, will you stay in hospital?

Q *What's the best time to make a plan? I am four months pregnant. Is it too soon?*

A Most women wait until later in their pregnancy, when they have had time to read and think about pregnancy and birth and have grown used to the whole idea of being pregnant.

If you plan too soon – before you have attended antenatal classes, for example – you might find that you want to make changes later. (Obviously, if circumstances change, you are free to change your plan accordingly.) On the other hand, if you leave it until too late, you may not have time to think through all the issues. Aim to complete your plan about four to six weeks before your due date.

When you meet your midwife or doctor to make your final plan, arrive with a few notes ready and be prepared to be flexible. Have a list of questions, too, so you don't forget any issues you meant to raise.

Q *It all sounds very formal. Is there a special form that I should use?*

A In some hospitals, the birth plan follows a set format so that your wishes on important points are covered. But if you find that the form doesn't cover something that is important to you, add it on a separate sheet of paper. Some doctors prefer that you write a letter stating your hopes, in any case, because labour and delivery are too personal to be adequately covered by a standard form.

Q *What happens to the plan once we have written it?*

A It's a good idea to make two copies. Keep one, and have the other filed with your notes. Sign and date the plan and have your doctor sign it as well. A doctor may wish to include some disclaimer in the event that last-minute changes to your plan are medically necessary.

Q *Won't I feel bad if I can't stick to the plan? What if I have a caesarean section, for example?*

A When birth plans were new, their detractors argued that women's expectations would be set too high, and they would feel bad about themselves or their birth experience if they couldn't adhere to every aspect of the plan. But the plan is not intended to set out a blueprint for the labour and birth. It reflects the fact that your feelings and choices are important. A birth plan avoids the "production-line obstetrics" once common, but there are occasions when medical considerations intervene. A woman whose plan proves unworkable in the circumstances can feel confident that she and her partner will be consulted and informed of what's happening. She'll know why she had to have a caesarean, for example; it won't just be "done" to her.

Q *How do I go about making a plan?*

A Tell your doctor, midwife or someone else closely involved in your care that you intend to make a birth plan. Say you'd like this person's help, support and opinions. Arrange a time when both you and your partner (or birth companion) can meet, preferably when there will be enough time to sit down together – not hurried at the end of a routine antenatal appointment, when you may be aware that there are other mothers-to-be waiting.

QUESTIONS TO ASK

If a caesarean proves necessary, can my partner be there? Can he hold the baby while I recover from the anaesthetic?

What forms of pain relief are available at this hospital?

Is there an anaesthetist on duty at all times?

I think I'll be more relaxed if I can have some of my favourite music in the labour room. Is that possible?

Can I be sure that an episiotomy will be avoided if at all possible?

Will I be able to hold my baby immediately after the birth? Can I have a water birth?

The eighth month

FOR YOU

You may be thinking about leaving work during this month, but if you feel well, you are active, and your job is not too physically arduous or stressful, there's no health-related reason to leave. On the other hand, you may want some free time at home, to prepare for your baby's arrival. If you want to keep working, check first with your midwife.

The top of your uterus is well up into your rib cage, and your navel may have popped out.

From now on, your antenatal visits will be more frequent. You may also have an ultrasound scan at some time during this month if the placenta looks low or if the doctor suspects other problems. A placenta that lies low in the uterus, or even across the lower part, is known as placenta praevia (see pp. 176–77). In such a case, your doctor will decide in the ninth month whether you will have to give birth by caesarean section – that is, if the placenta blocks the way for the baby to get out.

Are these real contractions?

The uterus, which is in fact a large muscle, contracts all the way through pregnancy. But you probably won't start to feel these contractions until the eighth month and possibly later. They're sometimes called "practice", or Braxton-Hicks, contractions (after the doctors who first observed them).

Braxton-Hicks contractions tone your uterus for delivery, adjust your baby's position for the birth, and help efface your cervix in preparation for labour contractions. You will occasionally feel your abdomen harden, and if you are taking a bath, you will see your abdomen become taut and remain tense for a number of seconds. The contractions are rarely painful, but may be uncomfortable. They give you, of course, an excellent opportunity to practise your breathing exercises (see pp. 56–57). It often helps to change your position, too, standing up and moving around if you have been lying down. If you are very active, you may hardly notice the contractions at all.

Towards the end of a first pregnancy, it can be difficult to tell whether these contractions are labour or not. Generally, however, Braxton-Hicks contractions tend to be irregular, usually short in duration (between 30 and 60 seconds), and intermittent. They also tend not to increase in length, intensity or frequency over a period of a couple of hours. If contractions occur more than five or six times in an hour, time them. Ask your midwife how to monitor them, and ask when you should call for advice.

FOR YOUR BABY

Your baby's position in the uterus becomes increasingly significant from this stage on. Until the beginning of this month, babies tend to lie in any position in the uterus. They move around a lot, but at "rest" most are breech – that is, feet or bottom towards the vagina. By the end of the eighth month, most – 95 percent – have turned around, to be in a better position for birth. This head-down position is known as vertex, or cephalic. There is no cause for concern, however, if your baby is still breech at this stage; he still has time to turn. Some doctors attempt to turn the baby manually, using ultrasound guidance, by a process known as external cephalic version.

Skin
Extra fat makes the baby plumper and rounder, and his skin becomes less wrinkled.

Hands and feet
The fingernails and toenails are fully grown. Movements at the end of this month will feel like strong kicks.

Eyes
The baby's eyes will have colour, almost always blue in fair babies and brown in darker-skinned babies. Their colour may change in the months after the birth.

Size
The baby measures about 43 cm (17 in) and weighs 2.1–2.6 kg (4½–5½ lb). The additional weight comes from extra fat rather than an increase in length, which is comparatively slight.

Hair
Some hair is normal in all babies, and many have a lot, although it will change in colour and texture during the baby and toddler years. Lanugo on the baby's face and body has started to disappear, but the vernix remains (see pp. 97 and 103).

MAJOR PURCHASES

While it's true that babies' needs are very basic, it's a good idea to get your home ready in advance and to buy some of the equipment you will need.

One of the most sensible things you can do before planning a shopping trip for baby equipment is to ask friends with babies what they have found useful. Some items are used only in the first three months or so: a baby bath, for example, soon becomes too small, and a changing table that has no safety straps is hazardous for a wriggling baby of four or five months. You may find that you can borrow such items from people whose babies have outgrown them. But bear in mind that anything that makes your life easier and more comfortable in the first few months may be worth buying.

Baby capsules and car seats

The safest way for a newborn to travel is in a rear-facing baby capsule. When your baby outgrows the capsule, switch to an approved car seat. To use a car seat, he must be able to sit and easily hold his head upright. Never use a capsule or car seat in the front if you have a passenger air bag.

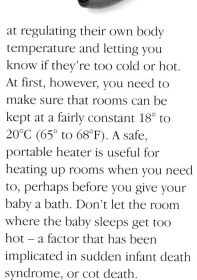

THE BABY'S ROOM

If you plan to make a special room for your baby, now's the time to get it done, even if you don't complete every aspect of it just yet. Check the temperature of all the rooms in which your baby will spend much time. Healthy babies are soon good at regulating their own body temperature and letting you know if they're too cold or hot. At first, however, you need to make sure that rooms can be kept at a fairly constant 18° to 20°C (65° to 68°F). A safe, portable heater is useful for heating up rooms when you need to, perhaps before you give your baby a bath. Don't let the room where the baby sleeps get too hot – a factor that has been implicated in sudden infant death syndrome, or cot death.

Somewhere to sleep, both during the day and at night, is vital – your baby may spend up to 18 hours of every 24 asleep. His pram is fine for the first few months, but it will be too small for long sleeps after this time. You may want a cot or carry basket, and most parents like to have one

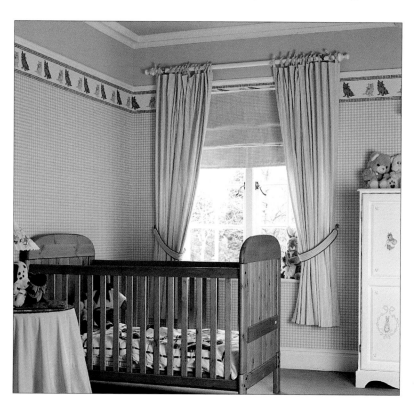

Although you may decide to have your baby sleep with you at night – initially at least – before the birth is still the best time to get his room ready. Leave one or two finishing touches to be made to celebrate his arrival.

from the very start for night time, keeping the pram for daytime naps. Alternatively, you can put your baby into a full-size cot. The bars of the cot should be no more than 6 cm (2½ in) apart. Ask for the latest information on mattress safety, and make sure the mattress fits snugly – with no gap that could trap a tiny hand or foot. Choose layered bedding – sheets, one or two thin blankets, and a light eiderdown – so that it is easy to take off a layer if the baby seems hot to you. Babies under a year should not have a pillow.

A baby bath is not essential but lets you bathe your baby in any room. Leaning over to bathe a tiny baby in the family bath can be backbreaking (it's easier to take him in the bath with you). You will also need two towels and two face washers.

TRANSPORTING YOUR BABY

The law requires a baby capsule when you travel with a baby in a car. The capsule must be the right size for a newborn and should be placed correctly in the car in time for the journey home from the hospital. It's safer to buy a new one, although a secondhand one in good condition – with no cracks in the shell or buckle and a harness that shows no signs of wear – can be a good buy.

There are various types of pram. Some are built so that the top lifts off the wheels, and the chassis folds up for easy storage. Traditional carriage prams with large wheels give a smoother ride, although babies do not seem too concerned about this as long as they have a comfortable mattress; smaller ones are lighter to push and easier to manoeuvre.

You may choose a sturdy stroller with a seat-back that folds down flat: a young baby must be able to lie flat.

A front pack or sling is a good idea if you travel often by public transport. Once a baby can hold his head up, one that fits on your back may be more comfortable – and gives your baby a better view.

SECONDHAND OPTIONS

There is often a good market in secondhand baby supplies. But be sure to check prams, strollers and cots for safety and strength. Look at wheels, screws and frames to make sure that they're sturdy. Have them repaired or reconditioned if you have any doubts. It's always best to buy a new mattress.

Changing mat
A plastic-covered changing mat allows you to change your baby anywhere in the house and protects carpets, upholstery and bedding.

Towels
You can, of course, use the family's towels for your baby, but make sure they are soft and fleecy: a newborn's skin is delicate.

Bath
The disadvantage of a baby bath on a stand is that you may have to carry it full of water. One that fits in the bath is easier on your back.

YOUR BABY'S NEEDS

Once you have made the major purchases, you can start to attend to your baby's more personal needs – and do some advance planning.

Before you rush out to buy lots of baby clothes, a roomful of toys and several packs of nappies, ask friends and family if they have any baby clothes or toys they can pass on to you, and which nappies they recommend. Now is also the time to think about how you want to feed your baby.

NAPPIES

In the last few years, parents have switched to disposable nappies in a big way. Although disposables are expensive, they are easy to use, fit well, and do not involve time- and energy-consuming washing and drying. Cloth nappies cost less, even after taking into account the costs of washing and drying, liners, plastic pants and pins. And one baby is unlikely to wear them out, so you can use them for a second child. Using a nappy service – a company that takes away dirty nappies, washes and dries them, and delivers them to your home – costs about the same as using disposables.

Apart from their laundering requirements, cloth nappies are environment-friendly. Disposables use up resources at every stage. And, despite their name, they are difficult to dispose of. So far, there is no way to recycle them.

An alternative is reusable nappies. These shaped cloth nappies are used with liners, as normal cloth nappies are. But their shape and availability in several sizes give them almost as good a fit

as, and the comfort of, a disposable. Some parents use cloth nappies most of the time, and disposables or reusables when travelling or on holiday.

Babies can be cleaned with cotton wool dipped in water that has been boiled to kill any bacteria, then cooled, but packaged wipes are convenient, especially when you are travelling. A barrier cream may be useful, but most professionals do not recommend baby powder because the fine particles can aggravate breathing problems in some babies.

CLOTHES

Keep your baby's clothing simple and designed for easy nappy changing (front fastenings, wide necklines and press studs up the insides of the legs, for example). Avoid anything with drawstrings or lace in which small fingers could become trapped. And buy

only a few first-size items.

The following basics will see your baby through the first three months and prevent the need to wash a load of baby clothes more often than every other day or so: five all-in-one stretch suits; five singlets; three cardigans or jackets; a baby blanket; a warm hat for a winter baby, a sunhat for a summer baby. Make sure that everything you buy is machine washable and dryable, and colourfast.

Baby clothing is outgrown before it's outworn, and good-quality clothing can be passed on to several babies before it starts to look shabby. Remember: the most unexpected people may send or give you baby clothes.

FEEDING YOUR BABY

Breast-feeding requires no equipment, although you may find breast pads useful. If you want to express milk – a skill that allows you to take a few hours off from the baby (see p. 207) – you'll need a pump and bottles with teats. If you plan to return to work, an electric breast pump

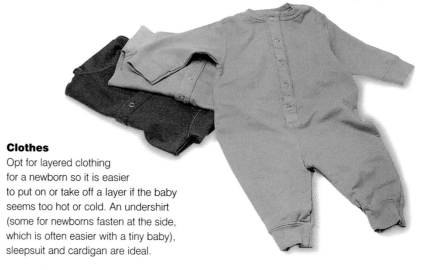

Clothes
Opt for layered clothing for a newborn so it is easier to put on or take off a layer if the baby seems too hot or cold. An undershirt (some for newborns fasten at the side, which is often easier with a tiny baby), sleepsuit and cardigan are ideal.

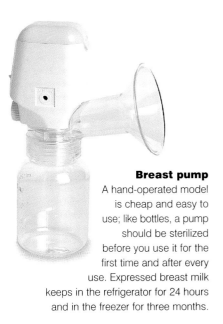

Breast pump
A hand-operated model is cheap and easy to use; like bottles, a pump should be sterilized before you use it for the first time and after every use. Expressed breast milk keeps in the refrigerator for 24 hours and in the freezer for three months.

may be useful. You can rent or buy one. A sterilizer is not vital for the odd bottle – just boil it in water for 10 minutes – but you will need a bottle brush to be sure that you have removed all traces of old milk.

If you are going to bottle-feed, you will need half a dozen bottles with teats, plus sterilizing equipment. Some professionals argue that the high temperature of the water and air-drying in a dishwasher make sterilizing unnecessary. If you plan to put bottles in the dishwasher, check that they and their nipples are dishwasher-safe.

You don't have to buy a high-chair until later, when your baby will start eating solid foods. Still, it's worth budgeting for one now.

TOYS

A new baby does not need many toys, but she will like one or two small ones – she will not be able to focus on anything large – that become familiar from the start.

Check that toys conform to safety standards and are suitable for a newborn. Anything with sharp edges or small, detachable pieces is a hazard.

Planning ahead

You may feel an almost physical "nesting instinct" in these last few weeks, an urge to make your home just right and comfortable for your baby. If you feel a surge of energy as the birth draws near, use it profitably to complete any light household repairs or garden tasks you've been meaning to do "when you get around to it".

Plan to do as much housework ahead of time as you can, to cover the two weeks or so following the birth. You'll be pleased at the extra time this gives you to spend with your baby, and you'll appreciate the chance to catch up on your rest and sleep, as the baby allows.

Shopping

Eating well is as important after the birth as it was before, but you may have less time to cook and be too tired to do so. Cook in bulk now and stock the freezer with meals you need only to heat and serve. Stock up on cupboard items (pasta, pulses, grains) and household supplies.

Safety

Think about safety while you still have time to do something about it. You may never need them, but it's worth learning baby CPR (this is essential if you have previously lost a baby to cot death). Ask your midwife or doctor for advice on where to go. Some hospitals offer courses, and instruction videos are available. Make safety measures second nature before the baby arrives. Run the cold water into the bath first, then add hot. Turn the thermostat down a couple of degrees. Shield fires and radiators. Remove rugs and fix any loose carpets, particularly on stairs. Fit locks on cupboards containing medicines or chemicals.

With a little planning, you should be able to arrange your shopping so that all you need to buy in the first couple of weeks is fresh fruit, salad and vegetables.

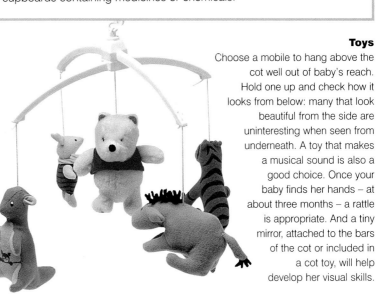

Toys
Choose a mobile to hang above the cot well out of baby's reach. Hold one up and check how it looks from below: many that look beautiful from the side are uninteresting when seen from underneath. A toy that makes a musical sound is also a good choice. Once your baby finds her hands – at about three months – a rattle is appropriate. And a tiny mirror, attached to the bars of the cot or included in a cot toy, will help develop her visual skills.

FOR YOU

If you have chosen to stop working by now, these weeks may seem to pass slowly; you have more time to think about the baby and the birth. But things are happening. In week 36 or 37, your baby's head is likely to engage, which eases pressure on your diaphragm. Engagement happens later with second and subsequent babies because after a woman has a baby, her pelvic

When the baby's head engages, you will feel less pressure on your ribs. You will find it easier to breathe, although you may need to urinate more frequently as pressure on the urinary tract increases.

bones are arranged slightly differently. Don't worry if your baby's head does not engage: in about 10 percent of first pregnancies, engagement doesn't occur until the start of labour.

Occasionally, the pelvis is too small for the baby's head, so it can't engage properly. This is usually spotted before labour begins, and the diagnosis of cephalo-pelvic disproportion is suspected. In clear-cut cases, you'll be advised to have a caesarean. But in most cases, your doctor will advise you to wait and see. He or she will allow labour to start and progress to see whether a vaginal delivery is possible.

How your baby may lie in your uterus

The position your baby adopts in the uterus is known as his presentation, or lie. The presenting part is closest to the birth canal and will therefore be born first. Most babies are vertex, or head down. They are also occiput anterior: the occiput – crown – faces your front, slightly left or right. If the baby is occiput posterior, his crown is towards your back, again slightly to the left or right. More rarely, a baby lies breech, in which his legs or bottom may be the first part to emerge. The impact of these positions on your labour and delivery is discussed on pp.166–67.

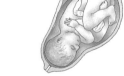

ROP: Right occiput posterior
The baby is head down with his face towards your front and his crown slightly to the right.

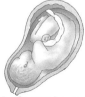

LOA: Left occiput anterior
The baby is head down with his face towards your back and his crown slightly to the left.

FOR YOUR BABY

The baby's head sinks down into the pelvis in preparation for birth. In the last few weeks of pregnancy, your baby gains about 200 g (7 oz) a week, with a final acceleration of weight gain in the last couple of weeks. He also grows about 10 cm (4 in) in length.

It is usual for your baby to move less, but tell your midwife if you feel that movement has ceased for several hours. Your baby quite naturally has sleeping hours and wakeful times, and a quiet period may mean no more than a long nap. But if you are concerned, your doctor can listen to your baby's heartbeat for reassurance.

Arms and legs
There is now so little room in the uterus that the baby's movement is restricted, and distinct jabs from arms and legs are less common than earlier.

Size
At term, the average baby is 53 cm (21 in) long and weighs 3.2 kg (7 lb).

Eyes
The baby's eyesight develops rapidly after this time, and he can differentiate between light and dark.

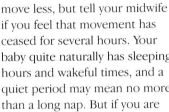

Breech
The baby is sitting in the pelvic cavity so that his bottom is the first part out.

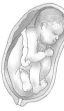

Footling breech
The baby is sitting in the pelvic cavity with one or both feet extending towards the cervix.

Mouth
From about 36 weeks on, the baby can coordinate his sucking and swallowing efficiently, and he has a powerful sucking instinct.

Lungs
Although there is no air in them, the baby's lungs are maturing, and he practises light breathing movements. As a result, amniotic fluid passes into the airways from time to time, and he gets an occasional bout of hiccups, which you'll feel as a series of light, rhythmic movements.

Skin
The amount of vernix and lanugo (see pp. 97 and 103) covering the baby's skin diminishes during these weeks; a baby born at or after term is likely to have little of either.

COMMON DISCOMFORTS

This is the time in which many minor problems diminish, although increasing fatigue may have an impact on how you feel.

Some problems are more common at the end of pregnancy than at the beginning. Almost all of them relate to the size of the baby or to the effect of your extra weight on your circulation. You can do a great deal to avoid many of these problems.

STRESS INCONTINENCE

This has nothing to do with emotional or psychological stress. It simply refers to the stress placed on your pelvic floor muscles when you cough, sneeze or run. In later pregnancy, the weight of the baby can cause these muscles to be lax, which allows the bladder to leak urine on occasion.

The best prevention is to be meticulous about doing your pelvic-floor exercises (see pp. 44–45) to keep the muscles toned and taut. (You should continue to do them after the birth to restore the muscles' tone and efficiency.) The only solution if stress incontinence becomes a problem is to increase the frequency of your exercises and to wear a pad, if necessary, to keep you comfortable. Change pads often.

Frequent, persistent leakage when you do not cough or sneeze could signal a leakage of amniotic fluid and should be reported to your doctor.

OEDEMA

Some swelling of the ankles, legs, fingers, face and hands, due to fluid retention in the tissues of these areas, is normal in later pregnancy and relates to the extra fluids circulating in your body. To minimize discomfort, lie down or sit with your legs raised whenever you can; make sure that your shoes are comfortable; and avoid anything tight – such as elasticated socks – around your legs and ankles. Support tights may make you more comfortable. Drinking water will *not* increase swelling, nor will restricting salt intake decrease swelling.

The majority of cases of oedema are not dangerous, but report swelling at your next antenatal check-up, since it is one of the warning signs of pre-eclampsia (see box on next page).

A very few women suffer a condition called carpal tunnel syndrome, in which fluid collects in the wrists and produces a tingling, sometimes painful sensation in the fingers. Raising the hands above the head for several minutes helps, by allowing the fluid to drain away.

Lying in a warm bath takes the baby's weight off your pelvic floor, reducing stress there. It also eases pressure on the diaphragm, allowing you to breathe more easily. A warm bath can also promote peaceful sleep. You should, however, avoid hot baths or hot tubs.

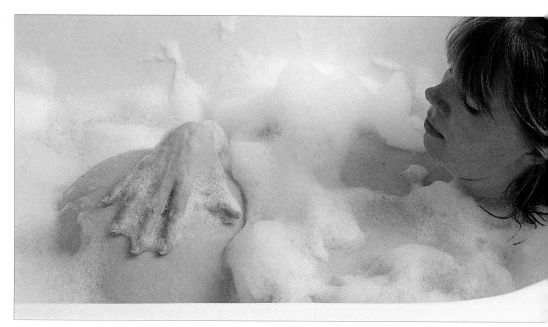

Pre-eclampsia

The condition known as pre-eclampsia is unique to pregnancy. Its symptoms are consistently high blood pressure (after 20 weeks of pregnancy, a reading of more than 140/90 is high; one of 160/110 is serious), especially after 30 weeks; oedema of the face, hands and ankles; and protein in the urine. In more severe cases, sufferers experience headaches, blurred vision, gastric pain, vomiting and confusion. If left untreated these symptoms can accelerate and eclampsia may develop, causing convulsions and, occasionally, coma.

Since the symptoms of pre-eclampsia are easy to spot, a woman's blood pressure and urine are checked at each antenatal visit.

Pre-eclampsia is more common in first pregnancies, in teenagers and older women, and in women who are carrying more than one baby or have a history of chronic hypertension. It also has a tendency to run in families.The

cause is not fully understood, and the links between the three main symptoms are unclear. But what seems to trigger them is vasospasm, or constriction of blood vessels throughout the body.

A healthy diet helps to prevent high blood pressure, as does exercise. (Pre-eclampsia seems to be more prevalent among under-nourished women, indicating that a healthy diet is advisable.) Many women have found that yoga helps to reduce raised blood pressure.

High blood pressure is dangerous because it can affect the functioning of the placenta and the flow of blood there. If the baby is not getting enough food and oxygen, his growth may be slowed.

The treatment of pre-eclampsia depends, first, on the stage of the pregnancy. Before about 28 weeks, doctors are reluctant to deliver the baby – unless he is in great danger – in order to give the baby the best possible chance of survival.

Rest is usually prescribed, often in the hospital, so that the woman's body can make the best use of the available blood supply. Drugs may also be administered. Low-dose aspirin may prevent pre-eclampsia in high-risk pregnancies by preventing vasospasm.

In milder cases, rest with or without drugs may keep the condition under control until labour begins. Since the placenta starts to function less well after 40 weeks in all pregnancies, most doctors are unwilling to allow a pregnancy affected by high blood pressure, which may further undermine the functioning of the placenta, to proceed beyond this time.

In more severe cases, however, once doctors are satisfied that the baby's lungs are mature enough, or if the mother is sick enough, they usually induce labour or perform a caesarean to deliver the baby. Since an epidural generally lowers blood pressure, the doctor may recommend its use.

Splints to keep the fingers upright may also be suggested. The condition normally goes away after delivery.

SHORTNESS OF BREATH

This very common condition can begin early in pregnancy and lessens when the baby's head engages in the pelvis (see pp. 140–41). Until then, the growing uterus presses against the diaphragm, squeezing the lungs so that they do not completely fill with oxygen when you breathe in.

Adjusting your posture may help. Stand up straight, if standing is necessary, and sit straight, rather than hunched over or slumped forwards. If you find that

breathlessness is a problem at night, try sleeping almost upright, propped up with pillows.

HEARTBURN

A burning sensation around the breastbone, heartburn is caused by a regurgitation of stomach acids and foods, which "burn" the lining of the oesophagus on their way up. This occurs during pregnancy because the muscle between the oesophagus and the stomach relaxes under the influence of hormones.

Eating only small amounts at a time often helps, since it prevents overloading the stomach at a time when space in the abdomen is at a premium. Avoid lying down for one hour after meals.

GESTATIONAL DIABETES

Diabetes related solely to pregnancy occurs when the body does not produce enough insulin to cope with the raised blood sugar levels of pregnancy caused by placental hormones.

Eating well and avoiding excessive weight gain are the best ways to reduce the odds of developing gestational diabetes. If you develop this condition, a healthy diet is crucial for keeping it within safe limits. Your doctor will be able to advise you on modifying your diet and monitoring your blood glucose levels, and your baby's growth will be checked carefully. Eat regularly and avoid sugary snacks. Insulin use may be required.

THE EMOTIONAL IMPACT OF THE LAST MONTHS

As the magical date nears, it becomes more difficult to think about anything other than the baby's birth, but keeping up other interests is important.

Antenatal teachers leading classes in the last weeks of pregnancy find it difficult to get the class to focus on "life after birth". Issues such as feeding, crying and how to be a parent provoke less interest and discussion than do topics wholly concerned with giving birth.

There is probably a certain amount of self-protective superstition in this, a fear that to buy lots of baby clothes and equipment, or to consider in any real depth what life might be like with a baby, is to tempt fate. But planning for life with the baby will keep you and your partner close. In addition, most women find that the days drag during the last month or so; keeping busy helps to pass the time.

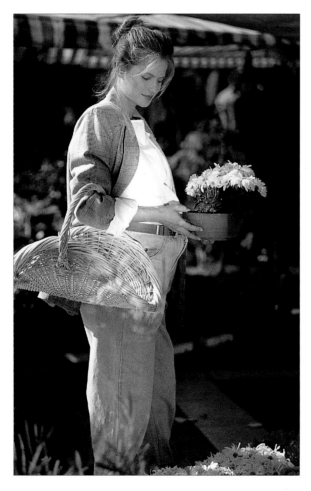

Shopping may provide an enjoyable outlet, and it will certainly be easier to get around now than later, when you are trying to cope with your baby's schedule. Wear comfortable shoes and don't carry heavy loads. If you drive, be sure to wear your seat belt. Position it between your breasts and across your thighs, below your tummy. Even if it feels uncomfortable to you, it won't harm the baby.

YOUR CONCERNS

It is likely that you will be less worried than before about your baby's health (see pp. 108–109), in part because you can feel your baby moving and kicking. But you may be concerned about whether you will know when labour really starts (you will) or if you will get to the hospital in time (almost certainly). If you go beyond your due date, you may worry about whether induction will prove necessary. Or, if your baby is very large or in a less than perfect position for birth, you may be anxious about the prospect of a caesarean.

As always, talk about your concerns with your partner and your medical advisers. Practise relaxation techniques (see pp. 50–51) and enjoy these last expectant few weeks.

PRACTICAL CONSIDERATIONS

Babies do occasionally arrive early, so it is worth making a few preparations. Pack your bag for hospital (see pp. 150–51). Make sure that you can always reach your partner. Keep all important telephone numbers next to the phone – doctor, midwife, taxi company. The last is in case your partner doesn't have time to get home. But remember that you can always call an ambulance if things happen fast. Even in early labour it is not safe to drive yourself. And make sure that there is always petrol and a couple of pillows in the car.

WHAT YOU CAN DO

Some women, of course, work almost to the end of their pregnancy and in this way manage to avoid boredom. But if you have stopped work in order to get everything ready and take a break before the demands of new motherhood take over completely, there is a lot you can do to make the most of the last few weeks.

Staying busy keeps you from getting too impatient for the birth, and keeping active may help you to cope better with labour. Try to keep moving: go for a walk or a swim as often as you can. Don't exhaust yourself shopping, but make sure you have at least a few basic pieces of equipment and some clothes for the baby (see pp. 136–39).

Many couples choose not to make social arrangements just in case the baby is early and they have to break the date. But this can be a mistake. If you find it relaxing to cook, invite some friends over for a meal (they will understand if you have to cancel); if you are not too tired and are comfortable sitting for a couple of hours, go to a film or a play. Remember that your social life may be on hold for some time once the baby is born, so make the most of it now.

Learn a new skill. Choose something you can make strides in reasonably quickly, such as a foreign language at a simple conversational level. Or start an absorbing book by an author you've always meant to read.

If you have a mobile phone, make sure that you keep it charged; if you don't have one, consider renting one, or rent a pager. Consult classified ads in parenting magazines for the names of companies offering this service.

Overdue?

It is common for a pregnant woman to count down the last couple of weeks until the day the baby is due, only to have the day come and go like any other. As do the next day and the one after that. Friends phone to see if there is any news, expectant grandparents can't keep away, neighbours express surprise that you are still around.

The practice of giving mothers a precise date on which to expect their baby is misleading, as fewer than 5 percent of babies actually arrive on that day and 30 percent of them come after it. The fact is that any baby who is born between 38 and 42 weeks of pregnancy is neither early nor late. This four-week spread is an average time span in which your baby could arrive. Some couples get around the potential stress of being "overdue" by telling themselves and others only that their baby is due "in late March" or "at the beginning of June".

If you do find that week 40 has come and gone, there is plenty of anecdotal evidence that sexual intercourse can get a slow-to-start labour under way (see p. 110). Providing your cervix has not dilated (see p. 163), sex certainly can't do any harm, so try it if you feel like it.

Your midwife will refer you to an obstetrician once week 41 arrives, and he or she may wish to attach you to a foetal monitor for a time to check the baby's heartbeat. An ultrasound scan may also be suggested to check on the baby's size and on the volume of amniotic fluid in the uterus: a decreased volume may be a sign that the placenta is working less well. Few doctors let pregnancy proceed past 42 weeks. If you get to 42 weeks, induction will normally be suggested.

As week 40 turns to week 41 and you still haven't had the baby, time may start to hang heavily on you. Try to keep busy; if you are too uncomfortable to keep moving, keep your mind occupied. Whether you go into labour spontaneously or not, your pregnancy is unlikely to last many more days. The end of pregnancy is inevitable!

IN UTERO TREATMENTS

Pioneering work is now being carried out in some hospitals around the world to treat babies at risk with drugs or surgery before they are born.

Medical intervention to treat a baby in the uterus is not new (see box, right). But increasingly, doctors specializing in in utero treatment are able to intervene surgically if a problem is detected.

OPERATIVE TECHNIQUES

When the flow of fluid in the body is blocked, the organs in front of or behind the blockage may be damaged. Inserting a tube at the site of the blockage to drain this fluid can prevent lasting problems.

This procedure has been used with success for babies in whom the outflow of urine is obstructed or when fluid has built up in the lungs. It has been less successful in cases of fluid on the brain. In such operations, the baby remains in the uterus. In other cases, however, the baby may be lifted out for treatment, remaining attached to the uterus through the umbilical cord and the placenta. (This technique is known as marsupialization.)

WHAT SURGEONS CAN DO

Surgeons have corrected babies' hernias of the diaphragm, in which a loop of intestine escapes from the abdominal cavity into

the chest cavity through a defect in the diaphragm, the muscular partition between the two. In severe cases this can interfere with lung and heart function and cause possibly fatal breathing difficulties.

Tumours of the lower back and lungs have been removed while the baby was still in the uterus, and heart pacemakers have been fitted in foetuses whose hearts were beating too slowly. Some cases of spina bifida (the incomplete closing of the backbone around the spinal cord), as well as obstructions to the blood flow through the heart and trachea (the air passage to and from the lungs),

have also been treated in utero.

A blockage in the connections between the blood vessels of twins within the placenta can also be removed surgically. When twins suffer from this condition, known as twin transfusion syndrome, the circulation of one baby pumps blood into the other one. This results in one baby having too much blood and the other one having too little. At best, this results in twins of widely different sizes at birth – one may weigh as much as double the other – and the small twin may have all the problems associated with low birth weight; at worst, it can kill both babies.

THE RISKS

The risks of surgery while a baby is still in the uterus are high, and

Once foetal surgery has taken place, babies are usually delivered by caesarean rather than undergoing a possibly stressful vaginal birth. Almost all then spend some time in intensive care, where they can be monitored closely (see pp. 208–209).

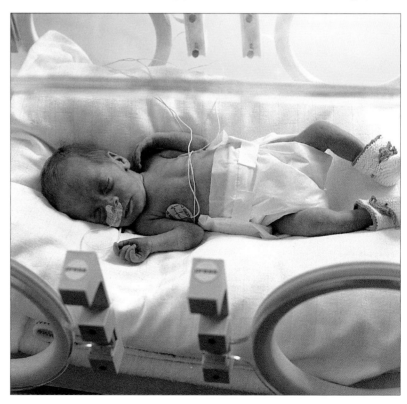

foetal surgery is still in the pioneering stages, available in relatively few places worldwide. The greatest risk is that in utero surgery will stimulate premature labour. The pregnant uterus's natural response to surgery is to begin contracting.

Drugs that combat this response are being developed all the time, and it is likely that drugs that are more effective at preventing premature labour, or at least delaying it, are likely to emerge in the future.

THE BENEFITS

As with any type of surgery, the risks have to be balanced against the benefits, which can be great. Foetal surgery is used when the baby's condition threatens his life either before birth or soon afterwards (for example, to correct a severe heart defect). Foetal tissue heals without scarring, which is a great potential benefit. As a result, conditions like cleft lip and/or palate, which often cause feeding problems in babies, can be corrected in utero. This will help the baby from the start and offers cosmetic benefits as well.

THE FUTURE

Work is still being done to decide which mothers and babies are likely to benefit from in utero surgery. Doctors are developing criteria to establish when the advantages of in utero surgery outweigh the considerable risks of premature labour or of harming the pregnancy. In some cases, waiting until after the birth – which may be induced early and done by a caesarean section – then surgery and intensive care, is less risky.

Medical conditions

Medical treatment while the baby is still in the uterus may be advised either to prevent problems from becoming worse – and perhaps affecting your baby's chances of survival – or to avoid more difficult or hazardous treatment after birth. Genetic counselling after the birth of a baby, or after the loss of a pregnancy due to factors that could recur, can lead to treatment in a subsequent pregnancy, if it's discovered that the same problem has arisen.

A deficiency in the production of red blood cells, for example, may respond to a bone marrow transplant, because bone marrow contributes to the formation of red blood cells.

In the case of rhesus disease (see p. 24) or to prevent or treat anaemia, a blood transfusion may be recommended. A congenital shortage of platelets, which can cause bleeding in the foetus, can be corrected by a platelet transfusion. Thyroid hormones, which regulate the metabolic rate of the body's tissues, may be administered if a deficiency is detected (the child of a mother with a thyroid deficiency may be affected). Drugs can also be used to regulate abnormal heart rhythms.

Steroids may be given to a foetus to improve lung function if it's clear that premature labour is about to start or if the baby has to be delivered before his lungs are mature enough, to avoid breathing difficulties.

Drugs can be given to the foetus by injecting the appropriate medication into the amniotic fluid. This is the usual procedure when giving drugs that affect the thyroid gland. Other disorders, including some heart malfunctions, are treated by giving drugs that cross the placenta to the mother and, therefore, to the foetus.

The air spaces in the lungs resemble the branches of a tree. Although the basic structure of the lung is laid down by the 26th week of pregnancy, many more subdivisions are needed before the baby can breathe air well. These are formed between weeks 26 and 38.

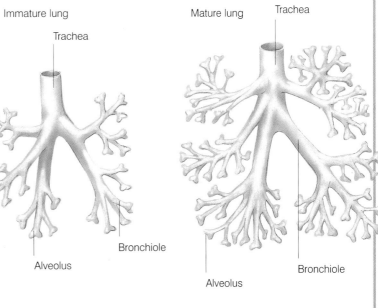

Immature lung

Trachea

Bronchiole

Alveolus

Mature lung   Trachea

Bronchiole

Alveolus

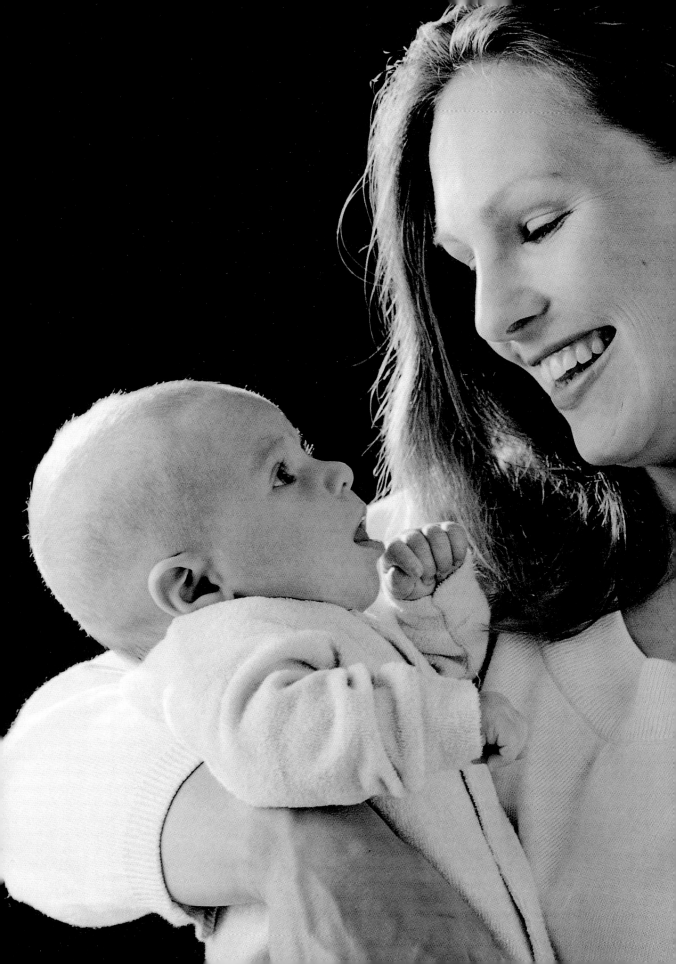

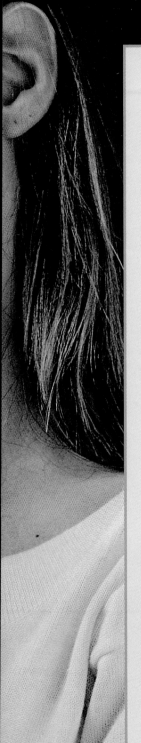

Giving birth

FOR MONTHS NOW, *you and your partner have focused more and more on the preparations and your expectations for your baby's birth day. You have probably:*

- *Thought about what labour and delivery will be like*

- *Prepared yourselves mentally and physically for the life-changing event of giving birth*

- *Planned how you want to labour and give birth, and discussed the circumstances under which your plans may have to change*

- *Considered some of the joys and challenges of parenthood.*

Your baby's birth is a unique event. You will remember small details, conversations and a range of feelings and emotions forever. No one else has ever given birth in the same way, with the same responses to the same extraordinary new person. That's the power – and the magic – of childbirth.

WHAT TO TAKE TO HOSPITAL

Packing your bag for hospital is every bit as thrilling as packing to go on holiday, with the bonus that your baby will accompany you on your return.

Some women wait to pack their hospital bag until the early stages of labour and find it a good way to pass the time before they actually have to leave for the hospital. Most women, however, like to pack ahead of time, just in case the baby arrives early. Two to three weeks before your due date is usually about right.

YOUR LABOUR BAG

The most important consideration in labour is your comfort. Many women find that they suffer extremes of temperature during labour, shivering one minute and perspiring the next. To keep you cool and refreshed, take a water bottle with a fine spray nozzle. Put it in the refrigerator when

you arrive. Include a soft flannel cloth for wiping your skin, and lip salve to prevent your lips from becoming dry.

To keep warm, pack a pair of thick socks and a small hot-water bottle (fill it with hot water when you get to the hospital) or thermal pack. Wrapped in a towel, the heat packs can be used to relieve aches in your back or legs. Massage is good for aching muscles as well, so pack some massage oil or light moisturizing body lotion.

Pack some drinks and snacks for you and your partner. During a long labour, you are both going to get hungry. Some doctors still recommend not eating anything in labour, just in case you need a

general anaesthetic, but check with the hospital. Mineral water, fruit juice, honey (for energy, since it keeps your glucose levels up), crackers and crispbreads can be packed in advance. Leave space to add a small thermal bag at the last minute filled with cold drinks and a bag of ice cubes or crushed ice. Transfer them to the fridge in the labour room, if there is one, when you get there.

To help to pass the time, you may want to take some music tapes and a cassette player. Take a variety of tapes so that you can select music to match your mood and your needs. If you plan to use visualization as one of your strategies to deal with pain (see p. 55), you should pack the photograph or other treasured object you have chosen as your focal point. Also include pens and paper – or your pregnancy notebook – for making notes, recording events and times, and taking the names of any helpers to whom you may want to send a note of thanks. Take a mirror for your partner to hold so that you can see the baby being born (or check whether the hospital can rig up a mirror for you). A camera (or a video camera if you have space in your bag) allows you to record the baby's first few minutes.

YOUR HOSPITAL STAY

Obviously, you need clothes and underwear – large, close-fitting pants (to hold sanitary towels) and at least one nursing bra. Your milk will come in after birth in about three or four days, when

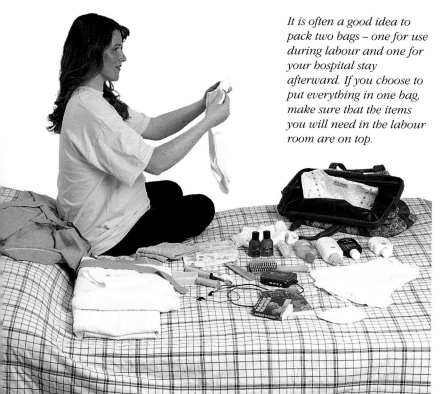

It is often a good idea to pack two bags – one for use during labour and one for your hospital stay afterward. If you choose to put everything in one bag, make sure that the items you will need in the labour room are on top.

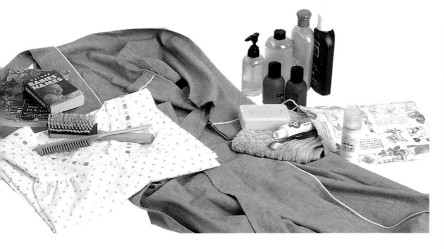

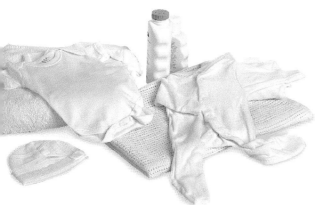

For the labour room, you will need a nightgown, T-shirt or one of your partner's shirts to give birth in, a dressing gown, plus personal toiletries. Ask what you will need for the baby. You may prefer that he wear his own clothes throughout your stay.

Partners: what you can do

Your first responsibility is to get to the hospital safely. If you have not already done so (see pp. 144–45), get a pager or mobile phone and make sure that it is always charged.

Do you know the route to the hospital? If it is not familiar, make a "dry run" during peak hour so that you know how long it might take and whether there are any road works that might slow your progress. Plan an alternative route in the event of unexpected delays. Find out where you should park. And make sure the petrol tank is always full.

Have a list of the phone numbers of the family members and friends you need to call after the birth to spread the good news, plus coins or cards for the phone. Mobile phones can interfere with medical equipment, so you will be asked to switch yours off if you have one.

your breasts will be full and heavy and need the support of a good bra. You may, however, feel more comfortable wearing one before then. Pack some nursing pads to absorb leaks.

You should pack toiletries, make-up and a hairbrush. Include a couple of soft towels if you prefer to use your own for bathing or showering.

Most first-time mothers overestimate how much time they will have "lying around" in the hospital. In the round of feeding and changing your baby, welcoming visitors, trying to rest and being examined by medical staff, you probably won't have a great deal of time to yourself. It doesn't hurt to pack some reading material. If you want to send friends news of the birth,

pack announcement cards, stamps and a pen.

Hospital food has a bad reputation, often undeserved. Meals and drinks usually come at regular intervals, however, which may not suit you if you are periodically awakened during the night to feed your newborn. Pack nutritional snacks, high-fibre breakfast cereal, fruit juice and spring water. Remember that most hospital stays are only 24 to 48 hours.

Every hospital is different, with some supplying practically everything and others relying on you to bring most things with you. A change in hospital management can mean a change in policy, so don't rely on what friends have told you. Ask beforehand what policies are.

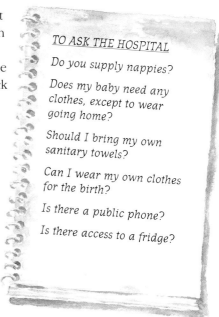

TO ASK THE HOSPITAL

Do you supply nappies?

Does my baby need any clothes, except to wear going home?

Should I bring my own sanitary towels?

Can I wear my own clothes for the birth?

Is there a public phone?

Is there access to a fridge?

PREPARING FOR A HOME BIRTH

Most professionals argue against home birth for first babies. But you have a right to a home birth if you want one, and it can be a rewarding experience.

Q *I had an epidural for the birth of my first child. Can I have an epidural for the home birth of my second baby?*

A No. A midwife cannot give you an epidural because these injections must be administered by an anaesthetist. However, other forms of pain relief are available at home. You can use TENS or have an injection of a painkiller (see pp. 170–73).

Many women find that their need for medication diminishes considerably between their first birth and their second, even if they are in the hospital both times. In second and subsequent births, they often need less relief and only later in labour. In addition, a lot of women who give birth at home, particularly after a vaginal delivery with a previous baby, find their need for pain relief much diminished. This is probably because they know what to expect of labour and birth and know that they can cope with it. This reduces the fear of the unknown (how much worse is this going to get?) that makes pain worse.

The fact that home birth takes place in familiar, stress-free surroundings may also be a factor. You may feel freer to move around at home, which can speed your labour along. And you may discover that you use relaxation, breathing and visualization techniques far more successfully at home than in a hospital.

Q *Where should I actually give birth. Is my bed okay?*

A You should give birth (and handle labour, for that matter) anywhere you feel comfortable. You don't have to use a bed, although this is easier for your midwife than if she has to get down on the floor to check on your progress. But you could cover a mat with towels or sheets and give birth on the floor, or even use a firm chair or sofa, or a table if you prefer. Discuss your options with your midwife; she will be happy to go along with whatever you want.

Giving birth in one room and moving to your own bed once the baby is born is also an option. You'll be in a clean, comfortable bed getting to know your baby uninterrupted, while others are doing any last bits of cleaning up.

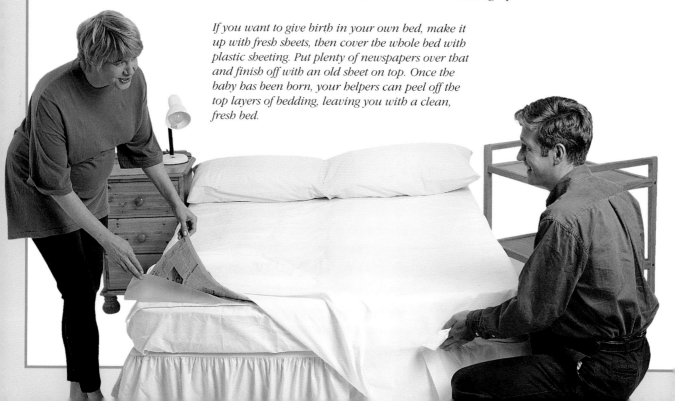

If you want to give birth in your own bed, make it up with fresh sheets, then cover the whole bed with plastic sheeting. Put plenty of newspapers over that and finish off with an old sheet on top. Once the baby has been born, your helpers can peel off the top layers of bedding, leaving you with a clean, fresh bed.

Q *My eight-year-old son wants to be at the birth of his baby brother or sister. Should I let him?*

A As birth becomes more family centred, more children are attending the birth of a sibling. This is an intensely personal decision for you, your partner, and your child. Some children may be frightened by the noises and actions of labour; others are more perturbed by knowing that something is going on behind closed doors. Some are fascinated by every tiny detail; others are bored by how long the whole business can take.

Talk it over among the three of you and make sure that you give your son an idea of what to expect, in terms he can understand. If you really don't think he is mature enough to be present for the whole of your labour, it's best to say so. A compromise might be to let him be there for the birth itself, so that he, too, can welcome the baby into the world.

If you allow him to be there for the whole time, it is a good idea to have someone to look after him and answer his questions openly as they arise. Most children will accept explanations like "Mummy can't talk at the moment. She has to concentrate, because ...," but you and your partner may be too wrapped up in what is happening at some point to be able to explain properly. If he gets bored with it all and wants to go and do something else instead, you need the reassurance that he is safe and that someone is taking care of him.

Q *I'm certain that I want my baby at home. But under what circumstances might I have to be transferred to hospital?*

A Your midwife would recommend your transfer to hospital if there were any signs that your labour was not progressing as it should, or that you or the baby were in distress.

For example, if your labour progresses slowly, and such simple measures as moving around and changing position do nothing to speed it up, your midwife may suggest moving you to hospital – especially if you become very tired, dizzy or faint – where you and the baby can be monitored more closely. Bleeding from the vagina might also indicate that you would be better off in hospital, where your condition could be assessed and measures taken if necessary. (Consider travelling time to the hospital when deciding whether to have your baby at home. You must be able to transfer quickly in an emergency.)

Foetal distress – that is, the baby is not getting enough oxygen (see pp. 174–75 and 177) – makes a move to hospital imperative.

It is unlikely that your midwife would find out during delivery that the baby was not in a good position and that a caesarean was necessary. But a caesarean might be recommended if the baby was showing signs of distress, or if you were overtired.

After the birth, a move to hospital would be needed only if the baby was having trouble breathing, if there was a long delay in delivering the placenta, or if you started to haemorrhage.

Q *How should I prepare the room in which I intend to give birth?*

A Your midwife will advise you on this and will bring with her anything that she needs. She may ask you to supply a table or trolley on which to place her equipment. She will probably request that the bed be placed so that she has access from both sides. You should also provide a comfortable chair for her to rest in, should your labour be protracted.

In addition to the things you would have packed in your labour bag for hospital (see pp. 150–51), you will need some clean face washers and towels in the room (keep them covered in plastic until you need them so that they stay clean). Have some clothes for your baby close at hand, too.

Home birth is no messier than a hospital birth. Your midwife will advise you on protecting your bed and furniture (or she'll do this herself) with pads or disposable sheets. Place some rubbish bags in the room for disposing of these and other throwaways. Make sure there are cold drinks on hand and snacks for the midwife and other helpers.

The midwife will also need a couple of bowls, a kettle so that she has plenty of cooled, boiled water when she needs it, and a good light. This does not have to be a bright overhead light; an anglepoise or spotlight is fine. The most important thing is that your midwife must be able to see what she is doing at all times.

WHEN LABOUR STARTS

With your first baby, labour can be slow to start and slow to progress, which can make you uncertain about whether you are really in labour.

It is difficult to pinpoint exactly when labour starts. For some women, everything begins to happen quite quickly, and they move seamlessly from one stage to the next. But for others, the first indications that labour is beginning may be spread over a couple of weeks, sometimes with no indication that anything is happening for days at a time.

Towards the end of pregnancy, the baby's head is likely to engage (see illustration), and you will probably be aware that this has happened by the greater ease with which you can now breathe. You may also lose some weight: it is not unusual to lose 1–1.5 kg (2–3 lb) in the last couple of weeks. Some women experience a rush of energy shortly before labour starts; others are highly fatigued. Any of these occurrences may indicate that you do not have long to wait.

THE SHOW

The show is the release of the mucus plug that seals the opening of the cervix. In some women, it comes away as a blob of pinkish jelly; in others it is a series of smaller pieces. Its release tells you that the cervix is beginning to stretch a little, in preparation for labour. You may notice it on your underwear, or on toilet paper when you wipe yourself. Several days may pass between the show and the start of true labour, or just an hour or

When the head engages

In a first pregnancy the baby's head may engage in the upper part of your pelvic cavity two to four weeks before delivery. (Or it may not engage until labour starts.) As labour progresses, the head descends farther into the pelvis.

so, or anything in between. A show accompanied by slight vaginal bleeding may be a sign of early labour.

You will be asked when you first report the start of labour whether you have "had a show" or not. If you haven't – or haven't noticed it – don't worry; you may still be in labour.

THE WATERS

Another sign of labour's onset is the rupture of the membranes that form the bag, or amniotic sac, of fluid inside the uterus. When the membranes rupture, amniotic fluid may escape. This can happen in a rush, which you will feel as a sudden gush of

liquid down your legs. More usually, however, it will trickle out – if the baby's head is engaged in the pelvis, there's no room for large quantities to leak out at once. Sometimes, a trickle slows, then ceases, which may indicate that the rupture wasn't complete and has sealed itself. Sometimes, in first pregnancies, the membranes do not rupture until labour is well established.

If fluid continues to escape and you don't go into labour within a few hours, telephone your midwife or the hospital. If the membranes rupture and labour doesn't start within a day or so, the baby is vulnerable to infection. If the baby's head is not engaged

A Case in Point
When Labour Starts Slowly

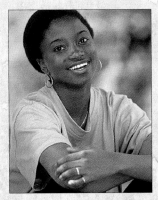

JULIE, 28, WAS TENSE IN THE LAST COUPLE OF WEEKS OF HER PREGNANCY.

"After about 38 weeks, every time I went to the bathroom I was looking for a show. And every time I felt a twinge of discomfort in my back or my abdomen, I thought it could be labour starting and noted the time. I was terrified to go out in case my waters broke and everyone looked at me. I didn't know that they probably wouldn't gush in any case. David didn't help; he was sure that it would all happen quickly and we wouldn't get to the hospital in time. We live in a city, but I think he had visions of having to deliver our baby alone on an isolated country road!

"By the time my due date arrived, I was so stressed and worried that my blood pressure soared. I couldn't believe that time could pass so slowly, and yet part of me didn't actually want labour to start. Finally I decided to use all my energy to finish painting the baby's room. I even invited some friends over for a meal and spent a couple of days planning what to cook for them. I made a few dishes to put in the freezer for us to have when I got home. This took my mind off the long wait.

"In the end, the first real sign I had was the show – it was quite obvious, and I immediately felt calmer. I waited a couple of hours, then called David. I think the fact that I sounded so relaxed calmed him, too. He came home, we had something to eat, and we started to watch a video. I felt the beginnings of contractions about six hours after I'd seen the show. We finished watching the film, I put the last-minute things in the bag for the hospital, and we drove there slowly. To my surprise I was already 5 cm [2 in] dilated."

when your waters break, the rush of fluid can bring the cord with it; compression of the cord can affect your baby's oxygen supply.

CONTRACTIONS

Contractions are a sign of labour if they increase in frequency and strength over a period of an hour or two and last longer than 40 seconds each. You will feel them as a tightening sensation across your abdomen and into your back, beginning gently, building up to a peak, and then fading away. Pain that intensifies when you move probably means that you are experiencing labour contractions.

Contractions are caused when the muscles that form the uterus shorten, exerting an upward pull on the cervix and downward pressure at the top of the uterus.

The muscles lengthen again as the contraction dies away. But with each contraction, the muscles shorten a little more, leaving the cervix slightly more open and pushing the baby a little farther down.

You may also find that your stomach is upset. A bout of sickness and diarrhoea is by no means unusual (and is one reason that routine enemas are no longer given – most women's bodies have already accomplished the task).

SIGNS OF FALSE LABOUR

You may experience some of the above symptoms yet still not be in labour. A show that is brownish rather than pink may be a sign of false labour. As the cervix starts to dilate and thin (or efface), blood capillaries may rupture, which tinges the show

pink. Either intercourse or a vaginal examination can dislodge the mucus plug, but in those circumstances, it will not have fresh blood in it, so it is more likely to be brown.

In established labour, contractions get longer and stronger over a period of a few hours. If your contractions remain irregular and do not increase in either intensity or frequency, chances are that you are not in labour. If contractions cease or subside when you move around, again you are probably not in labour.

It can be difficult to pinpoint the exact site of any pain, but generally, if the pain at the height of a contraction seems to be in your lower abdomen rather than spreading into your back, you are probably not in labour yet.

WHAT TO DO WHEN LABOUR STARTS

Your initial reaction once you are sure you're in labour may be to head for the hospital, but you may be more comfortable at home.

If your contractions start to come close and strong early in labour, an early move to the hospital will be necessary. But for many women, a first labour starts slowly and gently. You may have contractions for several hours before they are strong enough for you to report to the labour ward. Make sure you feel the baby move during early labour: an absence of movement could indicate foetal distress and should be checked.

Some women have mild contractions for 48 hours or more before hard labour begins – the contractions feel like vague, wave-like pains that come and go fairly regularly. You can put them in the back of your mind and do other things. (But stay close to home – they could get stronger quickly. Have important phone numbers handy.)

More typically, you may have a day or night with contractions that prevent you from concentrating even on a film or a book. In that case, make a hot drink, listen to relaxing music or browse through a newspaper while you wait.

WHAT YOU CAN DO

Try to eat something filling and nourishing. You will need all the energy you can get for the next half day or so. But don't force yourself to eat if you don't feel hungry. Some women are too excited to eat; others are too apprehensive. It won't hurt you to fast. Whether you eat or not, drink plenty of fluids and remember to empty your bladder regularly. A full bladder may interfere with the progress of your labour.

Get as much rest as you can; the next phase of labour will be tiring, and you may have no opportunity to rest. If labour begins in the middle of the night, try to sleep. Avoid lying on your back, which constricts your large blood vessels and may limit blood flow across the placenta. (Don't worry about "missing" the next phase – you won't.) If you can't sleep, get up and move around rather than lying in bed timing

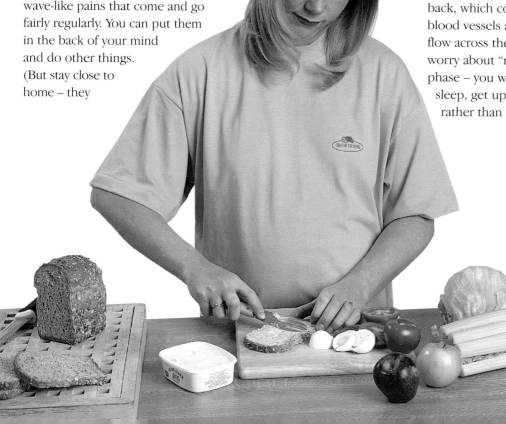

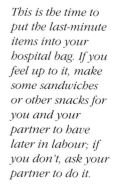

This is the time to put the last-minute items into your hospital bag. If you feel up to it, make some sandwiches or other snacks for you and your partner to have later in labour; if you don't, ask your partner to do it.

Going to hospital

Time the duration of your contractions using a watch with a second hand, and see how close they are. The right time to take action will depend on the distance you have to travel to get to the hospital, and the time of day or night you're going. If you are no more than about 15 minutes away from the hospital, for a first baby you can safely wait until you are experiencing contractions three times every 10 minutes, with contractions lasting about 50 to 60 seconds. If you experience a lot of pain, or if you feel you can't cope without help, you may want to go in sooner.

Travelling by car can be uncomfortable when you are in labour. You'll need as much room as possible, which may mean sitting in the back seat with the front passenger seat pushed as far forwards as it will go. Put a couple of pillows in the car to support your back or to hold onto during contractions, and throw in a blanket (you may feel cold). Take along a small bowl in case you become nauseated. It is also important for your own safety to fasten your seat belt (loosely under the bulge), no matter how uncomfortable this may feel.

Your partner should drive smoothly and safely, avoiding lurches or swerves that could make you more uncomfortable. Relaxation can really help: breathe slowly and regularly, and consciously release the tension in your shoulders and your hands.

If you experience bleeding (other than light spotting), or if, when your membranes rupture, the amniotic fluid is green, go to the hospital straight away – phone to say you are on your way. The fluid coloured green may be meconium (see p. 177); it is one of the signs that your baby may be in distress.

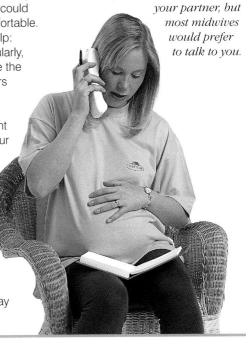

If you are in any doubt about whether to go to hospital, call and ask. It's best to do this yourself so that you can describe accurately what is happening – where the pain is most acute, how bad it is, and so on. Of course, you could relay all this to your partner, but most midwives would prefer to talk to you.

contractions. If it's daytime, try to get some rest, too. Watch TV or read a magazine. Distracting yourself a little will help you to pass the time and lighten the niggling pain you probably feel.

Take a warm (not hot) shower or a bath, as long as your membranes haven't ruptured. A bath may help you to relax, and a shower will refresh you. Both may take your mind off the contractions.

Call your partner, if he is not at home already, and let him know what is happening. Although he may not need to leave for home immediately – unless you want him with you – he needs to be on standby.

PARTNERS: WHAT YOU CAN DO

Your biggest task in these early stages is to keep your labouring partner relaxed, for which you, too, have to remain calm. It's understandable if you feel apprehensive – you also have a challenge ahead of you – but now is probably not the time to communicate your concerns to your partner. Remember that her body has been preparing for the next few hours for nine months and is ready to give birth.

Watch for signs of tension in your partner's face and neck, but don't alert her to tension (which may make it worse). Instead, if she is tense, offer her a massage – either a whole-body massage if she can get comfortable enough to relax and enjoy it (see pp. 58–59), or just her neck and shoulders. For many women, touch is instantly calming.

Try to distract her from the contractions. Talk to her, watch TV together, or play draughts or Scrabble. Every so often, time contractions for a short period as practice for when they are coming closer together and lasting longer. Contractions are timed from the beginning of one to the beginning of the next. Your partner will be able to tell you when it starts, or you can place your hand on her abdomen and feel it tightening.

EMERGENCY BIRTH

First babies rarely arrive so fast that you can't get to the hospital; if they do, it's usually because the mother's body and the baby are working perfectly together.

If you don't have time to reach the hospital, you have to rely on whoever happens to be with you at the time to help you, or – less probable – give birth alone. In the unlikely event of an emergency birth, you and your partner should know what to do. By learning what a helper can and should do, you will be prepared to instruct someone on how to help you.

Remember that when labour makes very quick, effective progress like this, it's likely to end with the happy birth of a healthy baby. It's a sign that your body and your baby are working together as well as is possible. Remain confident and relaxed.

PARTNERS OR HELPERS: WHAT YOU CAN DO

You can help by giving emotional support, by keeping the mother as comfortable as possible, and by doing the basic, practical tasks that help the birth to go smoothly. Call an ambulance, even if you are confident that you can manage and know that it will arrive too late. The professionals will need to check that all is well, and in the unlikely event that something does go wrong, their presence may make a critical difference.

Wash your hands and scrub your fingernails, then wash the mother's perineum and anus with clean cloths and cooled, boiled water (it will cool faster in a very cold, shallow bowl). Use a clean sheet or towel to cover the place where the mother is sitting, kneeling or lying. If you have time, help her to move onto a higher surface, such as a bed, settee, or

If you are waiting for help and the baby's head hasn't appeared yet, help the labouring woman to raise her legs and buttocks; this can take the pressure off the perineum and may slow things down.

Do's and don'ts

Do be prepared: Have emergency telephone numbers beside each phone at home and in your handbag.
Do stay calm: Your body knows what it is doing.
Do boil some water: A supply of boiled, cooled water is useful for washing the mother's perineum before and after the birth and for washing the baby.

Don't panic: It's natural to be anxious, since this is not the birth you have planned. But remember your relaxation techniques and breathe slowly and regularly.
Don't cut the cord: Leave it until the ambulance crew or doctor arrives. If the cord is very short and the baby won't reach the mother's breast, place her on her stomach.
Don't pull on the cord: This could dislodge the placenta prematurely and cut off the baby's oxygen supply before her lung breathing is well established.

desk. If she is comfortable on the floor, leave her there. Lying flat with her legs raised or kneeling with her elbows on the floor and head on her arms may slow things down. Panting should reduce the mother's need to bear down.

You will see the head crown (see pp. 182–83). As it does, tell the mother to pant. The head will emerge gradually with the next couple of contractions. Cup it gently with your hands so that it doesn't "shoot" straight out, but don't pull it to try to help it out. Once the head is out, check that the umbilical cord – it looks like a dark rope – is not wrapped around the baby's neck. If it is, work it gently over the head. With your fingertips, wipe any mucus or fluid away from the baby's nose and mouth (stroke outwards from the nose, down from the mouth). Another couple of contractions should bring the first shoulder out, and another the second. After that, the baby will slip out very easily. Be careful: she will be slippery.

Don't wipe any vernix off the baby's body (it will help to keep her warm), and wrap the baby in something warm – a warmed towel is ideal. She will lose heat from the top of her head, so make sure it is covered. Then give her to her mother; if the cord is not long enough for her to reach the breast, put her on her stomach.

Don't cut or pull on the cord. Without drugs, the placenta is not likely to emerge for about 20 minutes, but put a bowl or some newspaper down to catch it. If it emerges before the ambulance gets there, keep it so that the crew can check that the entire placenta has been delivered.

IF YOU ARE ALONE

At home, try to reach a phone and dial 000 (or 111 in New Zealand). If you can't, attract attention by breaking a window or, if you have close neighbours, banging on the floor or a wall. Go somewhere comfortable, clean and warm (or a room that can be heated quickly when help arrives).

Find a comfortable position. Remove your pants, shoes and any clothing that might get in the way. Push when you feel the need to. When you see or feel your baby's head, pant, so that the head comes out more slowly.

Sometimes, the cord is around the baby's neck as she comes out. Ease your finger between the neck and the cord and lift the cord over the head. You may see some membrane over the baby's face; wipe it away, so she can breathe. As she emerges, use your arms to "catch" her. Don't get cold. Wrap your baby, then wrap both of you in a quilt or blanket. Don't cut the cord.

If you are out alone, go to where there are people, such as a shop; if you are driving, stop a motorist and ask him or her to get help.

A Case in Point
A Helpful Neighbour

FIRST-TIME MOTHER SARAH, 25, ASSUMED SHE WOULD HAVE TIME TO LABOUR AT HOME.

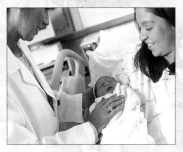

"After an hour of contractions, I realized that the baby was on its way. I dialled an ambulance and my husband, Tom, and then a neighbour, Jenny, who was there in minutes. She said she could see the top of the head and asked me where I wanted to be. I was still sitting on the stairs where I'd made the calls. I couldn't move, so she left me there, hanging onto the banisters. She got a load of clean towels, put a couple under me, and turned up the heating. I could feel the baby's head with my hands. Jenny knelt at the foot of the stairs and told me to pant while she cupped the baby's head. She had just said the head's out when another contraction pushed the baby out. She slid into Jenny's hands. Jenny wrapped her in a towel and gave her to me.

"The ambulance arrived, and a paramedic cut the cord and checked the baby – she was obviously okay, wide awake and pink-cheeked – while we waited for the placenta. Then they helped us into the ambulance. Tom was there in time for us to go to the hospital together. He was disappointed he'd missed the birth but relieved that we were well.

"When I look back, I wonder at how calm I was. But Jenny radiated confidence – although she later confessed that she had been terrified. But once I knew the baby was coming and there was nothing I could do, I wasn't frightened. I knew we'd be okay."

ADMISSIONS PROCEDURES

Before you are left with your partner to continue the labouring, a number of checks will be made on your health and on your baby's well-being.

Q *Will the hospital admit me at any time of the day?*

A Of course – babies come when they want to! It's always a good idea to call the labour ward, to let them know you are on your way. In the time it takes for you to get there, the staff will have prepared a room for you.

Some hospitals have different parking arrangements and different entrances at night, so it is worth asking about these in advance. If you haven't, don't worry – but remember to ask about them when you call to say you're on your way.

Q *What happens when we get to the hospital?*

A You may be asked to go into a special admissions room. A midwife will ask about your contractions, about any other symptoms of labour, and about whether you have experienced any bleeding. Some points in your notes will be confirmed – such as whether this is your first baby and what problems, if any, you have had in your pregnancy. Your plans for your labour may be discussed, with reference to your birth plan.

A vaginal examination will tell whether you are really in labour, how far you have progressed, and whether your membranes are intact. Between contractions, your midwife will insert one or two fingers into your vagina to feel the cervix. She will tell you how dilated (open) your cervix is after each exam. Before labour, your cervix is closed; for the baby to be born, it needs to have dilated 10 cm (4 in). At admission, with a first baby, you will probably be 2 to 4 cm (¾ to 1½ in) dilated.

Q *Are there any other routine checks?*

A A midwife will take your blood pressure and ask for a specimen of urine to check for traces of sugar and protein.

Contractions will be timed for length and frequency, and the midwife will listen to your baby's heart and check her position. You may be hooked up to a foetal monitor for a period of 10 to 20 minutes (see pp. 174–75) so that the midwife can listen to the baby's heartbeat during contractions and make sure she is getting enough oxygen.

You may be invited to take a bath or a shower, which can be pleasant and relaxing for you. Some hospitals prefer you wear a hospital gown; others will allow you to wear your own clothes. Your partner will not have to wear a surgical gown unless you are having a caesarean.

You can help your midwife if you are able to give a record of your contractions and details of any other signs – such as a show or your membranes rupturing. If you can't talk through a contraction, your partner can answer any questions.

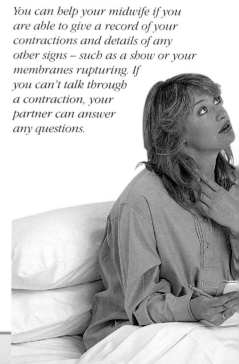

Make sure that you are familiar with the hospital in advance, or ask for a map. A building can look different in the middle of the night, and there may be fewer staff around to ask for directions.

Q *The thought of a stranger shaving my pubic hair distresses me a great deal. Is this really necessary?*

A Hospitals have discontinued this practice, but if the thought really bothers you, confirm that this is the case. Shaving used to be done in the (mistaken) belief that pubic hair harboured bacteria that could harm the baby.

If an episiotomy (see pp. 186–87) becomes necessary to facilitate the birth, a small area may be shaved to make the cut and repair easier. Again, few doctors consider this necessary and simply push the hair out of the way as they stitch. Ask what the hospital's policy is and make a note in your birth plan to make sure your wishes are heeded. Itchy regrowth of hair, coupled with healing stitches, is uncomfortable.

Q *I'm sure I'll be able to cope with labour as long as my partner can be with me. Will he be able to stay throughout?*

A Again, this is an area in which practices have changed. It used to be that your partner would be asked to wait outside while these preliminary checks and discussions went on, and he was sometimes asked to step outside during internal exams. But partners are now asked if they'd like to stay. A father-to-be has an important role to play as your helper and support. Some find it all fascinating – and remember details you missed – and most women are more relaxed if their partners are close by. If you prefer to be together, there's no reason you shouldn't be. If your partner is squeamish about such procedures as the vaginal examination, he can look away.

If he is asked to leave and you want him to stay, say so. If he is satisfied he is in the way and does leave, he should ask how long he should wait outside and come back in as soon as that time has elapsed.

Q *What if I am in hard labour when we arrive?*

A No one will delay getting you the help you need for "procedures". A vaginal examination will be done immediately to assess how far along you are, and you will be taken to a delivery room. In this situation it is unlikely that your partner will be asked to leave the room.

Q *Does the vaginal examination hurt?*

A No, but women sometimes find it uncomfortable, especially if they are tense. Relax and breathe deeply. If you are having a contraction, ask the midwife to wait until it's over before examining you.

Most women welcome these internal examinations as proof that the contractions are making something happen, but you should remember that dilatation is not steady: it is common to progress only by 1 to 2 cm (½ to ¾ in) in what can seem like hours, only to find that the next 3 or 4 cm (1¼ to 1½ in) are completed quickly.

Q *What if my waters haven't broken?*

A In the process known as ARM – artificial rupture of the membranes – the amniotic sac (the bag of waters) is pierced with a hook-like instrument, which allows the amniotic fluid to escape from the vagina.

Medical opinions on this procedure change quite frequently. Some doctors and midwives believe that it is best to let nature take its course, as long as you and your baby are well. But recent studies of amniotomy have shown that ARM can help to move labour along if it is clear that labour is well established and the baby's head is not too high in the pelvis. In some cases, such aggressive measures can actually lower caesarean rates.

If the decision to speed up your labour is made and your membranes have not ruptured, ARM will be performed (see pp. 168–69).

THE FIRST STAGE

In the first – and longest – stage of labour, your cervix will gradually open to allow your baby into the birth canal.

Once labour begins (see pp. 154–55), the first stage typically lasts 10 to 12 hours with a first baby; with second or subsequent babies, the first stage of labour is likely to be shorter.

WHAT IS A CONTRACTION?

Labour starts under the influence of hormones. At term, the placenta starts to work slightly less efficiently. In response to this, the baby's pituitary gland releases oxytocin which crosses the placenta into your bloodstream. Your body's response to this oxytocin is to produce oxytocin itself, which stimulates contractions. In addition, when the baby's adrenal gland is mature, it secretes the hormone cortisol. This crosses into your bloodstream and alters your levels of oestrogen and progesterone; as a result, you start to produce hormone-like chemicals called prostaglandins. Prostaglandins soften the cervix, and this softening also stimulates the uterus to start contracting.

Each contraction has two effects. First, it restricts the space in the uterus for the baby (and the amniotic sac, if it hasn't ruptured yet), forcing her into the area where there is least resistance, that is the softened cervix. Second, each contraction shortens the muscle fibres attached to the cervix and pulls them upwards, away from the opening. (This is called effacement and is measured in percentages. You will be 100 percent effaced at the end of the first stage.) At the same time, the muscles around the cervix are widening the opening (dilatation). With each contraction, the baby is forced farther down towards this enlarging opening.

You'll experience contractions as a hardening of your abdomen. Each contraction comes gradually, rising to a peak, then fading away. Contractions may feel like intense period pains, although some women experience them as a sharper pain or a rush of energy. Generally, however, you are likely to feel pain at the peak of a contraction and be able to relax before and after.

HOW LONG DO THEY LAST?

During the first stage of labour, the uterus contracts at increasingly shorter intervals,

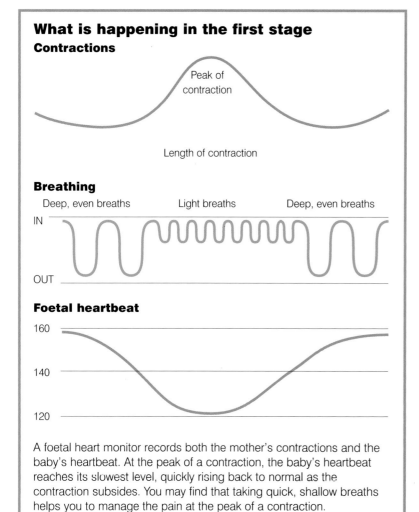

What is happening in the first stage
Contractions

Peak of contraction

Length of contraction

Breathing

Deep, even breaths   Light breaths   Deep, even breaths

IN

OUT

Foetal heartbeat

160

140

120

A foetal heart monitor records both the mother's contractions and the baby's heartbeat. At the peak of a contraction, the baby's heartbeat reaches its slowest level, quickly rising back to normal as the contraction subsides. You may find that taking quick, shallow breaths helps you to manage the pain at the peak of a contraction.

while the contractions gradually become longer. At the start, you may be feeling one contraction of 40 to 50 seconds every 10 minutes. At the end, each contraction will last longer than a minute, and there will be a gap of no more than a minute between each one, giving you very little time to rest between them.

Every single contraction helps the cervix to open up and pull back. By the end of the first stage, the cervix is completely effaced and fully dilated, ready for the birth of the baby.

Labour often progresses slowly at first. There may be several hours where nothing seems to happen at all. You may feel contractions, and feel them getting longer and stronger, yet you may not dilate more than half a centimetre. This is normal. Once you get to 7 to 8 cm (3 in), your baby's head will descend further.

What is happening to your baby

During the first stage of labour, your baby continues to receive oxygen and nutrients across the placenta. He has been experiencing contractions while he has been in the uterus, and at the beginning of the first stage of labour the contractions will not feel any different. Some babies appear to sleep through some of the early stages of labour. But as your contractions increase in intensity, your baby will feel the uterine walls pressing against his body and the pressure of the cervix on the bones of his head.

The baby's response to the effects of contractions can be seen when he is monitored. When the uterus is contracting, the blood flow through the placenta is slowed down. It normalizes as the contraction passes. In response to the lower volume of blood, the baby's heart beat may slow, with a dip at the peak of each contraction. When the contraction fades away, the heart rate speeds up once more. This dip in heart rate causes no problems at all to a healthy baby who's ready to be born.

An average heart rate for a baby in the first stage of labour is usually about 120 to 160 beats per minute, although your midwife is unlikely to be concerned if it falls as low as 110 or rises as high as 170. A graph of a healthy baby's heart rate shows minor variations most of the time, as the heart responds to such stimuli as a change in your position, ingestion of food or drink, or a massage of your abdomen, in addition to the stimulation of contractions. These variations show that the heart is functioning well, responding to the stresses of being born by adjusting its rate to cope. Persistent decelerations which do not rise again may be a sign that your baby is not tolerating labour well; you may be given oxygen or your position may be changed.

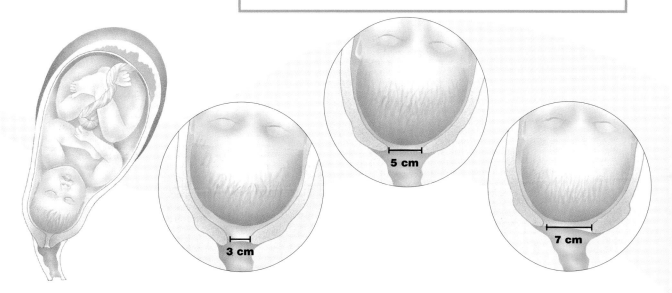

5 cm

3 cm

7 cm

1 At the end of pregnancy, the cervix is closed, although the os (the hole at the top of the cervix) has stretched and softened enough for the mucus plug (operculum) to have come away (see p. 154).

2 At the start of labour, contractions begin to open the cervix slightly, pulling it upwards and outwards.

3 At 5 cm (2 in), someone caring for you will be able to feel the top of the baby's head. You are halfway to full dilatation. The second 5 cm (2 in) may be accomplished more quickly.

4 At 7 cm (3 in), it will be easy for someone caring for you to feel the top of the baby's head through the open cervix during an internal examination.

WHAT YOU CAN DO

The first stage of labour is the hardest and most exhilarating work you may ever do. For part of it, you will be able to move and to manage the pain.

Contractions can be painful, but between them you won't feel pain. As you feel a contraction coming, try to relax. Release the tension in your shoulders, face and hands. Tension in your body transmits itself to all your muscles, including those of your uterus, and increases pain.

Concentrate on your breathing. As a contraction begins, breathe deeply and slowly, using your abdomen, in through your nose and out through your mouth. This delivers oxygen to all parts of your body and across the placenta to your baby. With each exhalation, you are expelling tension. As the contraction peaks, take shallower breaths in and out through your mouth. As it subsides, revert to deep breathing. Don't resist the contraction – it increases in intensity, reaches its peak, and starts to fade.

Between contractions, relax. This will help you to conserve your energy when your contractions are coming close together. You will need all your energy later to help push your baby out.

Take frequent sips of water or fruit juice, and if you are hungry and feel like eating, ask if you can have a snack. Some women find the thought of food nauseating; others are too involved with breathing and relaxing to notice that they have not eaten for some hours. You may find it refreshing

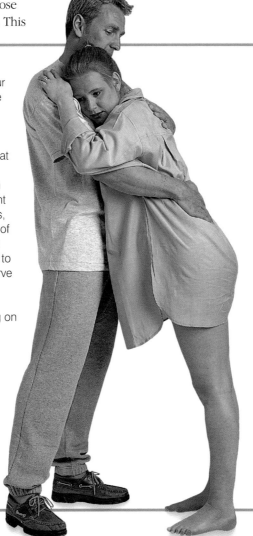

Staying upright

Most women manage labour best if they are free to move and find a position that is comfortable. You will probably find that different positions work best for you at different times.

Studies have also shown that women who stay upright tend to have shorter labours, since keeping the pressure of the uterus on the cervix can speed dilation. If you prefer to lie down, perhaps to conserve your energy or gather your strength, lie on your side, rather than your back. Lying on your back, especially on a hard surface, may restrict blood flow to the baby.

Stand, leaning against a wall or your partner. Be sure that he can take all your weight if necessary.

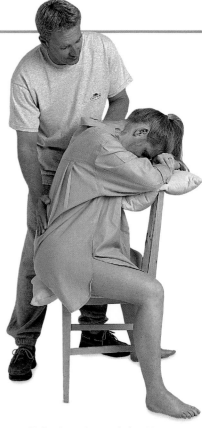

Sit backward on a chair, with your arms and head resting on the back. Use pillows to increase your comfort.

to suck on some crushed ice. Urinate frequently – a full bladder is very uncomfortable during contractions.

If you experience backache during your labour, ask your partner to massage you, but ask him to stop if it breaks your concentration during a contraction.

PARTNERS: WHAT YOU CAN DO

The most important thing is for you to be there, comforting and encouraging your partner, but you can also carry out many practical tasks to help your partner through this tiring stage.

If your partner is being monitored electronically, ask the doctor or midwife to interpret the

1 AM Contractions too strong to sleep through; once every 10 mins. We watch a video.

4 AM Hospital says come in. Need help to get in the car. Contractions every 5 mins, can breathe through them.

5 AM Exam: 3 cm dilated.

7 AM Contractions strong, but bringing me closer to seeing my baby. Coping.

8 AM Tired. Contractions every 2 mins; hard to relax between them.

9 AM Dejected: only 7 cm dilated. Want to be alone.

9.30 AM Can't stand the pain. Tired and weepy. Advised to wait ½ hour for pain medication.

10 AM Contractions every minute, but almost 10 cm. Will see my baby soon.

record for you. If it helps her, tell your partner when a contraction is coming and fading. (Some women find that knowing helps them feel in control, others that it makes them tense, so ask her if it is helpful.) If she is not being monitored, use a watch with a second hand to time the length and frequency of contractions for short intervals. Every half an hour for 5 to 10 minutes is probably enough. If she wants you to, place your hands on her abdomen so that you can feel the contraction and breathe through it with her. If she loses her rhythm, this will get her back on track.

Help her to be comfortable, whether that means asking for another pillow, getting her a drink, rubbing her back, holding her, or cooling her face and neck with a sponge or water spray. Use a sponge to wet her lips. And if she tells you to leave her alone, don't take it personally. Stand by to help when she wants you.

Reassure her that all is well; the fact that it may be taking a

Record the milestones of your labour or ask your partner to do so. Once your baby is in your arms, you may find it hard to remember the details of labour, but you will enjoy having this record to remind you.

long time is normal. Tell her how well she is doing and remind her of how many contractions are behind her. Don't tell her it is almost over unless the midwife says so. Although you may be able to empathize with her, don't tell her you know how she feels, because you don't.

Be her intermediary with the health professionals. Answer any questions they may pose yourself, if you can, so that your partner can concentrate on what she is doing. If she wants medication, or more medication, communicate her request. And be prepared to tell her gently if the professionals think that pain relief is not a good idea: if she is nearly fully dilated, they may not recommend it. At that point, concentrate on the fact that she is almost ready to start pushing.

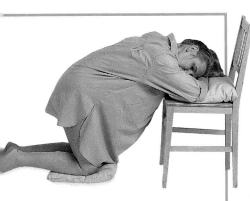

Kneel, leaning forward on a chair, the end of a bed, a beanbag, a pile of pillows or on your partner's lap.

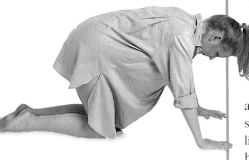

Kneel on all fours, rocking your pelvis during a contraction. If it helps, try arching your back in this position too.

THE BABY'S POSITION

How your baby is lying in the uterus can have an important impact on your labour and on whether you are likely to need surgical intervention.

The ideal position for your baby to be in when you go into labour – for both of you – is head down, or cephalic (see pp. 140–41), and with the head engaged (see p. 154). When the baby's head engages, it is a good indication that your baby "fits" and that labour will progress smoothly. In the last few weeks, babies can change their position, but an average-size baby doesn't have much room to move around.

Women rarely go into labour with an undetected feet-first, or breech, baby (see pp. 140–41), since a midwife can usually feel if the baby is head or bottom down. The midwife should also be able to tell whether your baby is posterior or anterior (facing your front or back) by feeling the outline of her body from the outside.

Complicated delivery positions are rare. At term, about 96 percent of babies are head down with the crown as the presenting part – the part that will be born first. Between 3 and 5 percent are breech. Transverse and oblique lies, along with face and brow

If your baby is occiput posterior, backache may be severe. Lie on your side to relieve pressure on your back, and ask your partner to massage your back vigorously.

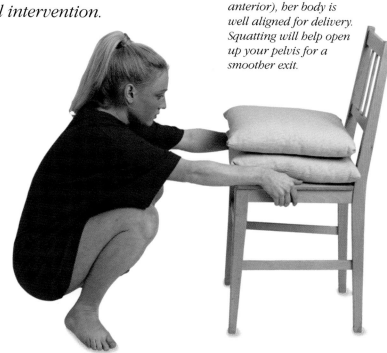

If your baby's head faces your back (occiput anterior), her body is well aligned for delivery. Squatting will help open up your pelvis for a smoother exit.

presentations, account for only 1 percent of deliveries.

OCCIPUT ANTERIOR
If your baby is left or right occiput anterior (head down, facing your back, and slightly to the left or right), you have an excellent chance of having a straightforward labour. Her chin is tucked into her chest, so that the presenting part is the crown. This is the narrowest part; the soft, cartilaginous skull bones can be shaped and moved by the birth canal for a smooth exit.

OCCIPUT POSTERIOR
If your baby is occiput posterior, she is facing your front. This is not as efficient as an anterior lie, because the head is less well flexed. The narrowest part is not the first to emerge, and the uterus has a harder job of pushing the baby out. For this reason, labour may take longer. Your baby's spine may press against yours; there is more chance of backache during and between contractions. Strong pressure on your back may help to relieve the pain.

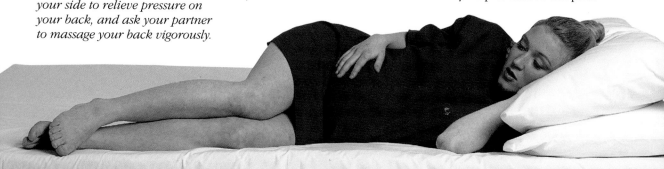

Most posterior babies turn around at the end of the first stage for the descent down the birth canal; if your baby does not turn, the second stage of labour may be long, and the baby may need forceps or a caesarean section to help her emerge.

BREECH

Most breech babies lie bottom down, some with their legs flexed and tucked in (a complete breech), some with their legs pointing straight up (a frank or extended breech). During labour, one leg may drop down, so that the foot becomes the presenting part (a footling breech). A properly managed breech birth can have an excellent outcome, especially if you arrange delivery by someone who has confidence in, and experience with, vaginal delivery for breech babies. There are, however, a couple of potential problems for the baby.

A small risk exists that the umbilical cord will drop into the birth canal and become trapped. Your practitioner will watch out for this. It is also possible that the baby's bottom will not dilate the birth canal enough for the head to pass through easily as there is no time for moulding to occur. For this reason, most breech babies delivered vaginally are those where the doctor or midwife knows – through X-ray – that the mother's pelvis is adequate. If the baby is premature, her head will be especially delicate. Many doctors advise a caesarean if you go into premature labour with a breech baby.

Most women opt for an

In a breech presentation, it is important that the head is born in a controlled, gentle way (rather than shooting out in the wake of the legs and trunk). Your helpers will assist you in choosing a comfortable position that minimizes this possibility.

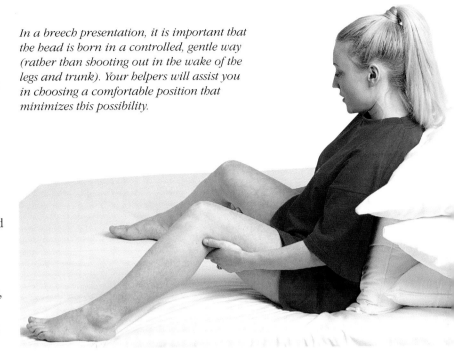

epidural if their baby is breech; otherwise, a local anaesthetic may be needed to relieve pain in the vagina once the baby's bottom begins to distend the perineum. An episiotomy may be necessary, and forceps may be used to help the head out.

About 60 percent of breech babies are delivered by caesarian.

BROW PRESENTATION

The baby is head down in a brow presentation, but the head is tilted backwards and the forehead is the presenting part. Since the brow is wider than the crown, labour may not progress and you may need a caesarean. Sometimes, however, babies who present the brow at the start of labour manage to flex the head into a face presentation as labour progresses, and a vaginal delivery is possible.

FACE PRESENTATION

This happens when the head is tilted even further back. As the face is not much larger in diameter than

the crown, labour should progress normally. In rare cases, forceps or a caesarean may be needed.

OBLIQUE OR TRANSVERSE LIE

A few babies lie diagonally (oblique), so that a shoulder is the presenting part, or widthwise (transverse) across the uterus. These positions are more likely if the baby is small and has more room in which to move around at the end of pregnancy. They may also occur if a woman has had several children already and her uterus is unusually stretchy (allowing the baby to move more freely), or if the placenta is low-lying. These positions also occur in twin deliveries.

In a single pregnancy, an oblique- or transverse-lying baby will be delivered by caesarean. If the baby is the second twin, the doctor will try to turn her either before labour begins or after the birth of the first baby so that she, too, can be delivered vaginally.

INDUCTION

If labour has not started naturally by the 41st or 42nd week, your doctor may suggest induction. If it progresses slowly, augmentation may be suggested.

Most labours start naturally at term (after 37 weeks) and progress over a period of hours to the delivery of the baby. In some cases, though, this doesn't happen. Labour may not start when you expect, or there may be sound medical reasons for delivering the baby sooner rather than later. Alternatively, labour that has started naturally may be slow. It may even seem to stop. Contractions may cease, or they may continue without being strong enough to do the work of opening the cervix and pushing the baby out.

You can sometimes jump-start a slow labour by walking around or changing your position. Be patient and don't lose heart. If you become tired, or if your baby shows signs of not dealing with the stress of labour, you may be asked to consider accelerating or augmenting your labour. If labour shows no sign of starting within 12 hours after your membranes rupture, your doctor may suggest induction.

WHAT IS INVOLVED?

Induction or acceleration can be done in one of three ways: by introducing into the vagina prostaglandins, hormone-like substances that soften and "ripen" the cervix and may induce labour

A Case in Point
Choosing Induction

CLARE, 30, FOUND HER MANAGED INDUCTION A REWARDING EXPERIENCE.

"Our first baby was born a month premature and showed signs of foetal distress during the birth. I waited too long to be given a painkilling injection, and there was no time for an epidural. Fortunately, it took some time for them to locate an anaesthetist for an emergency caesarean, and I progressed to the point that Louise arrived with the help of forceps. The birth I had wanted was not the birth I got: it was long and painful. Our anxiety over how Louise was faring overshadowed her actual arrival, and she spent a month in the hospital awaiting surgery for a heart problem (which had caused the distress). We finally took her home when she was 10 weeks old, after which she thrived. But I couldn't summon up a single positive thought about her birth.

"When I was pregnant with Nicola, we were monitored carefully. Because she seemed rather large, and I am not a large woman, my doctor suggested a managed induction. I wasn't sure, but the thought of trying to deliver a baby who was much larger than Louise frankly frightened me. My husband and I talked it over and we agreed. We chose the day ourselves and discussed in advance the possibility of my having an epidural, since the induced contractions would come fast. The first stage was fine; I walked around until the doctor decided that the suppositories hadn't worked as well as he would have liked. He wanted to rupture the membranes. At that point they set up the epidural.

"An hour later I was ready to push, and the epidural was wearing off – not enough to allow me to be upright but enough to let me feel when to push. Nicola was

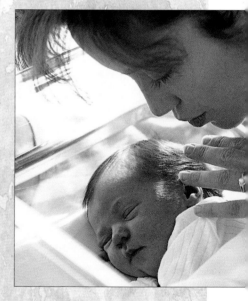

born 15 minutes later, just four hours after we had checked into the hospital.

"Because it wasn't painful, and we felt in control, in spite of all the medical intervention, I have only positive thoughts about Nicola's birth. Induction isn't ideal, but for me it was so much better than I could have hoped, and so much more fulfilling for me than Louise's 'natural' birth."

by stimulating the uterus to contract; by ARM (artificial rupture of the membranes); or by means of a hormone drip. Usually these methods are tried progressively; that is, if prostaglandins alone do not induce strong enough contractions, ARM may be attempted; if labour is still not progressing, a drip will be set up.

Prostaglandins provide the least invasive method. One dose or more is inserted into the vagina. The prostaglandins are contained in a gel that is placed in the vagina or, more rarely, inserted into the cervical canal. The prostaglandins do not enter the amniotic sac, which contains the baby.

If the hormones are not effective, contractions may be stimulated by ARM. This is commonly known as breaking the waters. The membranes are loosened slightly with the fingers (called a membrane sweep), and the sac is pierced with a small hook. The amniotic fluid then leaks out. This releases prostaglandins, which start the labour process.

The use of prostaglandins, followed by ARM, is the most common method of induction, but it can be supplemented with a hormone drip. In this method, syntocinon – a synthetic form of the hormone oxytocin, which is produced by the body throughout pregnancy, plays a role in triggering labour – enters your bloodstream directly. A catheter, attached to a drip stand with a solution of hormone in it, is inserted into a vein. The drip administers the hormone, and the dosage can be increased or reduced as necessary.

When induction is justified

The most common reason for inducing labour is that your pregnancy has continued for longer than 40 weeks. This can lead to problems of postmaturity, caused by the aging placenta's failure to nourish the baby adequately. Many doctors prefer to induce by the time the baby is 10 days overdue; some wait for two weeks. During the wait, your baby may be monitored for a short period to check that he or she is showing no signs of distress (lack of oxygen) or poor growth. The amniotic fluid level may also be assessed.

Twins are often induced after 38 weeks, because by then the babies are mature, and allowing them to continue growing in the womb may cause problems and discomfort for you. Similarly, if an ultrasound scan at 37 or 38 weeks shows that your baby is very large, you may be offered induction to avoid the necessity of a caesarean later. This is controversial, in part because estimated weights may be inaccurate.

Certain medical conditions in you or the baby may make induction advisable. Rhesus disease (see p. 24) and some heart conditions that need treatment may prompt doctors to induce labour. Induction may also be recommended if you suffer from pre-eclampsia, high blood pressure or diabetes, which could affect your health or that of your baby if the pregnancy continued (see pp. 127 and 142–43).

ARE THERE DISADVANTAGES?

Induction should be carried out only when it is medically necessary for the mother's or baby's benefit. Some risks are associated with induction: induced labour may be more painful than spontaneous labour; and induction sometimes fails, and labour ceases to progress, which can lead to a caesarean that might otherwise not have been necessary.

These risks have to be balanced against the risks of waiting for labour to start on its own. Basically, you and your doctor need to feel sure that your baby is better off out than in or, if the induction is proposed because of your health, you both need to be confident that it is necessary.

Even when it goes smoothly, induction can be uncomfortable. Induced contractions are almost always stronger and follow each other more rapidly than in spontaneous labour, and you don't have the gradual build-up that helps you become accustomed to them. Labour that has started and is then speeded up can stimulate strong contractions, too. This is, of course, the aim, but their strength can come as a shock. If you have an intravenous drip, you are less mobile than you'd probably like to be. You may also need more pain relief than you would otherwise have wanted.

The risk exists of adverse consequences for your baby, too. The baby and the hormone drip must be carefully monitored. If the contractions induced by oxytocin are stronger than is technically necessary, they may unduly reduce the oxygen supply to the baby. All contractions impede the baby's oxygen supply, but because induced contractions are rapid, there is less time for him to "recover" between them. Foetal distress occurs more frequently during this form of induction if the baby is not carefully monitored.

NATURAL PAIN RELIEF

Labour and birth involve pain, and pain-relieving drugs may have side effects; fortunately, many ways exist to control pain, with or without drugs.

You can lessen the pain of labour by preparing yourself beforehand and learning how to handle it. Many women who prefer to do without drugs (see pp. 172–73) choose to reduce pain through breathing, relaxation or the use of complementary therapies. These approaches are grouped together under the heading of "natural pain relief".

The main objective of natural pain relief is to reduce the impact and intensity of the pain (it can't completely eliminate it) while leaving you aware and able both to make decisions and to assist in the birthing process. You will experience labour and birth to the fullest, which many women find meaningful and satisfying.

Natural pain relief also speeds your recovery after the birth. Although you are certain to feel tired, your energy is likely to return sooner if you don't have the after-effects of drugs to

contend with. You will also sleep better and more naturally.

There are benefits for your baby, too. Nothing artificial reaches him. A baby born without the secondary effects of pharmacological pain relievers is more likely to be alert and responsive in the first half hour or so after birth. He breathes well, and his skin colour and skin tone are good. He can look at you with wide-open eyes, because he is not sleepy or listless. The first breast-feed goes better since the sucking and swallowing instincts are not dulled by drugs.

The following are the most commonly recommended forms of natural pain relief.

BREATHING
This is the time when the breathing exercises you can practise throughout pregnancy become useful (see pp. 56–57). As much as possible, respond to

your body's needs by altering the pattern of breathing to suit the phase and intensity of labour you are experiencing. Try level 1 breathing in early labour, when your contractions are relatively mild and short; level 2 as labour progresses; and level 3 in the final stages, when contractions are long and intense.

Focus on remaining relaxed. Don't tense your shoulders, face or hands – all common places to hold tension without realizing it. Don't breathe too hard or too fast: this may seem like a natural response to stress, but breathing out too much carbon dioxide can make you light-headed. Your partner can help you by breathing with you through a contraction.

RELAXATION
Practise relaxation techniques (see pp. 50–51) during pregnancy, so that you are able to relax quickly and recognize when and in which part of your body you are tense. Have some favourite music playing (unless it interferes with your ability to concentrate). Music that has pleasant associations – something you heard while on holiday or during a special evening out, for example – can aid your relaxation by reminding you of calmer times.

Work on these techniques in different positions – lying, sitting, squatting, standing or kneeling. If you have chosen the position in which you would like to give birth, concentrate on it, but don't neglect the others – labour is an individual event that can never be planned to the last detail.

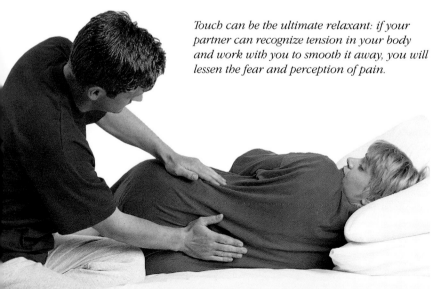

Touch can be the ultimate relaxant: if your partner can recognize tension in your body and work with you to smooth it away, you will lessen the fear and perception of pain.

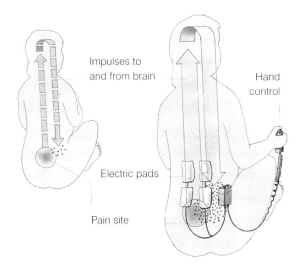

Impulses to and from brain

Electric pads

Pain site

Hand control

Pain signals are transmitted via the brain (far left). In theory, with TENS, the current sent to the brain is relayed back down a different nerve path. When this current meets the pain signal on its way to the brain (left), endorphins are released. These act in a similar way to morphine, reducing pain.

VISUALIZATION TECHNIQUES

Visualization is a form of relaxation by which you concentrate on something pleasant. One theory suggests that focusing on something that brings a sense of achievement after a period of struggle – such as running a race or climbing a mountain – encourages you to believe in your own ability to get through labour. In more general terms, the subject doesn't matter, as long as it makes you feel good, and helps you to relax.

You may also be helped by being distracted during labour – especially during late labour, when you may find it more difficult to concentrate on breathing. Counting down from 100, thinking of girls' and boys' names through the alphabet, reciting a nursery rhyme or repeating a difficult tongue twister can all be useful.

HYPNOSIS

Hypnosis and self-hypnosis have been shown to be effective at reducing pain during labour and delivery. These methods appeal to many women because they allow you to remain awake and aware without feeling pain. Hypnotherapy is not for everyone, however. Some people do not respond at all. Others respond so well that they are able to undergo caesarean sections with no anaesthetic other than hypnosis.

Self-hypnosis techniques are best learned in early pregnancy from a qualified hypnotherapist. Word-of-mouth recommendation is the best way to find a therapist. If this is not possible, make sure the practitioner you choose is a member of a recognized professional organization.

TENS

TENS stands for transcutaneous electrical nerve stimulation. It works via a small power box with electrodes which is placed on your back. By adjusting the controls on the box, you control the emission of a low-level electrical current. Two theories exist as to how TENS works. One claims that the signal travels to the brain, stimulating it to produce endorphins, the body's natural painkillers. The other supposes that nerves can carry only one signal to the brain at a time; the TENS current overloads the nerves, thereby blocking the pain signal from the uterus. The fact that you control the current gives you a sense of being "in control". TENS produces no known side-effects, but it is not usually effective against severe pain.

Ask your doctor, hospital or antenatal teacher about renting a machine – you can usually acquire one beginning at about 38 weeks – and practise using it beforehand.

PHARMACOLOGICAL PAIN RELIEF

A number of commonly used drugs can safely and effectively ease the pain of childbirth.

Despite the arguments in favour of natural childbirth (see pp. 170–71), there is no virtue in avoiding pharmacological pain relief if you feel you need it. Everyone has a different pain threshold, and what one woman will endure without much strain, another may find intolerable. In addition, every labour and delivery is different.

If you are concerned that you will not be able to manage labour, talk to your midwife about the options. This is not an admission of failure on your part – you are not in any form of competition, and if you become too tense or tearful, you may hinder the progress of your labour. Some studies show that medication for pain relief can actually speed labour and lower caesarean rates by enabling women to cope better, making "failure to progress" less likely. Everyone's wish is for you to safely deliver a healthy baby: how you achieve that is your decision.

You should be aware, however, that drugs used for the relief of pain in labour have an effect on your baby, as well as on you. This is because the drugs cross the placenta and enter your baby's bloodstream. The effect is usually short-term and, in most cases, slight. The chart at right explains what to expect from the most commonly used forms of pain relief, for you and for your baby.

What is it

Pethidine

Pethidine is a powerful, synthetic analgesic, similar to morphine. It is most effective when administered in one of two ways, either by a one-shot intramuscular injection, usually into the buttocks (this can be repeated after two to four hours), or, less commonly, through a catheter into the epidural space.

Pethidine is not usually administered until labour is well established; it takes about 20 minutes to start taking effect.

Entonox

Sometimes referred to as "gas and air", Entonox is a mixture of oxygen and nitrous oxide, which you breathe in through a face mask or mouthpiece you hold yourself.

Entonox does not take away all the pain, but it can make it easier to bear. The fact of being in control of the mask makes many women able to manage pain better. And, since it needs only about 15 seconds to start taking effect, you can breathe it in as you feel a contraction coming and stop when the contraction has peaked.

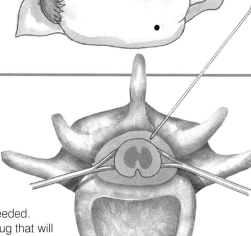

Epidural anaesthesia

This is a popular form of pain relief. An anaesthetic drug is injected into the epidural space at the side of the spinal cord. A catheter is left in at the injection site so that more anaesthetic can be given if needed. You are usually given an IV drug that will prevent your blood pressure from falling too low, then asked to lie on your side while the anaesthetist inserts the epidural.

Some doctors now administer low doses of the anaesthetic together with small doses of an analgesic. This works more quickly than anaesthesia alone and allows you to feel the urge to push and retain the ability to do so. Such so-called walking epidurals seem to combine the best of both worlds – pain relief and active participation in delivery.

Effect on you	Effect on your baby
● Pethidine may make you drowsy or "woozy" but won't normally interfere with your contractions or – later – your ability to push. ● Women react to pethidine in different ways, some finding it relaxing, others disorienting, which makes managing more difficult. ● You may experience nausea and vomiting (which can be controlled with further drugs), a feeling of depression, and/or a drop in blood pressure.	● This varies according to the strength of the dose and the timing (the nearer to the birth the dose is given, the greater will be the effect on the baby). Your doctor will keep the dose as small as possible. ● Your baby may be drowsy and have difficulty sucking. ● In rare cases, a baby may need additional oxygen for a few hours to help her to breathe.
● There are no lasting side effects on you. ● Some women find Entonox makes them feel drowsy, sick or lightheaded. However, since you control the dose yourself, it is easy to stop using it, and once you do, you soon start to feel normal again.	● Entonox has no side effects on the baby.
● A standard epidural offers total pain relief to most women (a very few experience relief on one side only). ● You will have no feeling from the waist down, which – depending on dose and timing – may make it harder for you to push in the second stage of labour. Some studies have shown that this increases the likelihood that forceps will be needed; others refute that. ● You will be numb for several hours. ● You may experience a violent headache for some days, usually the aftereffect of fluid leaking from the epidural space.	● On rare occasions an epidural can slow the baby's heartbeat, so your baby will be monitored continuously. ● Some studies have shown that babies born after an epidural are more likely to be drowsy. ● The breathing problems associated with analgesics and tranquillizers do not occur. ● The baby may require forceps or vacuum extraction for delivery.

PERCEPTIONS OF PAIN

Whether or not you want to take pain-relieving drugs, you can help yourself by being aware of and minimizing the psychological factors that make pain worse.

Choose a sympathetic but practical birth companion. You are more likely to succumb to fear or self-pity if you are on your own, or if your companion is over-anxious on your behalf. Be aware of the power of ignorance in fostering fear. Find out as much as you can about what is likely to happen and take each stage as it comes. And be positive. Every pain is doing good; it is bringing the arrival of your baby closer.

Labour is aptly named. It can be hard work. If you go into labour exhausted, you may find it more difficult, because fatigue heightens pain. Practise relaxation and breathing techniques so that you can manage contractions and conserve your energy between them.

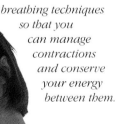

FOETAL MONITORING

By monitoring your baby electronically, your carers can be sure that he is not placed under unnecessary stress during the birth.

Q *My doctor is in favour of continuous foetal monitoring. What exactly does this involve?*

A Foetal monitoring is a way of assessing your baby's health and strength throughout labour and delivery, by checking the pattern of his heartbeat. All mothers receiving care in labour will have some form of foetal monitoring.

Some health professionals use a Pinard stethoscope; this looks like a trumpet and is placed against your abdomen to pick up the heartbeat better than the ear by itself. The Pinard is non-invasive, and it has no effect at all on the baby. It can't be used continuously. Although it doesn't pick up the heartbeat well during a strong contraction, an experienced user can learn a lot from listening through it.

There are two forms of electronic foetal monitoring. In external monitoring, a portable machine uses ultrasound to monitor the baby either intermittently or continuously. A small transmitter-receiver placed on your abdomen picks up the baby's heartbeat and measures the strength of your contractions.

Internal foetal monitoring uses a tiny electrode, clipped to the baby's scalp (or bottom, in a breech baby). This picks up the heartbeat, which is transmitted through a wire to a machine, usually positioned close to you. The machine traces the heart rate on graph paper.

Telemetry – which is not yet widely available – uses the same sort of scalp electrode, but the signal is sent via radio waves to the receiver. You are not attached to anything with this form of monitoring and are free to move around as long as you stay within range of the monitor.

Q *Is electronic foetal monitoring painful or uncomfortable?*

A No, but the fact that you cannot move around when you might want to, may be frustrating (telemetric monitors do not preclude movement). However, the insertion of the scalp electrode means your waters have to be broken artificially if they haven't already broken naturally. This can make contractions stronger earlier than they would otherwise be (see pp. 168–69).

Studies have shown that external foetal monitoring, when performed by the same midwife throughout labour, is as effective in detecting foetal distress as internal monitoring. Ask for external monitoring, but agree to internal if the doctor or midwife suspects a problem or can't hear the heartbeat well (if the baby is in an awkward position, or you are very overweight).

Q *When might continuous foetal monitoring be offered?*

A You will be monitored when you are first admitted to the hospital for about 20 to 30 minutes. Depending on the preferences of your midwife or doctor, and on whether your labour is considered high or low risk, you will be monitored continuously or at intervals of 15 to 30 minutes thereafter.

You may also be monitored during second stage labour. If monitoring is not continuous, the baby's heart will be listened to after each contraction. Some doctors believe that monitoring interferes with concentration at this stage and discontinue it.

Q *What are the advantages of electronic foetal monitoring?*

A Electronic foetal monitoring (EFM) allows continuous monitoring of the baby. This can be important if the baby is at risk, or if your doctor already knows that there could be a problem.

In the second stage of labour, when contractions come close together and you may be unsure when to push and when to conserve your strength, the monitor will signal the beginning and end of a contraction, helping you to maximize your efforts. In a longer than average second stage, EFM alerts the medical team instantly if your baby is becoming distressed so that they can take action – perhaps an assisted delivery or caesarean – immediately.

Q *How can I be sure that EFM is safe?*

A There is no evidence that EFM harms you or your baby, although – as with any invasive procedure – a theoretical risk exists with internal monitoring of introducing infection into your body. In rare cases, a baby develops a rash after the birth where the electrode has been attached to the scalp.

Q *Are there any disadvantages to EFM?*

A Opinions are divided about whether EFM is useful in low-risk labours, mainly because interpreting the reading – the machine produces a continuous printout – of the monitor requires great skill. Studies have shown that even experienced obstetricians differ about what might constitute a normal reading and what might give cause for concern. In addition, the machine can divert attention from the mother and her baby. Because the machine can also be unreliable, it can increase anxiety in the mother, her partner and those caring for her. This in turn can lead to unnecessary caesarean sections or forceps deliveries. The consensus in many hospitals is that continuous EFM is not needed for routine, normal labour, especially not in the first stage.

Q *What happens if the monitor picks up a problem?*

A There are several courses open to you and your carers. Most simply, the baby may not be getting enough oxygen because you are lying on your back, interrupting the flow across the placenta; if you move, the machine's printout may return to normal. Giving you oxygen – through a mouthpiece or mask – may also help.

The midwife will quickly review your notes to see if an underlying condition of yours may be causing the irregular reading.

If foetal distress is suspected, your doctor will check for other signs to confirm the diagnosis. These may include examining a sample of amniotic fluid for traces of meconium, or taking a sample of blood from the baby to check its pH levels. If the diagnosis of foetal acidosis is confirmed, a caesarean will be performed as soon as possible.

Q *Everything I've read about EFM inclines me to refuse it. Can I do that?*

A Yes, although it is obviously wise to take advice from the professionals looking after you. If your baby has shown signs of foetal distress, if he's known to be small, or if any other potential problem has been identified, you should consider continuous monitoring, so that any problem is spotted immediately. You still can't sidestep the issues of different interpretation, machine failure and anxiety levels, but it may be that the immediate availability of the information outweighs these other aspects.

If you and your carers expect everything to be normal, ask if you can have the less invasive forms of monitoring – intermittent monitoring with ultrasound or a Pinard stethoscope. You'll probably find your baby's heart is listened to every 15 to 20 minutes, and after most contractions during the second stage of labour. If you want to move around, ask if telemetry is available.

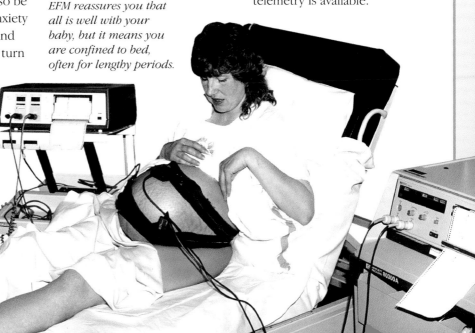

EFM reassures you that all is well with your baby, but it means you are confined to bed, often for lengthy periods.

WHEN YOU NEED A CAESAREAN

If vaginal delivery proves difficult or impossible, having a caesarean is a quick, safe way of bringing your baby into the world.

A caesarean birth means that your baby is lifted from your body after surgery involving an incision through the abdomen and into the uterus. A caesarean may be necessary if there are doubts about your ability to deliver vaginally, or about your baby's health and well-being.

Some detractors have suggested that doctors are hasty to advise women to have a caesarean because they are concerned about court action – that is, they want to be able to show that they did everything possible to avoid any labour-related birth problem. Some mothers ask for a caesarean, perhaps because they fear the pain of childbirth, or because they have had a bad experience in labour. But a caesarean, however safe, is a surgical procedure, not to be undertaken lightly. All else being equal, your body will also recover far more quickly from a vaginal birth than from a caesarean.

ELECTIVE CAESAREANS

You may know that your baby will be born by caesarean section before you go into labour. In this case, you will be given an appointment at the hospital before your expected date of delivery. Such operations are called "elective" because, on your doctor's advice, you choose to deliver by caesarean.

One reason for an elective caesarean is a diagnosis of cephalo-pelvic disproportion. Your baby is too big to fit through your pelvis, or your pelvis is of a shape that won't allow the baby to be born without distressing her or making your labour long and painful. If the baby is vertex, however, most doctors still advise attempting a vaginal delivery.

Your baby's position may make a caesarean necessary (see pp. 140–41 and 166–67). Some doctors and midwives prefer to deliver breech babies by caesarean because a vaginal birth can be problematic. With the right care and control over the delivery, however, breech babies can be born vaginally without undue risk (see pp. 166–67).

Placenta praevia is a condition in which the placenta attaches itself at the bottom of the uterus.

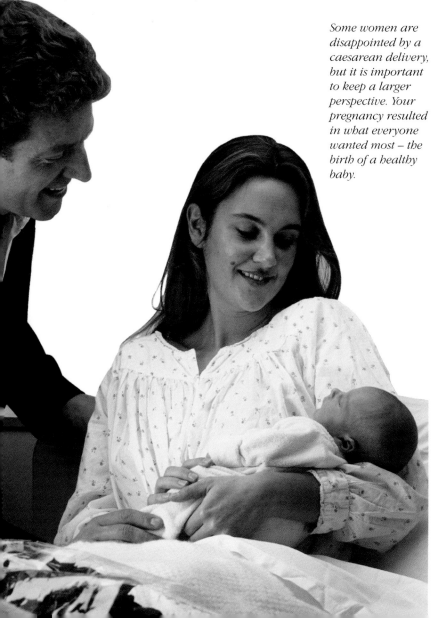

Some women are disappointed by a caesarean delivery, but it is important to keep a larger perspective. Your pregnancy resulted in what everyone wanted most – the birth of a healthy baby.

Vaginal birth after a caesarean

It was once commonly believed that a woman who had had a caesarean birth would be unable to deliver a subsequent baby vaginally. The theory was that the stress of contractions on the incision site might cause the uterus to rupture, endangering mother and baby. This argument had validity when the most common incision was made vertically down the centre of the uterus, creating the scar in the weaker part of the uterus. Today, a lateral cut is almost universal, and only the lower, stronger part of the uterus needs stitching. Although the risk of rupture during a subsequent labour is less than one percent, most doctors advise a hospital birth after one caesarean to make sure you get immediate care if there's an emergency.

A second caesarean would only be necessary if your first was caused by a problem that has not gone away or has repeated itself (which is unlikely). If, for example, you suffer from severe heart disease, most doctors would be unwilling to let you try to deliver vaginally. A diagnosis of cephalo-pelvic disproportion does not indicate that a caesarean will be necessary second time around; depending on the size of your second baby, you may try a vaginal delivery. (Studies have shown that some women who were diagnosed as suffering from cephalo-pelvic disproportion in their first pregnancy, and gave birth by caesarean, actually delivered a larger baby vaginally with their next pregnancy.)

Pre-eclampsia foetal distress, placenta praevia and an awkwardly positioned baby are caesarean situations that are unlikely to repeat themselves. With good support and back-up, you may be one of the 75 to 90 percent of women who have a successful vaginal birth after a caesarean.

This will show up on an ultrasound scan in late pregnancy (an early diagnosis may right itself as the uterus expands during the course of your pregnancy) and will make an elective caesarean inevitable to prevent hemorrhage.

Multiple births are often delivered by caesarean, especially if the first baby is in a breech or transverse position. Some problems for which a caesarean is indicated are more common in a multiple pregnancy than in women carrying only one baby. These include placental insufficiency, high blood pressure, and pre-eclampsia (see pp. 127 and 143).

AN EMERGENCY CAESAREAN

Sometimes you go into labour expecting to give birth vaginally, but circumstances change and make a caesarean necessary. Although termed an "emergency" caesarean, this operation is rarely as dramatic and last-minute as it sounds.

So-called failure to progress is a common reason for a caesarean after you have gone into labour. This means that after labouring for several hours, your cervix has not dilated very far, the baby's head is not descending, and the doctor considers a caesarean preferable to your labouring on with little result. Some doctors recommend a caesarean after 16 to 18 hours, if little is happening. Others check on how you and the baby are doing; if you are still coping and no signs of foetal distress appear, the practitioner may decide to wait or suggest accelerating your labour (see pp. 168–69).

You may find the first stage so tiring that you have little energy left to push the baby out. If she is well down the birth canal, it may be possible to deliver her using forceps. In cases in which this would be difficult, a caesarean will be recommended. Similarly, a baby who is in a less than ideal position for delivery may get stuck in the birth canal, which makes a caesarean necessary.

Another reason for an emergency caesarean is foetal distress. The printout on the foetal monitor may show that the baby is getting too little oxygen, which depresses her heart rate (see pp. 174–75). Or your midwife may notice meconium staining in the amniotic fluid. Meconium is usually passed as your baby's first bowel movement a couple of days after the birth. Passing it early may be a sign that your baby is under stress. Although this indication alone may not be significant, if your baby is showing other signs of stress as well, your doctor will opt for a caesarean delivery.

Cord prolapse happens when the membranes rupture and fluid gushes out, taking the cord with it, through the cervix and sometimes into the birth canal. As the baby descends the canal, there is a risk of her pressing on the cord, reducing or even cutting off her oxygen supply. Cord prolapse is rare but is an indication that an emergency caesarean should be performed.

A CAESAREAN BIRTH

A positive attitude towards caesarean birth – elective or emergency – can minimize many of the problems some women experience.

The surgical procedure for a caesarean is the same whether the operation is performed under a general anaesthetic or an epidural. A local anaesthetic means that you can be fully conscious throughout. You and your partner can greet your baby as soon as he is born and can spend the time while you are being stitched getting to know each other. You may, however, prefer a general anaesthetic. A general anaesthetic will also be appropriate if the baby needs to be delivered immediately and an epidural is not in place. An epidural takes about 20 minutes to start taking effect; a general anaesthetic will put you to sleep in a matter of seconds.

WHAT THE SURGEON DOES

Your lower abdomen will be shaved, and a catheter will be inserted through your urethra into the bladder to keep it drained of urine. Your abdomen will be washed with an antiseptic solution and, if you are going to be awake, a screen will be placed over your abdomen so that you do not see the cut being made. Your partner can sit by your head and shoulders and hold your hand.

Once the surgeon is satisfied that the anaesthetic has taken effect, he will make a horizontal incision along your pubic hairline (the scar will be hidden when your shaved hair regrows). The cut follows natural lines in the tissues of your abdomen, which minimizes bleeding and means less pain and faster healing. The surgeon will then cut through the lower part of your uterus; again, cutting here minimizes bleeding and the risk of scar rupture in a subsequent labour. You may be aware of the cuts being made, but they will not cause pain.

The amniotic fluid will be drained – if your membranes have not already ruptured – which you will hear as a gurgling sound.

Then the baby will be lifted out, sometimes by hand, sometimes with a pair of forceps. You may feel this as a pushing or tugging, but again it will not be painful. From the first cut to the delivery of the baby takes between 5 and 10 minutes. The baby's cord is cut and clamped, and if all is well he is given to you to hold. (Ask in advance if, should a general anaesthetic prove necessary, the baby can be given to your partner to hold.) The placenta and membranes are delivered, and then the process of stitching up takes place. The layers of uterine wall and abdominal skin are stitched one by one, so this is time-consuming; it will take about 30 minutes. The stitches used will usually be the type that dissolve so you will not have to have them removed. If they are not dissolvable, they will probably be removed before you leave hospital.

AFTER YOUR CAESAREAN

In the first few days after your caesarean section, you will feel tired – probably more tired than after a vaginal birth – and the area around your scar will be tender. You may suffer from intestinal wind, which is common after any abdominal operation. Laughing or coughing will be painful, because they pull on your abdominal muscles: you will be shown how to support your scar to avoid undue pressure. Your scar will be checked regularly to make sure that it is healing well.

You will be given painkillers to

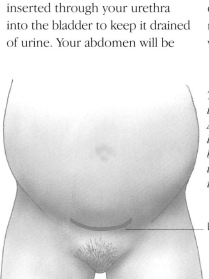

The cut in your abdomen may not be the same as the one in your uterus. Although most abdominal cuts are low and lateral, with a premature breech baby or in some cases of transverse lie (see p.167), a vertical incision may be made in the uterus.

Lateral cut

help with the discomfort. If you had an epidural, it may be left in place so that painkilling drugs can be given. If not, painkilling injections will be offered. You will have an intravenous drip in your arm for about 24 hours (or until you have recovered enough to drink as much as you want) to replace lost fluids. At first you won't be able to get up to pass urine, and you will either have a catheter in place or be helped to use a bedpan. You will, however, be encouraged to move around as much and as early as possible to help your breathing, improve healing and prevent blood clots from forming.

Breast-feeding your baby may take a little more patience than if you had had a vaginal delivery. You will need help to position your baby comfortably and to get yourself into a position that does not cause pressure or discomfort on your abdomen. Try raising your baby on a pillow across your lap or feeding him as you lie on your side (see pp. 206–207).

Once home, it is vital to get help with any heavy household tasks and to avoid lifting anything heavy. This may be a challenge if you have other children who need your attention or want cuddles. If no one is available to help you lift a toddler into a cot or highchair, consider other ways to cope for the time being. Could the child sleep on a mattress on the floor? Could you feed him or her at a low level, perhaps while you sit on a pillow on the floor? Can you hug together on the sofa?

THE EMOTIONAL IMPACT

Your physical recovery from a caesarean should cause no problems, although the scar will itch for a while: wear large pants that come up to the waist. Occasionally the surgery may trigger an infection, which can be treated with antibiotics.

Your caesarean may have a greater impact emotionally. Some women feel disappointed after a caesarean birth. If the baby is in good health, they may feel guilty about their negative reactions. People may not realize that you are concerned about the way your baby was born. But if you had looked forward to a vaginal birth, to have the baby delivered "for" you can make you feel that you have somehow missed out.

Talk about your feelings with your partner, with other mothers who have had caesarean births, and with your doctor, who can explain why the caesarean was necessary for this birth.

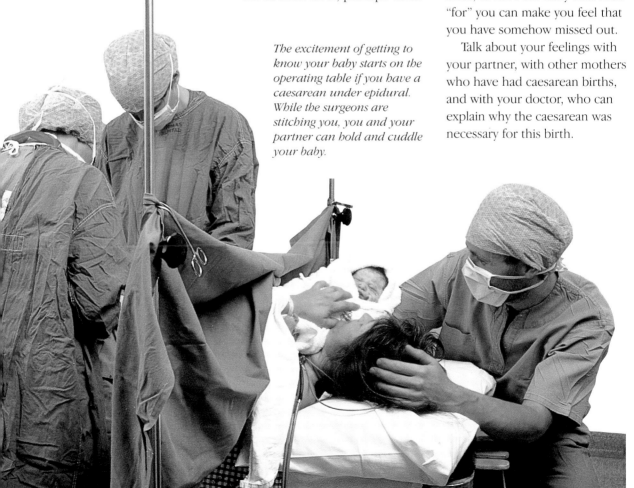

The excitement of getting to know your baby starts on the operating table if you have a caesarean under epidural. While the surgeons are stitching you, you and your partner can hold and cuddle your baby.

TRANSITION

The end of the first stage can be exhausting and emotionally draining, but transition is a labour milestone.

Most women clearly experience transition as different from the rest of the first stage. At this time, although your cervix is almost fully dilated, you may not feel the urge to push that comes with the contractions of the second stage; alternatively, you may feel an overwhelming urge to push but not be fully dilated.

Transition usually marks the last 2 to 3 cm (1 in) of dilatation and can last for as little as 15 minutes or as long as an hour. Physically, you may be too hot one minute and too cold the next. Your legs may tremble, or you may have cramps in them. A feeling of nausea is not unusual, and some women vomit. Since your baby's head is now well down, it presses on your rectum, making you feel

that you need to open your bowels. Your contractions will be strong, up to 90 seconds long, and coming every two minutes. Since they are long, intense and close together, you may be less aware of them coming, peaking and waning; they may seem to be all peak.

This intensity may affect you mentally, too. You may lose your ability to concentrate or to focus on anything at all except the next, or current, contraction. You may be impatient and tired, as well as exhilarated. It's also possible that you'll become angry, frustrated and irritable with your carers.

This is the time when some women start to have doubts about their ability to deliver their baby. Exhaustion may play a part in

these fears, but they may also be caused by the fact that transition is a psychological state as well as a physical one. You are near the end of one momentous experience – the demanding task of getting through the first stage, with increasingly strong contractions – and at the brink of another – the long-awaited arrival of your baby.

WHAT YOU CAN DO
Trust what is happening to your body and don't try to fight it. Take each contraction as it comes, rather than trying to think about how many more there might be.

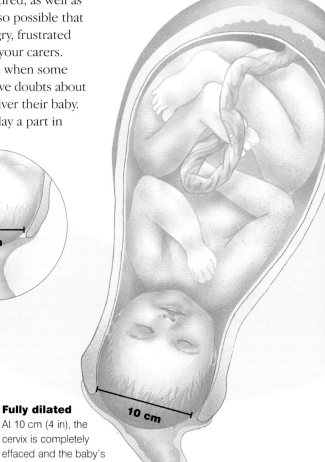

The first stage ends

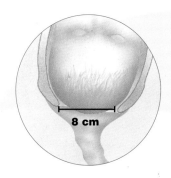

8 cm

8 cm dilatation
At 8 cm (3 in), a doctor or midwife will be able to feel a slight lip of cervix on each side of the baby's head.

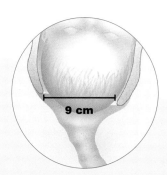

9 cm

9 cm dilatation
At 9 cm (3½ in), contractions will be coming very fast as the pressure of the baby's head works to complete dilatation.

10 cm

Fully dilated
At 10 cm (4 in), the cervix is completely effaced and the baby's head fits through.

A Case in Point
The Experience of Transition

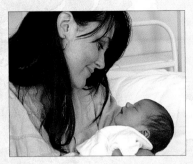

JILL, 35, WAS OVERWHELMED BY THE INTENSITY WHEN THE FIRST STAGE OF HER LABOUR ENDED.

"Transition was the time I lost my cool, physically and emotionally. My labour was induced because I'd reached 42 weeks. My waters were broken and a drip set up at about 3 P.M. The contractions then started to come close together, but I had had a painkilling injection, which took the edge off them. I could cope. I was kneeling, hanging onto Steve, who seemed to know what to do, one minute rubbing my back, the next wiping my forehead, sometimes talking, and at others just letting me get on with it.

"After about two hours of this intense labouring, I suddenly felt so hot I could hardly breathe. I had one of Steve's old shirts on and I had to take it off, but because of the drip I couldn't. I remember screaming at the midwife to cut it off me because I couldn't bear it another minute. It only took seconds for them to unhook the drip, but I shouted at Steve to rip the shirt off me if they couldn't get some scissors.

"Then I burst into tears and pushed him away, saying that I didn't want a baby and how could he have done this to me. I don't know how long I knelt there sobbing, but I remember trying to work out how I could get home. Then suddenly I had to push. The urge was overwhelming. The midwife said she wasn't sure – she had only checked me 10 minutes before when I was at 8 cm [3 in]. I swore at her and told her to check again. She said I was right; I was fully dilated. I calmed down and started to push. Ben was born at 5.59 P.M.

"The midwife came to see me the next day to check that we were okay. She seemed very young. I started to apologize for shouting and swearing at her, but she said I had done very well and that lots of women experienced very extreme emotions at that stage. It was odd because all the books seemed to make light of it, as just the end of the first stage, a time to get through. But for me it had a clear beginning and end. It was a definite phase in its own right."

If you can, relax between contractions and maintain your breathing pattern through them.

Find a position in which you are comfortable. Many women find that kneeling down with their head and arms on a pile of pillows helps them to conserve their strength. Above all, hang on. You are nearly there.

WHEN YOU CAN'T PUSH
The cervix sometimes dilates unevenly. As the midwife checks your progress, she will be able to feel a portion of undilated cervix between the baby's head and your pubic bone. Pushing against this "anterior lip" is ineffective, wastes your energy and can bruise the cervix, which will delay the birth. You may feel you need to push, but your carer tells you to hold off. Usually, another couple of contractions will be enough to complete the dilatation of the cervix. It may help you to pant, which will distract you from the urge to push and prevent you from doing so. You can also try kneeling with your head down and buttocks up. This will reduce the pressure on the lip of cervix, lessen the intensity of contractions and conserve your energy.

PARTNERS: WHAT YOU CAN DO
This is one of the most difficult stages for a birth companion, because the reactions of women to transition vary so widely, are unpredictable and can change from minute to minute. The most important thing is to be there, even if your partner pushes you away. She will want you soon. Take any insults or abuse without complaint. If she wants you close, hold her, to give physical support.

Remind your partner that she is in transition and that it will pass, probably quite quickly. Praise her for how far she has come, and offer lots of extra loving words of encouragement. If she is shivering, warm her feet and legs; if she is too hot, wipe her forehead with a cool sponge, or give her crushed ice to suck.

THE SECOND STAGE

Most women find the second stage of labour easier to handle than the first, since they can exert more control over what is happening.

Once your cervix is fully dilated, your baby's head can start to descend through the birth canal. This marks the beginning of the second stage of labour; it will end with the birth of your baby.

If you haven't had an epidural, you will know you have reached the second stage by the feeling that you want to bear down and push. If you have had an epidural, depending on the dose and timing, you may not feel the urge to push and will only know you are fully dilated when your midwife tells you. She will also tell you when to push; alternatively, you or your partner can feel contractions by placing a hand on your abdomen, or by watching the printout from a foetal monitor (if you are being monitored electronically).

WHAT IS HAPPENING TO YOUR BODY

At the start of the second stage, your baby's head may be visible during a contraction. Each contraction, and each push, helps it to move farther down the vagina. At first it disappears when the contraction ends, pushed back by the resistance of the pelvic-floor muscles. But progress has been made. The head doesn't go back as far as it has dropped. After a few more contractions, the resistance is overcome and the head does not recede again. It moves farther down with each contraction. When the top of the

Descending the birth canal

Once the cervix is fully dilated and effaced, the only resistance to your baby's birth comes from the muscles of your pelvic floor and vagina. Gradually, the contractions of the uterus and the pressure of the baby's head overcome this resistance.

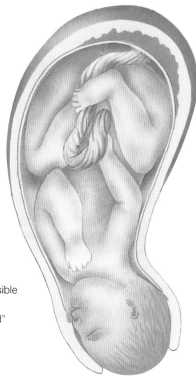

Crowning
As the top of the head becomes visible to your midwife, it appears "crowned" by the vulva.

head becomes completely visible at the vulva, the head is said to be "crowning".

The contractions of the second stage are different from those of the first stage. Part of the contraction is an urge to bear down, or push. Although second-stage contractions are painful (unless you have had an epidural), many women find them easier to manage than those of the first stage. To begin with, you can actually do something during them. And although they may still last up to 90 seconds, the intervals between them may be longer than those of the first stage, giving you more chance to rest.

The baby's head will press against the back of your pelvis and on your bowel, which you may feel as an urge to defecate. Some women worry so much

that they will actually excrete some faeces, their ability to push is impeded. It is normal to evacuate anything in your rectum or bladder; the medical staff will not be bothered by this and neither should you be. As the head descends the birth canal and this pressure diminishes, you will feel pressure instead on your pelvic floor and on the perineum and vulva as they stretch.

As the perineum stretches, you may want to watch in a mirror for your first sight of your baby's head; if you don't, your partner can perhaps tell you if he can see much of the baby's hair and what colour it appears to be.

You may be conscious of a burning sensation as the skin of your perineum is stretched thin. Your midwife will ask you not to push, if she thinks you risk

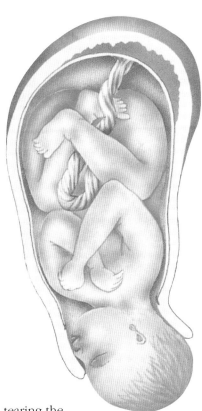

The head emerging
The tissues of the perineum are stretched to the utmost as the head continues its exit.

Birth
In a couple more contractions your baby's face is fully visible.

tearing the perineum. She will suggest that you breathe deeply, pant or push more gently. A warm compress held against the perineum will encourage the tissues to expand and may help you to avoid a tear. But if your midwife feels you are going to tear, you will be given an episiotomy (see pp. 186–87).

With the next contraction or two, your baby's head glides out (see pp. 190–91).

WHAT HAPPENS TO YOUR BABY

Your baby will be monitored throughout the second stage, although you may not be aware of this happening. Your energies and your concentration will be focused on pushing.

By the start of the second stage, the baby's head usually turns so that her crown is towards your front, allowing the widest part to fit through your pelvis. The head and neck extend around the pubic bone, and the head crowns.

The baby's head is compressed by her descent down the birth canal; the edges of her soft cartilaginous skull bones slide under and over each other to ease the journey. This process is called moulding, and it can make your baby's head look a little misshapen for a few days after the birth. If she has a tight fit through the birth canal, she may have a few tiny broken blood vessels.

None of us consciously remembers our journey into the world, but the reactions of some babies in the first few hours after birth indicate that some of them may find it frightening. Your loving hands and warm body will soon take away any fear.

How long does the second stage last?

With a first baby, the second stage of labour usually lasts about an hour. It is possible, however, for it to be over in a few contractions, each lasting a minute and with less than a minute between them. Second and subsequent babies may come after just one or two pushes in a single contraction.

A prolonged second stage – lasting more than two hours – is exhausting for you and may mean undue stress for the baby as you bear down. If your baby is still doing well, and you are coping and making clear – if slow – progress, your caregivers may allow you to continue. But if you are tired or the baby is showing signs of stress, your doctor may consider helping her out with forceps, vacuum extraction (see pp. 188–89) or even a caesarean (see pp. 176–79).

WHAT YOU CAN DO

Pushing your baby out is hard work, but most women are invigorated in the second stage of labour and want to help their baby into the world.

After a lengthy first stage and the unpredictable demands of transition, the second stage is time for working with your partner. It is rare for a second stage, even in a first labour, to last longer than two hours, and most couples' perception is that it passes quite quickly.

Get into a comfortable position in which you can bear down easily and effectively, and in which your pelvis can open to allow the baby's exit. Gravity will help you, but if you are too tired to squat

or semi-squat, try something else. There will probably be intervals between contractions, but you will need to conserve your energy rather than using it to shift position, unless you find that you are uncomfortable.

To make the most of every push, push only during a contraction. Breathe deeply as the contraction is building, then as it reaches a peak, push for about five seconds, or until you want to take a breath. Prolonged breath-holding can affect your

baby's oxygen supply and exhaust you unnecessarily, so hold your breath only as long as you are comfortable, then let it out. If the contraction is still peaking, take a few more deep breaths, then push again. The more you put into each push, the sooner you will see your baby.

You'll be guided about when and how long to push, but listen to your body and respond to your needs. You will probably feel the need to push three to five times in each contraction. Do it calmly and imagine your baby coming nearer and nearer each time you bear down.

The best position lets you feel comfortable between contractions, makes it easy to move your pelvis, and allows your midwife to see what's going on and to be able to reach the baby with her hands. You will need a clean, comfortable floor covering if you don't deliver on the bed. Mats with clean sheets over them are fine.

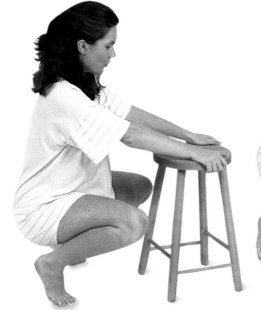

Squatting
If you can squat comfortably, this position allows your pelvis to open wide and your baby to be born with the help of gravity. Squatting can be difficult, if you are not used to it, and it is well worth practising it during pregnancy. You may need support for your upper body to help you keep your balance when you squat.

Supported squat
A chair makes a good support for squatting. Alternatively, your partner can support you from behind by holding you under your arms, although he will need to be strong enough to take all your weight as you bear down.

PARTNERS: WHAT YOU CAN DO

Your partner may need your physical support – to maintain a comfortable pushing position, for example – and she will certainly need your emotional support.

Tell her how well she is doing; encourage her to push when your midwife advises it (but if there are too many cheerleaders, talk to her quietly); let her squeeze your hand; give her crushed ice to suck; massage her back; tell her when you can see the baby's head.

Your other options

If none of the positions illustrated feels right to you, you have several other choices.

Sitting
This works against gravity and causes some compression of the pelvis, but it allows you to relax between contractions. You need plenty of pillows to support your back and shoulders.

Kneeling
Have a supporter on each side to help you keep your balance. This is a good position for keeping your pelvis open and helping the baby out.

Lithotomy
Traditionally, in the West, mothers have been asked to lie on their backs with their legs up in the air, their ankles supported by stirrups. For a normal delivery, this is uncomfortable, it makes you feel out of control, and it compresses some of the larger blood vessels, restricting circulation.

Birthing stool or chair
You may be offered – or could ask for – a birthing stool or a birth chair to support you in a semi-squatting position. You may need support for your back if you are on a stool.

All-fours
Some women find kneeling on all fours very comfortable. This position also allows a good view of the perineum and emerging baby for your midwife.

Head down
This position has all the advantages of being on all fours, and also allows you to rest in between contractions. It also reduces pressure on the perineum and may help you to avoid tearing or an episiotomy. It can be difficult, however, to bear down effectively if your head is low, so it is best kept for intervals between contractions.

Standing
You may be too exhausted to stand alone, and if you have had an epidural you are unlikely to be able to do so, but being upright allows gravity to help the baby out. Have a chair or stool to support you. You could also adopt this position to give your partner a break from supporting you in a semi-squat.

EPISIOTOMY

Many women tear a little during delivery, but if your doctor or midwife thinks that you risk a severe tear, he or she may suggest an episiotomy.

Q *What exactly is an episiotomy?*

A It's a cut made in the perineum, the area between the vagina and the anus, extending through the underlying muscles into the vagina. It makes the exit point wider for the baby, and allows the head to be born more quickly and easily. If necessary, it will be done when the baby's head is crowning.

Two types of incision are common: the first, called the midline, runs directly back towards the anus. The second, a mediolateral cut, starts like the midline cut, then goes to one side to avoid the anus.

Q *Why do some women need an episiotomy when others do not?*

A Sometimes it depends on what your professional carer's usual practice is. Surveys have shown that some professionals use episiotomy more than others. The clinical justification is twofold: to prevent a ragged, possibly deep and long tear in the perineum and vagina (which could be complicated to stitch up and difficult to heal), and to ease the delivery of the baby's head. If forceps are necessary (see pp. 188–89), you may need an episiotomy first.

Q *Is an episiotomy always better than a tear?*

A Research shows that small tears – that is, tears that do not involve several layers of muscle – heal more quickly and with fewer problems than episiotomies.

Larger, ragged tears, however, are more difficult to stitch well and may cause more problems than a neat cut that can be stitched easily.

Q *It sounds painful. Does an episiotomy hurt?*

A No. You will be given an injection of local anaesthetic before the cut is made.

If the episiotomy is done because it is necessary to use forceps to ease your baby out, and you have not been given an epidural, you will also be given a local anaesthetic.

The midline cut extends directly towards the anus; the mediolateral cut is made to one side to avoid the anus.

Q *Is stitching afterwards painful? My skin won't be stretched then, will it?*

A Stitching up, or suturing, is done after the third stage, the delivery of the placenta, and it can be painful. You will be given an injection of local anaesthetic that should deal with this. If the anaesthetic doesn't deaden all the pain, ask for another dose.

Stitching can take a long time since the doctor has to stitch through the vaginal skin, then muscle, then the external skin of the perineum, layer by layer. Your legs are likely to be in stirrups while this is being done so that the doctor has a good view of what he or she is doing.

Try to relax your head and shoulders – pillows will help here. Obviously, it helps if you and your partner can hold and cuddle your baby while this is happening, since the euphoria of greeting the new arrival and having a good look at him are likely to divert your attention from any discomfort.

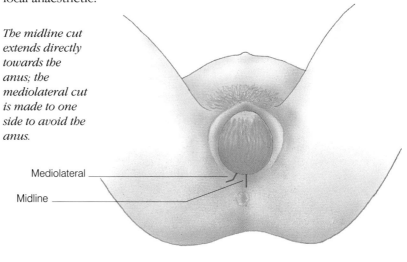

Mediolateral

Midline

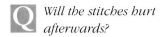 *Will the stitches hurt afterwards?*

 Yes. At best they will be uncomfortable; at worst, painful, particularly for the first week or so. You can ask for painkillers (although traces will get into your breast milk and may make your baby drowsy). If you are especially sore, ask for the scar to be checked. A stitch may have a knot in it that hurts you, or you may have been stitched too tightly. The knot can be snipped off, or you can be restitched. You may find that your stitches ache when you are tired, so try to rest.

An ice pack may help relieve discomfort: wrap a bag of frozen vegetables in a cloth and apply this to the stitches. The hospital may also suggest a foaming cream that should ease discomfort. And lavender essential oil (add 10 drops to your bath) is reputed to heal stitched and bruised tissue. You could also try salt baths or arnica tablets.

Sitting down is usually a little uncomfortable at first, although once you're actually seated you should be fine: sit squarely to avoid pulling on the stitches. Get in and out of chairs slowly and carefully.

Many women worry that they will burst their stitches when they move their bowels. You won't, but it makes sense to try to avoid constipation by drinking plenty of fluids and eating fibre-rich foods. If you are concerned, lubricate the anus with vegetable oil before a bowel movement.

Pelvic-floor exercises (see pp. 44–45) will improve the blood flow to the perineum, which will promote healing. And if you find it uncomfortable to dry the area with a towel, use a hairdryer on a warm setting (this can also be very soothing).

After four or five weeks, everything should be back to normal.

Q *Are there any long-term effects?*

A Most episiotomies heal without a problem. The stitches dissolve and don't need to be taken out. The skin knits together, leaving you just the same as you were before (although even after a year or so you will be able to see a faint scar if you really look for it).

In a few cases, however, mothers do suffer from after-effects, usually due to infection or poor suturing. Very rarely, a stitch may become infected, and this can be painful. Poor suturing can mean you are sewn up so tight that the healing process leaves your perineum and your vagina much less elastic than they should be. Sexual intercourse can be uncomfortable or even impossible. You should seek help if this happens to you; you may need to be recut and restitched (under local anaesthetic).

Occasionally, the fact that an episiotomy was performed becomes a focus for any negative feelings about the whole birth experience. If you find this is happening, talk to your doctor; he or she may recommend counselling.

Q *Will I need an episiotomy next time, if I have one this time around?*

A You may, as the skin of the perineum doesn't stretch as well where there is scar tissue. If you have had an episiotomy before, your carers may be more likely to perform an episiotomy to avoid tearing.

Q *I really don't want an episiotomy. Can I avoid it?*

A Tell the people looking after you that you'd prefer to avoid one, and put it in your birth plan. Skilled and careful professionals can try to control the delivery of the head. They will give you guidance on when not to push, which will prevent the head from being born too fast.

You can massage the perineum throughout pregnancy to keep it supple and stretchy, and better able to give with the pressure of your baby's head, without tearing or making your midwife think it is going to tear. Squat, lubricate one or two fingers with a vegetable oil, and insert them into your vagina, then press down on your perineum. Some experts recommend doing this daily from about six months on, gradually increasing both the downward pressure and the number of fingers. You can also increase the elasticity of the perineum by inserting both index fingers and gently stretching.

Giving birth in an upright or semi-upright position also helps by putting less pressure on the perineum. If you squat, the muscles of the perineum relax, making a cut or tear less likely.

ASSISTED DELIVERY

Sometimes a little extra assistance is needed at the time of delivery. About one in five babies is born with the judicious use of forceps or vacuum extraction.

Some babies, and their mothers, do not handle the second stage of labour well. In several situations, a little help may be a good idea. These cases fall into one of two categories: the birth seems to go on too long for you to deal with; or your baby is showing signs of distress.

If the situation is not so threatening that it necessitates an emergency caesarean (see p. 177) and the baby's head is well engaged, your doctor or midwife may decide to use forceps or vacuum extraction to speed the birth.

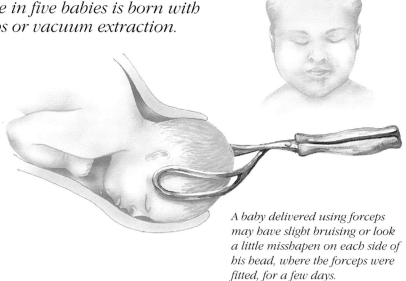

A baby delivered using forceps may have slight bruising or look a little misshapen on each side of his head, where the forceps were fitted, for a few days.

WHEN HELP IS NEEDED

One of the most common reasons for an assisted delivery is foetal distress, which occurs when the baby is short of oxygen. A diagnosis of foetal distress is made when the baby's heart rate slows in response to contractions but does not speed up again as it should. Another sign is that the baby opens his bowels and passes meconium (the contents of his rectum), which will stain the amniotic fluid a greenish colour. Blood oxygen levels from the baby's scalp can also be evaluated to help in the diagnosis.

Foetal distress may be caused by a poorly functioning placenta; a long, tiring labour; contractions that are too strong or too frequent; or prolapse of the umbilical cord, which can be compressed by the baby's

body, thus preventing sufficient oxygen from reaching him.

The baby's exit may be obstructed or hampered because he is in a poor position, such as face-up (occiput posterior), or because his mother's pelvis isn't able to open wide enough. Most doctors choose to use forceps to cradle the head of a breech baby during delivery.

Sometimes the contractions of the second stage are simply not strong enough to help push the baby out. The midwife may try an oxytocin drip to increase the strength of the contractions, but if this does not help, he or she will probably suggest using forceps or vacuum extraction. In another case, the mother may be too exhausted to help the contractions along by pushing when they are strong. The use of forceps is fairly common in women who have had an epidural. If the anaesthetic has

not worn off and the mother cannot feel the contractions, she may find it difficult to coordinate her pushing with them.

Finally, if the mother has a health problem, such as high blood pressure or a heart disorder, prolonged pushing may exacerbate the problem, and her doctor is likely to suggest help.

HOW HELP IS GIVEN

If you need an assisted delivery, you will be given an anaesthetic. If you have an epidural already in place, more anaesthetic will be administered; otherwise, a local anaesthetic will be administered in the perineum. Your bladder may be emptied with a catheter. You will probably need an episiotomy (see pp. 186–87) to allow room for the instrument to be inserted. You will lie down on your back, and your legs will be raised, with the ankles supported in stirrups, so that you are in the lithotomy position (see pp. 184–85): this may make you feel a little exposed, but it helps the doctor to see what he or she is doing.

There are different styles of forceps, but all are made of two separate halves that lock onto each other. Each half has a handle at one end and a scoop-like blade at the other. The doctor's choice of forceps may depend on whether the baby needs to be turned before being lifted out or simply has to be helped out. The forceps are inserted into the birth canal one blade at a time. Each blade goes around the baby's head, cupping it at each side and the handles lock together.

As you feel each contraction coming, you will be told to push, just as you were doing before, while the doctor will gently ease the baby towards delivery (there is no tugging or pulling involved). This part of the process usually takes just two or three contractions. You may be able to see your baby being born if you are slightly propped up. (There is no need for your partner to leave,

unless he wants to; if he would rather not watch, he can sit by your head.)

Vacuum extraction can also be used to turn and deliver the baby. The instrument, known as a ventouse, has a tube with a cup at one end. The other end is attached to a vacuum bottle and then to a small pump. The cup is applied to the baby's head, and the pump creates negative pressure that fixes it there. As the mother pushes with each contraction, the doctor helps with gentle traction on the cup. Again, the baby is usually born within two or three contractions. An episiotomy may not be necessary with vacuum extraction.

ASSISTED DELIVERY FOR YOUR BABY

Your baby will be able to feel the blades of the forceps or the vacuum cup on his head during the delivery and may be aware that force is being applied during contractions. Contractions are likely to last about a minute, but pressure will be exerted only while you are actively pushing.

Most babies delivered by forceps or vacuum extraction are fine. The few who need some time in special care immediately after birth usually do so as a result of the situation that led to the assisted delivery, such as foetal distress, rather than because of the style of delivery itself.

AFTER AN ASSISTED DELIVERY

You are likely to feel sore and bruised after an assisted delivery. If you have had stitches, follow the advice on pages 186–87. Some women feel a sense of disappointment that the birth of their baby was achieved in this way, but most accept that their baby's safe delivery was more important than the manner of that delivery. If you do experience any negative feelings, it may help to talk them over with the doctor who delivered the baby or with a professional counsellor.

If you have had an assisted delivery, it does not mean that you will need similar help during a second delivery. Your labour will probably be quicker next time, you may be less fatigued, and your baby may not become distressed. If delivery by forceps occurred because the baby was in an awkward position, a second baby may not assume a similar position. Even if he does, your contractions may be strong enough to help him out.

If you are anxious to avoid a second assisted delivery, you may want to avoid an epidural (or ask if you can have a so-called walking epidural – see pp. 172–73). It may help if you remain as upright as you can throughout the second stage of labour.

A baby delivered by vacuum extraction may have a swelling and bruise (sometimes called a caput) on the top of his head; this will disappear over the first few days following delivery.

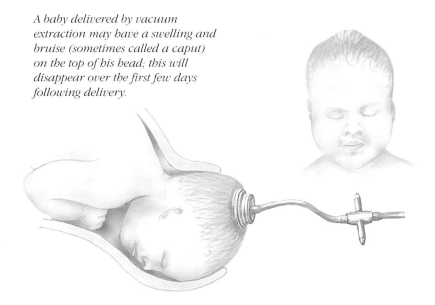

YOUR BABY IS BORN

From the crowning of the head to the delivery of the baby takes only a few minutes, but you will remember every second.

The hard work of labour is over. While your baby is being delivered, your uterus will continue to contract, and you will be asked to carry on pushing, usually more gently than before. You may be asked to pant to slow down the baby's exit, if your midwife thinks you risk tearing. You will almost certainly be less aware of pain or discomfort than at any time since you went into labour. But these last few minutes can seem to take a long time as your impatience to see your baby and finally hold her in your arms reaches a peak.

WHAT THE BABY DOES

During the second stage of labour, your baby's head turns 90 degrees, from a position where she's facing to one side to one where the back of her head moves towards your front. At the same time, she flexes her head, tucking her chin in towards her chest. As the head crowns (see pp. 182–83), a further contraction completes this turning process. Then, as the the baby continues her journey, her head follows the steep curve of the vagina towards the exit. To make this easy and smooth, the muscles at the back of the baby's neck begin to extend, lifting the head up slightly with the next contraction or two.

Your baby's head emerges face down. At the same time, her shoulders rotate so her body is sideways: one shoulder towards your front, the other towards your back. This position allows the shoulder towards your front to be delivered first, followed by the other one. While the shoulders are turning, the head – now able to move freely – turns once again to the side, so that it is in line with the shoulders. This movement is called external rotation and restitution, because it restores the head to the position it had at the start of the second stage.

After the shoulders, the rest of the baby's body slides out smoothly and easily, still attached to the placenta (yet to be delivered) by the umbilical cord.

PARTNERS: WHAT YOU CAN DO

Make sure your partner can see the head as it emerges, if she wants to. Prop her up, or adjust the angle of the bed, if necessary. She may also like to feel the top of the baby's head, so guide her hand. (This will also reassure her that she is making progress.)

Note the time. Once the baby is born, give her to the mother to hold and cuddle while you help her get into a comfortable position for feeding. You may want to take some photographs

Throughout labour your baby has moved her head and body to ease her passage. Now, the turning of her head to help the birth of her body is spontaneous.

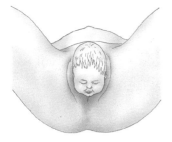

Whether you are lying upright, on your back, or on all fours, your baby's head is likely to emerge facing your back. Once the head has crowned, the rim of the vulva comes down first over the brow, then over the whole face.

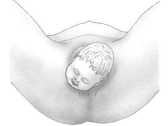

Once the head is out, the cord will be checked and, if it is around the neck, it will be looped over the head. The baby then turns her head about 45 degrees so that it is in line with her shoulders.

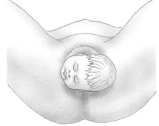

There may be a pause before contractions start again. When they do, the baby's shoulders descend to the vulva. Her whole body eases around so that her head and shoulders are at right angles to your body, and she is born sideways.

Starting to breathe

Your baby may begin to breathe through her mouth even before her shoulders and body are born; alternatively, her whole body may emerge before she draws her first breath. Most babies take their first breath two to three minutes after their mouths emerge through the vulva.

Your baby may gasp, splutter or even give a cry as the first rush of air enters her lungs. Don't worry if you do not hear a cry: some babies start to breathe without making a sound.

No one knows exactly what makes a baby draw her first breath, but the temperature of the air and the change in pressure she experiences once outside your body may be trigger factors. With her first breath, your baby's chest expands and draws air into the lungs. Until now, they have been in a collapsed state, rather like deflated balloons. The sudden expansion of the lungs causes a rush of blood to them, and the oxygen that has been inhaled is quickly absorbed into the baby's bloodstream. When this happens, the baby's circulation undergoes a dramatic change as it switches from receiving oxygen from the placenta to receiving oxygen through the lungs. The increased pressure of the sudden rush of blood sends blood to and from the heart and lungs through the pulmonary arteries. At the same time, the arterial system that fed blood to and from the heart and the placenta shuts down. Once the cord has been cut (see pp. 192–93), the ducts in the heart, which operated while the baby received oxygen through the placenta, close in response to the changes in pressure within the chambers of the heart.

Your baby will now breathe at a rate of between 40 and 50 breaths a minute, with perhaps a few odd gasps in between as the respiratory system is established. The oxygenation of her blood is responsible for your baby's colour change; from being a purplish blue when she emerges, she will turn pinker by the second.

These blood vessels wither once the baby starts to breathe in air.

Before the birth

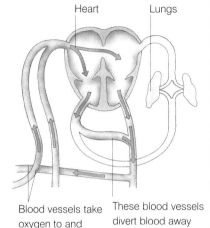

Heart   Lungs

Blood vessels take oxygen to and from the placenta.

These blood vessels divert blood away from the lungs.

After the birth

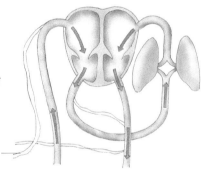

---

or video footage immediately, or you may prefer simply to hug the new mother and your baby.

Occasionally, there is a problem after the birth. Most commonly, some babies are born with too much mucus around the mouth and nose, and perhaps in the throat, to start to breathe without a little help. Usually, this can be suctioned off quickly and your baby will then take her first breath. You can watch as this happens and relay to the mother the fact that all is well. If your baby was suffering from foetal distress and the birth was accelerated through the use of forceps, or if the amniotic fluid had traces of meconium, a paediatrician will be on hand to check her over. Again, you may be better placed than the new mother to see what is happening and pass on reassurances.

WHAT YOU MAY NOTICE
If all's well with you and with your baby, she will be given to you to hold immediately. She may have vernix on her skin, and there may be a few streaks of blood on her head and body (your blood, not hers, from a tear or episiotomy). Her head may look slightly misshapen, due to the moulding of her skull (see pp. 182–83). Your baby may be alert and watchful. Your carers will be watching you and your baby quite carefully and making some initial observational checks (see pp. 202–3).

You may feel or even hear a rush of water as the hindwaters (the amniotic fluid behind your baby) leak out; these have been held back until now by your baby.

Once your baby is breathing well (see box), the umbilical cord will be clamped and cut (see pp. 192–93). There are no nerve endings in the cord, so this will not hurt your baby.

THE THIRD STAGE

With your attention fully focused on your precious baby, you may be almost unaware of the third stage of labour.

The last part of labour begins after the delivery of the baby and ends with the delivery of the placenta and membranes. It usually takes less than five minutes, but you will have to stay in the delivery room while any tears or an episiotomy are stitched.

For the overwhelming majority of women, the third stage passes totally uneventfully; in a few cases, however, a problem can arise even when everything's gone well beforehand.

WHAT HAPPENS TO YOU

In most Western hospitals, the third stage is managed – that is, medical interventions are routinely carried out with a view to speeding up the progress of this stage of labour, mainly to avoid haemorrhaging caused by a retained placenta.

When your baby is about to be born, usually when the first shoulder is emerging, you will be given an injection of oxytocin. You will get the injection in your thigh or buttock, or through the intravenous drip, if one is already set up, and you may not even notice it. When your baby has been delivered, the umbilical cord is clamped and cut. It is usual to wait until the baby is breathing well and the cord has stopped pulsating, an indication that the baby's oxygen supply is no longer dependent on the placenta. (The cord can, however, be left intact until after the delivery of the placenta.)

Oxytocin stimulates the uterus to contract strongly. The uterus becomes smaller, harder and tighter (you may feel these contractions, but you may be too

wrapped up in the baby and your partner to notice them). This results in the placenta's peeling itself off the inner wall of the uterus. The expulsive force of the contraction helps push the placenta down and out. You may be asked to give a push or two to help it along. The doctor or midwife may also speed the delivery of the placenta by a manoeuvre called controlled cord traction – that is, by pressing on the uterus with one hand while holding the cord taut in a small pair of forceps with the other.

At the same time that the placenta comes away, the blood vessels that were connected to the placenta close off under the force of the contractions. This prevents excessive bleeding.

You may feel the placenta slide down and out between your legs, followed by the membranes. They are usually delivered into a bowl so that the midwife can check that it is all there. Any

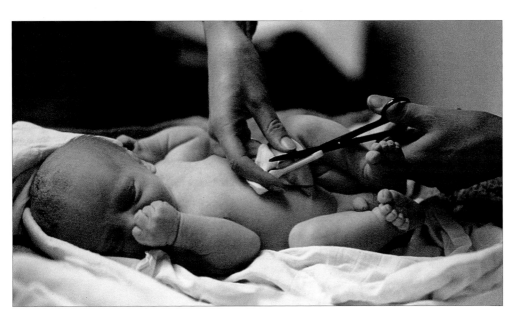

The umbilical cord is about 50 cm (20 in) long. After your baby's birth, it is clamped in two places to prevent blood loss, then cut about 25 mm (1 in) from the baby's body.

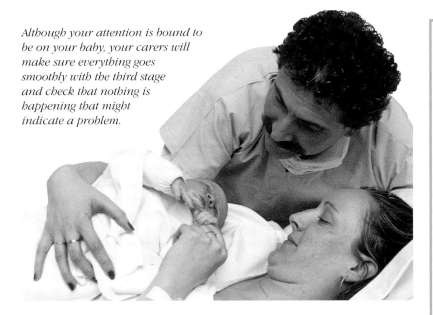

Although your attention is bound to be on your baby, your carers will make sure everything goes smoothly with the third stage and check that nothing is happening that might indicate a problem.

open or torn vessels on the placenta will indicate that a section may have been retained. It must be removed immediately. If pieces of placenta are left in the uterus, you may suffer from infection or heavy bleeding.

POSSIBLE COMPLICATIONS

The most common complications that can occur in the third stage are postpartum haemorrhage (excessive bleeding after delivery), retention of all or part of the placenta and inversion of the uterus.

Postpartum haemorrhage occurs when the amount of blood lost exceeds 500 ml (1 pint). It happens when the blood vessels torn by the separating placenta are not effectively closed off by the contracting uterus. This may happen because the placenta has not come away completely, thus preventing the uterus from contracting properly. It may also happen when the placenta has come away but the uterus has not stayed retracted – it has sprung back too far, either because muscle tone is poor

after a long delivery, or because it was excessively stretched (by more than one baby, for example).

If you haemorrhage, the doctor may try uterine massage or administer drugs to help the uterus to contract. If neither works quickly, the mother will be given intravenous fluids and drugs, but rarely a transfusion. If the condition is caused by a failure of the blood to coagulate properly, drugs to aid clotting will be administered.

Occasionally, the upper part of the uterus contracts very forcefully and retains the placenta before it has had a chance to come away properly. If this happens, the doctor will try to remove the placenta.

Inversion of the uterus occurs only when the placenta was attached at the top of the uterus; when the placenta is removed, the uterus folds back on itself. This can often be corrected manually: the doctor simply pushes the uterus back into place. In rare cases, surgery may be necessary.

A physiological third stage

Those who argue in favour of more natural childbirth claim that management of the third stage is unnecessary and that women should be allowed to deliver the placenta in their own good time, without drugs to stimulate contractions and without traction of the cord. The placenta will emerge, under the stimulus of naturally occurring uterine contractions, in about half an hour.

If the umbilical cord is not cut, it will continue to pulsate until the placenta detaches itself from the uterine wall.

Holding your baby to your breast, whether she sucks or not, releases oxytocin. This hormone naturally helps your uterus to contract, expelling the placenta and membranes. Oxytocin will also be released as you breast-feed your baby in the coming days, which will cause uterine spasms, or afterpains. The release of milk from your breasts triggers the production of more milk.

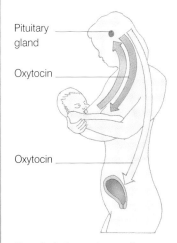

Pituitary gland

Oxytocin

Oxytocin

Your baby's rooting and sucking reflexes are strong in the first hour after birth (see p. 205). These actions stimulate your pituitary gland to produce oxytocin and prolactin (see p. 67).

BIRTHING TWINS

Many twin deliveries are uncomplicated and vaginal, but more potential complications exist in giving birth to two babies.

Twins are often born before 40 weeks. You may go into labour earlier, or your doctor may advise induction or a caesarean before 40 weeks. The average length of a non-induced twin pregnancy is 37 weeks, and about 20 percent of twin pregnancies do not reach the 36th week.

Doctors induce labour because a uterus that is overstretched may not contract efficiently. You may find your size exhausting, and you are at a greater risk of developing high blood pressure. In addition, one or both twins may be growing too slowly. Occasionally one twin takes the majority of nourishment crossing the placenta. This leaves one underweight while the other is of average size.

HOW TWINS LIE

The best presentation of twins is also the most common – in 45 percent of cases, both are head down. In 35 percent of cases, one is breech presentation; in 10 percent of cases, both are.

In 10 percent of twin pregnancies, one baby lies across the uterus, while the other is cephalic or breech. If the first baby is transverse, a caesarean is inevitable. Rarely (about one in every 1000 twin deliveries), twins can be "locked": the first baby is breech, while the other is cephalic (see pp. 166–67), and the head of the breech baby is trapped above the head of the other. In such a

One or two placentas?

Fraternal twins have a placenta each. For identical twins, if the bundle of cells splits in two soon after fertilization, each twin will have his own outer sac (chorion), inner sac (amnion) and placenta. If the cells do not separate until implantation, the babies will have their own amnion but will share a chorion and a placenta.

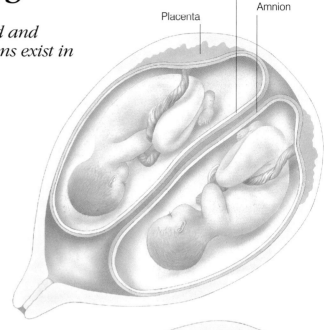

Fraternal twins

Placenta · Chorion · Amnion

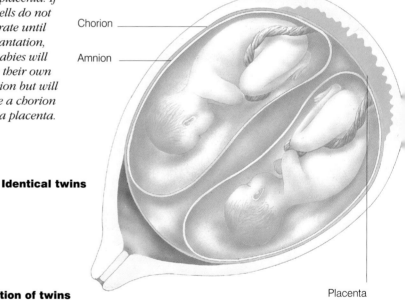

Chorion

Amnion

Identical twins

Placenta

Position of twins

By the end of most twin pregnancies, the first twin to be born is lying vertically, either head or bottom first.

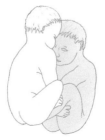

Breech and breech

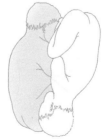

Vertex and breech

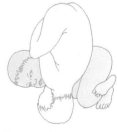

Vertex and transverse

case, a caesarean may be necessary. This can be done under epidural if the problem shows up in advance on an ultrasound scan; if it is discovered at the last minute, a general anaesthetic may be administered.

YOUR LABOUR

There are likely to be more people present at a twin birth: two or three midwives, a doctor, an anaesthetist and two paediatricians – one for each baby. The babies will be monitored separately throughout.

The first stage of your labour may be about the same length as that of a woman having only one baby. The extra pressure on the uterus may make the cervix efface more quickly, but neither baby may be in an ideal position to stimulate strong contractions, thereby prolonging dilatation.

The second stage in a vaginal delivery proceeds normally to the birth of the first baby, whose cord is clamped and cut. Attention will then shift to the second baby. If his heartbeat is normal and he is either vertex or breech, your doctor will wait for contractions to start again. (If he is transverse, he will be turned from the outside to bring his head or legs in line with the cervix.)

If any problems arise, the second baby's membranes may be ruptured, or drugs may be given to stimulate contractions (see pp. 168–69). Because the cervix is fully dilated and the birth canal has been stretched by the first baby, most second babies arrive naturally within 20 minutes of their siblings. If events slow down, your second twin may be helped out with forceps.

Breast-feeding your babies

Your body is capable of making as much milk as a baby needs, and, with twice as much stimulation as a mother of only one baby, your breasts will produce enough milk for your twins. Apart from the great benefits you are giving them, breast-feeding your babies – which you can't hand over to someone else – forces you to sit down for periods of the day.

You may need help teaching your babies to take the breast well (see pp. 206–207) and plenty of support from your partner and others around you (a mother who has successfully breast-fed twins may be the ideal helper; contact your local multiple-births association).

You will have to decide whether to feed the babies separately or together and, if together, experiment with ways to make yourself and both babies comfortable. Twins tend to differ in their feeding habits, just as any other two babies might, and coordinating feeding to keep them both happy is not always easy. One may be hungry and crying while the other is asleep and not interested. In this case, you can find that you spend almost all day – and most of the night – feeding.

If you feed them together, it is a good idea to have someone who can sit with you to help. One baby may need help latching on again, and a helper can take the first baby to finish from you, wind him and either settle him to sleep or keep him occupied while the second baby finishes.

Some mothers keep one breast for each baby so that the supply is individually tailored to their babies; others alternate them. Alternating may help at the beginning so that you always produce enough milk to satisfy the hungrier baby; once feeding is well established, it is less necessary.

In time, with support, lots of encouragement and belief in yourself, breast-feeding will become less difficult and a great deal easier than making up the necessary bottles of formula.

The third stage is the same as with a single baby, but with fraternal twins, there will be two placentas, which are delivered after both babies have been born.

AFTER THE BIRTH

Even if both babies are a good size and suffer no problems, you may find that they are taken to the special care unit for observation for a short time. Don't panic, but have your partner check that this is simply a precaution.

If one or both babies have to stay in special care, you will be encouraged to see them, touch them and hold them as soon as you have recovered from the birth. If they are too small to feed from breast or bottle, you may be encouraged to express milk that can be fed to them a drop or two at a time.

If the twins are premature, one baby may go home while the other stays in hospital. This can be physically and emotionally draining. Help is vital, especially if you are trying to express milk and visit the baby in hospital. Accept all offers of help, and realize that you and your partner can only do your best in less than ideal circumstances. There will be time to catch up on your relationship with your baby when he is home.

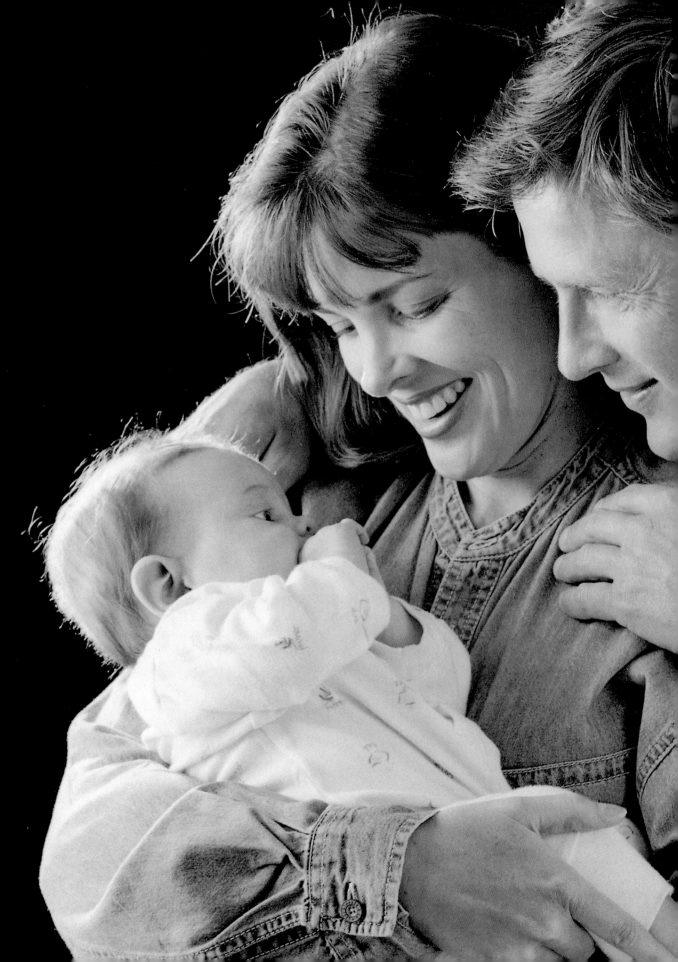

After the birth

THE WAITING IS OVER, and your baby is here. As you start to get to know her in the first few days of her life, you will probably:

- *Learn how to feed her and satisfy her most basic needs*

- *Get to know her cry and begin to interpret whether it is one of hunger or distress*

- *Introduce her to excited grandparents, thrilled siblings and family friends*

- *Watch as she is checked by doctors to make sure that all is well*

- *Begin to feel changes in your body as it starts to return to normal.*

The first few days and weeks with a newborn are exciting, if exhausting. As you and your baby get used to each other, make time to enjoy this special period in your life.

GETTING TO KNOW YOUR BABY

The hard work is over, and now you and your partner can get on with the important task of welcoming your baby into the world.

If your baby is healthy and breathing well, he is likely to be quite alert and responsive for an hour or so. Cuddle him against your skin as soon as you can. The delivery room is likely to be warm, but put a sheet or towel over him to be sure he doesn't get cold. Look at all his parts, and marvel at him. Talk to him softly – he has delicate hearing. Don't worry about what to say: the right words will come naturally.

You may receive help to get your baby latched onto your breast (see pp. 206–207). Then, if all's well, the hospital staff will leave the three of you to share these quiet, precious moments.

HOW YOUR BABY WILL LOOK

Although to you he is, of course, perfect, it is unlikely that your baby will emerge chubby-cheeked and smiling. Most newborns look nothing like the idealized image we all have of a "new" baby.

The first thing you are likely to notice is your baby's head, which will be disproportionately large (it averages a quarter of the baby's overall length). If you gave birth vaginally, your baby's head may be slightly misshapen. You may be able to feel or see ridges on the head where the bones of the baby's skull have slipped over and under one another as he descended the birth canal. If his delivery was assisted, he may have odd bumps on his head (see pp. 188–89). If you went into labour and then had a caesarean, your baby's head may still be misshapen; it won't be if the caesarean was planned. You will be able to feel the soft spot on the top of the baby's head and, perhaps, to see the pulse beating

What your baby will look like

Because newborns change so quickly, even second-time parents forget what a baby who is only minutes old looks like. If you are a first-time parent, he may not match your mental picture of a newborn.

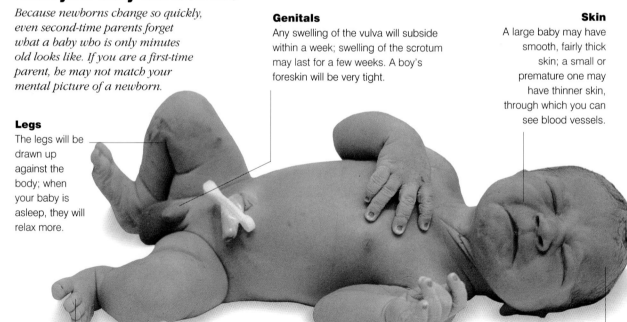

Genitals
Any swelling of the vulva will subside within a week; swelling of the scrotum may last for a few weeks. A boy's foreskin will be very tight.

Skin
A large baby may have smooth, fairly thick skin; a small or premature one may have thinner skin, through which you can see blood vessels.

Legs
The legs will be drawn up against the body; when your baby is asleep, they will relax more.

Hands and feet
Your baby's immature circulation may cause his hands and feet to remain blue or very pale for some minutes – sometimes even days – after the birth.

Head
The head may look squashed and misshapen. Any hair will be matted and may be streaked with blood (your blood, not your baby's).

there. Some babies are born with lots of hair, and others are bald; any variation between these extremes is normal.

A Caucasian baby's eyes are likely to be dark grey-blue; a darker baby will usually have brown eyes. The colour may change over the next few months. The eyelids will probably be puffy, and some babies look as if their eyes are crossed. This may be because they have difficulty focusing (see pp. 204–205) or because they can't make both eyes work together yet. The nose may be flattened, the chin receding, and the rounded cheeks bruised.

A premature baby's skin may be covered with lanugo (see p. 97), and even some full-term babies have traces of vernix on their skin. The skin of an early baby may be quite wrinkled. A postmature baby may have dry, flaky skin (use olive or almond oil as a moisturizer). Until breathing is well established (see pp. 190–91), skin tone may be patchy, and the extremities, in particular, may be pale. Skin tone may remain uneven for a few days. Your baby's neck will be all but obscured by folds of fat around the shoulders.

Just before birth, a surge of maternal hormones crosses the placenta. These can cause your baby's genitals (the scrotum in a boy and vulva in a girl) to look swollen. The breasts in both boys and girls may be swollen and may exude a milky fluid. There may be a milky or blood-tinged discharge from a girl's vagina. The legs will look spindly and the toes will be curled. The baby's fists may be clenched.

Bonding

In the same way that a duckling or gosling will follow until maturity the first object it sees (usually a parent), psychologists suggest that mothers and babies need to bond in the first few minutes after the birth in order to develop a close, loving relationship. Studies have shown that mothers find it easier to love and care for their babies if they have time to be close to the baby. Disrupting this process – unless there are sound medical reasons to do so – risks disturbing the adjustment process.

Bonding with your baby can start in the delivery room. The first few minutes of your baby's life can mark the beginning of a loving journey, launched with the wonder and relief of having your baby safe and healthy next to you. But bonding is a process, not an instantaneous happening. Holding your baby as soon as you can may help you embark on that process, but if you are tired, numbed, or shocked by the birth, if you have had a bad or distressing experience, if you have had medication, or if you are still being stitched, you may feel protective of your baby and relieved that labour is over without the overwhelming passion of maternal love.

The parent–baby relationship is not like glue. Some mothers do fall instantly in love with their babies, but many don't. If you have to be separated from your baby for a time, do not worry that all is lost and that you will never be as good a mother as you might have been. A separation doesn't mean that you can never get close, nor does the fact that you are too exhausted after the birth to pay any real attention to your baby. (Some experts, in any case, suggest that it takes about a week before your baby recognizes you, although he probably knows your smell before then.)

Give yourself time. A whole range of emotions arises during birth and afterwards. It may take a while to feel "normal" again. Intellectually, you know that this is your much-wanted baby, but emotionally you may feel that he is an over-demanding stranger. It is also normal to feel a sense of unreality or even detachment from other facets of life for a couple of days. You may suddenly experience a new intensity of feeling. Or it may be more gradual. You will warm to your son or daughter, getting closer and closer, and from there love will grow. Be reassured by the strong bonds that exist between adoptive parents and their children, and between some grandparents and their grandchildren. If it were vital to feel love from the moment of birth, such relationships would never thrive.

THE EMOTIONAL IMPACT OF BIRTH

Giving birth marks the beginning of enormous physiological, hormonal and emotional shifts in you, and great emotional changes in your partner.

Reactions to childbirth are as varied as the mothers and fathers who experience it. Whatever you and your partner feel in the first few hours and days after delivery is normal. Nothing you feel means that you will be a better or worse parent than anyone else; no reactions will surprise, shock or dismay the health team looking after you.

HOW YOU MIGHT FEEL

Your baby's arrival may take you to new heights of exhilaration and happiness. Many women describe feeling as if they were on cloud nine for the first day or so. This is probably partly due to the effects of the hormone adrenaline (see pp. 66–67), which has kept you going and is still circulating in your system. You may also feel unable to rest because you are so distracted, cuddling and feeding your baby, gazing at her for hours on end, bending over her cot to check that she is still breathing, making phone calls and receiving excited visitors. It's also common to experience a tearful day or two, often on about the third or fourth day.

The reasons for what many call "baby blues", or postnatal blues, are partly psychological. Your body is busy restoring balance after the huge event of childbirth, and you are realizing the great responsibility and changes ahead. You have had time to make your first attempts at caring for the baby, which may make you feel awkward and inept. You may sail through the first couple of breast-feeds, then find your baby can't latch on after all. From cloud nine, you come back to Earth with a jolt.

The blues may also be hormonal. The drop in progesterone that comes with the delivery of the placenta and the beginnings of the release of prolactin (the milk-producing hormone) may affect your moods. Physically, as the effects of any anaesthetics and other drugs wear off, and you have night after night of little sleep, you may be acutely conscious of bruising, soreness and stitches.

If all you need are love and understanding, tell your partner. But if you really need help (with breast-feeding, coping with afterpains, or crying), talk to the midwifery or medical staff. Now that your baby has arrived, having her with you around the clock – which you were sure you wanted – may seem like less of a good idea. If you are still in the hospital and want her to go to the nursery so you can have a break, ask. You are not failing by doing so. Pick a time after you have fed her, and ask for her to be brought to you when she next cries with hunger. Then get some rest. Don't fret that her needs won't be met: most nurseries are underused.

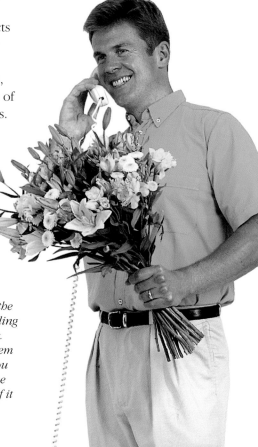

In the first couple of hours after the birth, you will probably start calling family and friends with the news. Perhaps now is the time to tell them the name you have chosen, or you may both want to try it out on the baby for a couple of days to see if it suits her.

PARTNERS: HOW YOU MAY FEEL

You are a parent – a father. The most emotionally draining – and fulfilling – day or so of your life has just ended. In the last 12 to 24 hours, you may have felt anxious, even fearful. Yet you will have felt strong at other times, and closer to your partner than you've ever felt before.

You've felt elation, pride and relief – pride in your partner, in yourself and in your new baby; and relief that it's over and that you have your longed-for baby. You may be aware that you will never be the same person, or live the same life, as you did before.

If you can't stay in hospital with your partner (such facilities are not widespread), once you have spent some time with your partner and baby, and both have settled down for a rest, you may be relieved to go home for some sleep. On the other hand, it's normal to feel a bit flat, especially if you are going home to an empty house. Your head is likely to be buzzing, and you will probably be restless and unable to concentrate on anything.

While your partner is in hospital (which may only be overnight), your routine will be dominated by visiting. Spend as much time as you can there, but be ready to cut a visit short if your partner is tired. She may still be exhilarated, or she may be somewhat weepy. Both are normal. Give her your love and support – being with you may be the only chance she has of expressing her feelings. Don't be disappointed if your baby is asleep when you get there: you have lots of time to catch up.

A Case in Point
A Friend Indeed

JOSEPH, 40, WAS EXHAUSTED AFTER HIS DAUGHTER'S BIRTH.

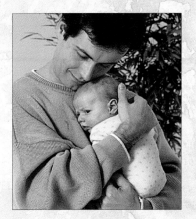

"Katie was born at 8 P.M. We had been at the hospital since early morning, and Clare had laboured at home most of the night before, so we were exhausted. I called many of our family and friends. One of them, Ben, said he'd come and get me because he felt that I shouldn't drive when I'd had so little sleep. When he arrived, he had his six-month-old son, David, on board; Ben had been trying to settle David for hours and he had finally fallen asleep on the drive over. We went back to his place, and while he put David to bed, his wife cooked an omelette for me and gave me a glass of wine. Then they made up the spare room for me. 'I'll never forget how miserable I felt the day David was born, coming home alone,' Ben said. 'Stay the night, and I'll take you back to the hospital in the morning.'

"I fell asleep immediately, but after a couple of hours I woke, knowing something amazing had happened, but not remembering quite what! Then, after three or four seconds, I realized – we had a baby. Clare and I were parents. I relaxed then and went straight back to sleep."

When you get the call to say that mother and baby can come home, make sure there's enough food for a couple of days and that the house is warm. Take some clothes for the baby if your partner didn't pack them, and include something loose-fitting for your partner to wear. Try to find something that is not part of her maternity wardrobe: she will want a change. A top with a front opening is ideal for breast-feeding. And don't forget some comfortable shoes.

WHAT YOUR BABY MAY FEEL

New babies' emotions are very basic and are linked to their powerful needs for warmth, food and security. When she cries, comfort her with gentle rocking and cuddling; when she's hungry, feed her. Remember that cold and hunger are new sensations; up to now, she has not experienced such feelings because the uterine environment met her needs perfectly. By responding as soon as she expresses her needs now, you teach her that she is safe and loved.

After the first hour or so, most babies tend to withdraw, probably because they are tired from the birth. Many babies sleep a great deal for the first couple of days and begin to take more interest in their new surroundings by day three or four.

CHECKING THE BABY

It takes a baby a few minutes to get used to life outside the womb, and your carers will be watching as he becomes accustomed to his new environment.

As soon as your baby is born, your carers assess his well-being while they are doing some routine tasks. His mouth and nose are cleared of excess mucus, and he may need to have some mucus gently sucked out of his mouth with an extractor operated by the doctor or midwife. His eyes are wiped with swabs.

THE APGAR SCORE

One or two formal assessments are made to give an Apgar score, most commonly at a minute and five minutes after the birth. In some hospitals, only one score – at two minutes – is taken.

The Apgar score is used primarily to help staff to recognize those babies who need immediate specialist care. Scores of 0, 1 or 2 are given on various aspects of the baby's appearance and health and then added up. Few babies achieve a maximum

of 10 because it takes time for the circulation of even the healthiest and most alert babies to reach all the extremities. A score of 7 is good; babies scoring 4 to 6 need help, such as suctioning of the airways and administering of oxygen; those scoring less than 4 (a rare few) need life-saving techniques (see pp. 208–209).

MEASURING THE BABY

Your baby's length, head circumference and birth weight will be recorded; these are useful baselines against which his future growth can be compared.

More than 95 percent of babies born at term weigh from 2500 g to 4250 g (5½ to 9 lb), with the average being 3400 g (7½ lb). Boys, on average, weigh 250 g (½ lb) more than girls.

Your baby's length, measured from crown to heel, will probably be between 46 and 56 cm (18 and

22 in); the average is 51 cm (20 in). His head circumference will be between 33 and 37 cm (13 and 14½ in); the average is 35 cm (13¾ in).

Your baby's mouth will be examined to check for cleft palate (usually a finger is put into the mouth to feel for this).

The doctor will listen to your baby's heart. Some heart disorders are indicated by the irregularity of the heartbeat or by the sound of the blood going in and out of the chambers of the heart. Heart murmurs are very common – as many as 50 percent of all babies have them in the first week. Within a few weeks, most are not heard anymore.

In most hospitals, vitamin K is given shortly after birth either orally or by injection to prevent a rare disease called haemorrhagic disease of the newborn, in which the blood fails to clot. Not everyone agrees that it is necessary. Ask your doctor his or her opinion.

Apgar scores

Sign	Score		
	2	1	0
Appearance, or colour	Pink (for a white baby); brown (for a black baby)	Pale or blue extremities	Pale or blue all over
Pulse, or heartbeat	Over 100 per minute	Less than 100	Not discernible
Grimace, or response to stimulation	Strong cry	Makes a face	No response
Activity, or muscle tone	Moves strongly	Limbs are flexed	Limbs are weak and floppy
Respiration, or breathing	Strong	Slow, or irregular	Absent

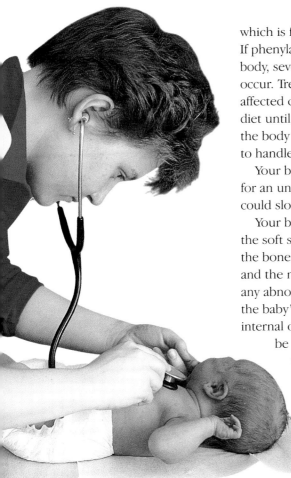

A baby's heart beats around 120 times a minute. As the paediatrician measures the heartbeat, she or he will also feel the chest to check that the lungs are expanding as they should.

which is found in many proteins. If phenylalanine builds up in the body, severe brain damage can occur. Treatment involves placing affected children on a restricted diet until puberty, by which time the body has acquired the ability to handle the amino acid.

Your baby will also be tested for an underactive thyroid, which could slow brain development.

Your baby's doctor will check the soft spots on the baby's skull, the bones of the arms and legs, and the neck and shoulders for any abnormalities, and will feel the baby's abdomen to check his internal organs. The genitals will be examined to make sure there is no sign of hernia. The doctor will pay particular attention to the hip joint to check for "clicky hip". He or she will manipulate each hip joint to check that the head of the femur (thigh bone) moves well within its socket and that it does not slip out. If it is dislocated – it slips out easily – or unstable, which

means that it is liable to become dislocated later, treatment involves using a splint or plaster to hold the femur in place as the baby grows.

You may notice after a couple of days that your baby's skin has a yellow tinge. In the early days of life, the liver does not always function well. As a result, bilirubin – one of the products of the breakdown of red blood cells in the liver – may spill into the bloodstream and build up there. This usually clears up after the fourth day, but if it persists, a blood sample will be taken to check the level of bilirubin. If levels continue to rise, the baby will be given phototherapy – treatment with ultraviolet light.

Your baby's heart will be listened to again before you leave the hospital and every time he has a check-up, at least until school age. This is a precautionary measure in case an abnormality has been missed and because some heart disorders become apparent only when the baby is older. Most problems can be treated if caught early.

LATER CHECKS

In the first week of your baby's life, several more checks will be made on his health.

A sample of blood will be taken by pricking his heel. The blood will be tested for phenylalanine, high levels of which indicate PKU (phenylketonuria), a very rare metabolic disorder that affects 1 in 15,000 babies.

PKU is an inability to metabolize the amino acid phenylalanine,

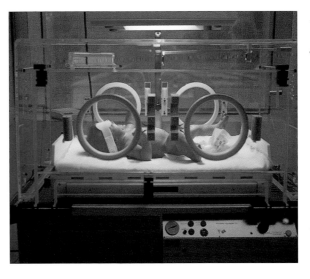

Phototherapy treatment for jaundice alters bilirubin so that it can bypass the liver and be excreted by the kidneys instead. The majority of babies sleep through this treatment. Bilirubin lights can also be prescribed for home use.

WHAT YOUR BABY CAN DO

She may seem helpless as she lies in her cot, but your baby is born with all the skills she needs to ensure her survival.

You need only watch, cuddle and talk to your new baby to appreciate how aware and responsive she is from the beginning. Your baby needs your help to develop her senses, but so many of her early reflexes and responses are guaranteed to capture your attention that a true synchrony will soon develop between your baby's needs and your reactions.

YOUR BABY'S SENSES

Newborn babies find it hard to focus on objects more than about 30 cm (12 in) away from their eyes, so your face is clear when you breast-feed, but a picture on the wall behind you is not. Her eyes will follow your face if you hold her up to your face and then turn your head, but her vision will not be fully developed until she is between three and six months old. Some newborns are very sensitive to light for a few days as they adjust from the semi-darkness of the womb, but most soon become acclimatized.

She can hear, and loud noises will make her jump. She seems to respond best to soft, high voices and to the sound of your heartbeat, which was the clearest sound she was aware of in the womb. If your baby seems miserable, she may respond to your holding her over your left shoulder, where she will feel the familiar rhythm of your heart-beat. It isn't necessary to tiptoe

around a baby for fear of waking her, or to try to get other members of the household to be especially quiet. Babies quickly become accustomed to normal household sounds and many are soothed by them. But it is important that no one makes a loud noise next to the baby's delicate ears or plays loud music that could damage them. If you can't talk comfortably over music, it's too loud. Turn it down.

Touch is your baby's most basic sense. The skin is the largest sensory organ, developed from the same part of the embryo as the nervous system six weeks after conception. Your baby will

Your baby will mimic a facial gesture within an hour of birth. Get her attention and make a face, several times if necessary, and she will make the same face back at you. Babies also quickly learn to watch your lips as you talk to them.

respond to your touch and be soothed by it, either through patting, rocking or massage.

YOUR BABY'S REFLEXES

A reflex is an involuntary action in response to a stimulus, and it is estimated that a baby has about 75 reflexes in the first few months of life. Some of these remain throughout life (blinking when a foreign body approaches the eye, for example); others disappear after a few weeks or months as the baby's nervous system develops and she begins to coordinate thought and action.

If you touch your baby's palm or place an object in it, she will grasp it tightly and hang on. Similarly, if you touch the sole of her foot, she will curl her toes as if she were searching for something to grasp.

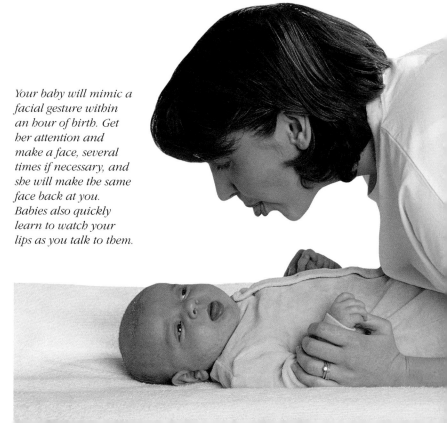

Rooting, sucking and swallowing

Your baby comes into the world with three very important reflexes that help her to feed. She roots when you touch her cheek gently, she turns her head to the side you touched and opens her mouth, looking for your nipple or something else to suck. If you stroke her on her upper lip, she opens her mouth, her lips start to move, and her tongue comes forward in a licking movement. You can sometimes see this reflex, which lasts several weeks, as you cuddle your baby: she tries to latch on to whatever is nearest to her mouth. If you have trouble getting your baby latched onto your breast, you may find it helpful to use this reflex.

The companion reflex to rooting is sucking. Once something is placed in your baby's mouth, she will suck on it strongly. You can feel this if you place your little finger in her mouth: put it in with the underside against her palate, and you will feel the pull as she puts her tongue up against it and creates a powerful vacuum.

When you breast-feed your baby (see pp. 206–207), she opens her mouth to make way for the breast. The nipple is taken far back into her mouth, and her tongue holds it in. Then she compresses the nipple and the breast tissue, squeezing milk from the ducts. The swallow reflex takes the milk down the oesophagus. Although the swallow reflex is present from birth, it takes most babies some time to learn how to coordinate swallowing and breathing. Don't worry if your baby splutters occasionally when she feeds, especially if your breasts are full: she is breathing and swallowing more than once a second, so some practice at coordination is essential.

These three coordinated reflexes aren't fully developed until about 32 weeks of pregnancy, which is one reason very premature babies find it hard or even impossible to feed.

The rooting, sucking and swallowing reflexes seem to be quite marked in some new babies in the hour or so after birth, which is why it's always worth offering the breast this early. Most babies aren't actually hungry at this point, and many don't really get a big appetite for a few days.

The Moro, or "startle", reflex is seen if you support your baby on your hand and forearm, and use your other hand to support her head. When she is relaxed, lower the hand beneath her head. She will fling out her arms and legs and throw back her head, then return to a normal position. She will also exhibit this response if a loud noise startles her.

You will witness the stepping reflex if you hold your baby in a "standing" position facing away from you on a firm surface, such as a table, with both hands around her chest. One knee bends and the foot extends, as if she were taking a step; her body and head tend to straighten at the same time. This reflex is hard to elicit after a few days.

The crossed extension reflex is seen when you stimulate the sole of one foot. The baby draws her leg away (flexing her toes, as in the grasp reflex) and then bends the other leg. Then she stretches her leg once more. If you stroke the sole of her foot, she will exhibit the Babinski reflex: her big toe will extend upwards, and her other toes will spread out. This reflex disappears at about the age of two, after which it is normal to curl all the toes in.

If you stroke your baby's back, following the line of her spine, she will curve her back. This is the trunk-incurvation reflex.

At this stage, too, urinating and defecating are reflex actions and remain so for more than a year, when they start to become increasingly voluntary.

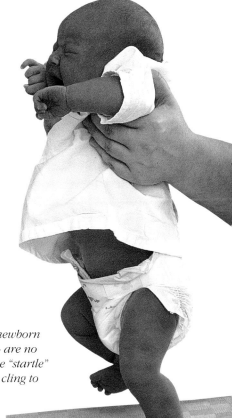

It is estimated that there are about 75 newborn reflexes, most of which – like stepping – are no more than curiosities. Some, such as the "startle" reflex, may be a search for someone to cling to for safety.

FEEDING YOUR BABY

For most babies, breast is best, but if you would rather not breast-feed your baby for any reason, bottle-feeding can give him a good start, too.

Breast milk supplies all your baby's food and drink needs for the first four to six months of life. It contains antibodies that boost the baby's immune response, so breast-fed babies tend to suffer fewer illnesses, gastrointestinal disorders and allergies. It may also lower the incidence of chronic childhood diseases such as diabetes. Breast milk is always of a high quality nutritionally and adapts perfectly to your baby's needs. Because it is easier for your baby to digest than formula, breast-fed babies are rarely constipated. And there appears to be a lower incidence of cot-death among breast-fed babies.

Breast-feeding is cheap and convenient: breast milk is always available. Above all else, breast-feeding your baby creates an unbreakable intimacy between you. It is the ultimate experience of bonding.

Breast-feeding is good for you, too. The hormones released when you breast-feed help your uterus to contract to its pre-pregnant size. And it burns kilojoules, so you will lose the weight you gained in pregnancy more quickly.

HOW TO BREAST-FEED

Breast-feeding is natural, but many mothers and babies have to learn to do it. You may need skilled help in positioning your baby in a way that doesn't hurt your nipples. Hold your baby chest to chest with you so that he doesn't have to turn his head or flex or extend his neck to take your breast. When his

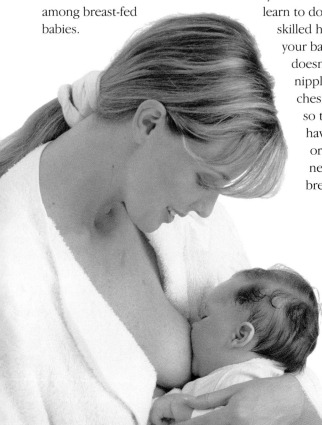

Breast milk is the ideal food for your baby, always the right temperature and drawing from your bloodstream the nutrients he needs. Breast milk even becomes more watery in hot weather.

mouth is wide open – as wide as a yawn – bring him gently onto your breast so he gets a good mouthful of areola. This is called latching on. If he has the breast properly, his bottom lip will be curled outwards, there will be more of your areola showing above his top lip than below his bottom lip, and he will create a vacuum with his tongue.

Avoid stuffing your nipple in or pushing his head on, and don't try to shape your nipple with your fingers. Any of these actions could make your baby grab only the nipple, which can lead to sore and cracked nipples and ineffective feeding. If you have inverted nipples, you may need extra patience and help to get your baby well latched on.

The baby's suck and the removal of milk from the breasts stimulate hormonal responses that tell your body to make more milk (see pp. 66–67). In fact, the more you feed, the more milk you make, which is why mothers of twins make twice as much milk. In addition, effective breast-feeding stimulates the let-down reflex, which pushes the milk stored inside the breasts down into the ducts and out through the exit points on the nipples.

Unrestricted, or "demand", feeding works better for most mothers and babies than scheduled feeding. Allowing your baby to establish the timing, length and frequency of feeds means that the right amount of milk is produced. Later on, when breast-feeding is established (after about six weeks), you will

Bottle-feeding

Some women choose to bottle-feed from the start; others switch to it later because they have problems with breast-feeding or they prefer the convenience of formula to expressed breast milk. Bottle-feeding allows your baby's father to take over some of the feeds from the start.

If you know that you do not want to breast-feed, no one should put pressure on you to do so. But if you are genuinely undecided, start breast-feeding and see how you manage. You can always switch to bottle-feeding later, but it takes a lot of support to switch to breast-feeding if you change your mind after a couple of weeks of bottle-feeding. (If you are taking medication, check with your doctor if you want to breast-feed; do not assume that medication means you must bottle-feed.)

Always use a baby formula (most are based on cow's milk, modified to suit a tiny baby's digestive system) and make sure that everything you use is scrupulously clean. Ready-to-use formula is convenient, especially when you are out, but it is expensive to use all the time; most parents use powdered formula, mixed with previously boiled water.

Making up a day's bottles at once saves time. Follow the manufacturer's instructions on quantity exactly. Put the stipulated amount of water in the bottles, then add the formula, levelling off the top of the scoop with a knife. Put the top on the bottles and shake thoroughly to dissolve the powder. If you are not giving the feed immediately, store it in the fridge and warm it before giving it to your baby by placing it in a bowl of hot water. Do not warm it in the microwave, since the heat-through is uneven and hot spots could scald your baby's mouth.

Check the temperature by shaking a drop on the inside of your wrist. You can keep reconstituted formula in the fridge for 24 hours.

---

probably find that your baby wants feeding in a more scheduled way. But in the early days and weeks, frequent feeds – 6 to 12 feeds in 24 hours – are normal.

In the first couple of days after the birth, your baby's sucking will give him colostrum, a mixture of water, protein and sugar that is rich in antibodies. Your milk will "come in" between days two and five, and you will feel when this has happened: your breasts will be full and heavy.

Colostrum is yellowish in colour; mature milk has a bluer tinge than cow's milk.

GETTING HELP

Many women do have minor problems with breast-feeding in the early days. It can be upsetting to find breast-feeding difficult. If you are still in hospital, ask for help there; if you are back at home, talk to the community midwife – she will call daily for 10 days – or contact a counsellor from one of the support organizations (see pp. 218–19) for encouragement. Almost all problems are surmountable with the right help.

Sore or cracked nipples are usually caused by incorrect positioning; a counsellor can show you how to position the baby and help you to treat your nipples. A baby who seems dissatisfied may not be getting enough milk; again, this may be a positioning problem – he has only the nipple in his mouth. Or, especially if he is small and sleepy, he may not be feeding enough to guarantee that you have a good supply. You may be advised to feed more often or express milk to keep your supply plentiful.

EXPRESSING YOUR MILK

Expressing is a useful skill to learn because it allows you to leave expressed breast milk (EBM) for your baby to be given by someone else. Wait until you and your baby are confident about breast-feeding before you give him a bottle. After six weeks or so, taking a bottle (which he sucks in a different way from the breast) should not confuse his sucking. EBM keeps in the refrigerator for 24 hours and in the freezer for three months.

If you express by hand, you may need practice to get it going. Choose a time when your breasts are naturally close to their fullest but you are at least an hour or more away from a feed; wash your hands and relax. Raise your breast with the flat of your hand, massage around it, stroking down towards the nipple and back towards your breastbone. Work around the breast with your fingers and thumb, but don't pull or squeeze the nipple. Once the milk starts to flow, catch it in a sterilized bowl.

You can also express milk from your breasts with a pump (manual or electrical), which works by creating a vacuum to draw the milk out. Follow the instructions supplied with the pump.

BABIES IN SPECIAL CARE

Hospitals are equipped with special cots in which your baby will receive the warmth, oxygen and nourishment she needs to mature.

If at birth your baby needs special care, she will be taken to the neonatal intensive care unit immediately. Depending on your condition, you and your partner may be able to go, too. This can be a confusing and distressing time, because the medical staff will act fast, often without consulting you, in order to get your baby the care she needs without delay. As soon as things calm down, ask for an explanation of the problem and how long your baby may need care. One in seven babies spends some time in special care, the majority for a couple of hours, some overnight. Most are there as a precautionary measure only.

WHY BABIES NEED CARE

Your baby may need special or intensive care if healthcare staff have to observe her closely (if she became distressed during the birth, for example); if she needs help with breathing; if she needs to be at a constant temperature; or if she needs continuous or frequent medication.

Most babies who spend longer than a couple of hours in special care are sick or premature. A small baby – one who weighs less than 2.5 kg (5½ lb) – will often be admitted to the intensive care unit. These babies are usually premature, born before or about week 36 of pregnancy, or suffering from intra-uterine growth retardation (IUGR) – that

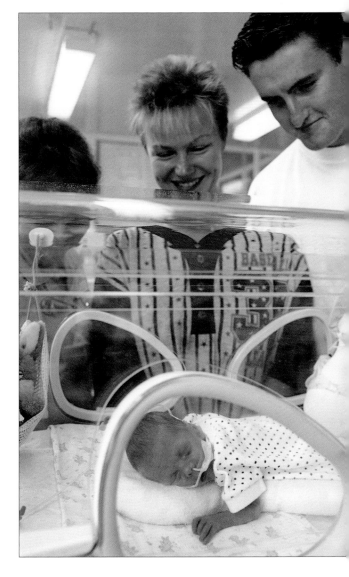

Ask staff to explain each of the machines to you. Some of them are not actually doing anything "to" your baby but simply measuring her responses and functions, such as her body temperature, heartrate and blood pressure.

is, they are considerably smaller than average for their gestational age. Placental insufficiency, which starves a baby of adequate food and oxygen, so that she suffers from IUGR, can be caused by maternal smoking or substance abuse, and by medical conditions of the mother such as raised blood pressure or kidney disease. Such a baby is more likely than others to suffer from respiratory problems, have trouble feeding, or be prone to jaundice, infection or hypothermia; but an average-size term baby suffering from any of these problems will also be admitted to the special care unit.

Babies born with congenital abnormalities that threaten their health will also be admitted to special care, as will those who have undergone surgery.

GETTING TO KNOW YOUR BABY

It can be hard to get used to loving a newborn if she is in an incubator much of the time, with electrodes and tubes attached to her tiny body. If your baby is very sick, or very premature, you may even be afraid to become too close to her emotionally, in case she doesn't survive. But getting close to her may in fact increase her chances of survival. Studies show that babies who are regularly stroked and touched put on weight more quickly than those who are not, so hold her whenever you can, even if it is only for short periods. Touching her, stroking her and talking to her are therapeutic. When you can take her out of the incubator, hold her as close to you as possible, with plenty of skin-to-skin contact. You may be able to carry her in a little pouch next to your chest so that she can feel and hear your heartbeat. If you find that you are holding back from loving your baby, ask the medical staff to give you an honest appraisal of her chances; more than 75 percent of babies who weighed only 1 kg (2 lb) at birth survive.

Intravenous feeding is necessary for babies whose gastrointestinal systems are too immature to digest breast milk or formula or who are too immature to suck (usually those born before 32 weeks). If your baby is too small or weak to breast-feed, you may be able to express your milk for her to take from a cup or, more usually, through a feeding tube passed up the nose and down into the stomach. (Expressing milk also establishes your supply so that you will be able to breast-feed your baby once she is stronger.) There will be an electric breast pump in the hospital that you can use.

Mother's milk is especially valuable for premature babies, since its antibodies help the baby fight infection. You may not get much milk at first, but tiny babies need tiny amounts. Your baby's doctor may want to know precisely how much your baby is getting, and he or she may advise supplements of premature-baby formula in addition to breast milk.

TAKING YOUR BABY HOME

Your baby will be allowed to go home as soon as she is strong enough to do well without medical intervention around the clock. If she has been in the hospital for any length of time, you may feel nervous about your ability to care for her, but be assured that she would not be allowed to come home if the doctor had any doubts about her ability to thrive. Your doctor or midwife will be available if you are worried at any time, and your baby is likely to do best in her family environment. Aim to keep the household calm and quiet for the first few days while you get used to each other.

She may still be small, and she may need special treatment for her routine care at home. You may be told to make sure the house is always warm and to feed her every three hours, or more frequently, whether she wakes or not. Small babies sleep a great deal but cannot be allowed to go for long without feeding if they are to maintain steady growth.

Your baby will change as she gets stronger. You may become used to having a sleepy baby for several weeks – and then be surprised when she starts to be more wakeful and demanding, to cry for more frequent feeding and to stay on the breast longer. These are the signs that your baby is doing all the things a newborn does after the first few days.

When will my baby catch up?

Once their small or premature baby is out of immediate danger, many parents want to know how long it will take for her to reach the same milestones as other babies of the same age. In trying to estimate when your baby will acquire a particular skill, work from her due date rather than her actual birth date, and for at least the first year, add a little to that. A baby who was two months premature, for example, may have at 14 to 15 months skills similar to those of a term baby around her first birthday.

Everything about your premature baby is in miniature, and all her organs are immature. She may need time for feeding to become established before she even begins to grow.

As long as your baby is well fed, cared for and loved, she will reach developmental milestones in exactly the same way that other children do – at her own pace.

YOUR FIRST DAYS AT HOME

While you are busy adapting to the demands of your newborn, your body is slowly beginning to return to its pre-pregnant state.

It takes time to fit your home life around your baby's needs, while making sure that your needs and those of the rest of the family are also met. Don't expect to have a smooth-running household immediately. If you can arrange it, have help around the clock for at least the first week. Don't aim to do anything but look after yourself and the baby – childbirth is demanding, physically and mentally, and you need time to recover.

GETTING SOME REST
If you are breast-feeding, you are unlikely to get more than four hours sleep in one stretch. Some parents find that they can sleep when their baby is asleep, perhaps in the afternoon or early evening, and catch up in that way. For many, however, sleeping during the day feels too odd.

Rest is a priority. Switch on your answering machine – or unplug the phone – and go to bed. You can take your baby into bed with you if he is not asleep or if he needs feeding. If he's restless and needs a loving pair of arms or the comfort of a pram ride, ask a helper to take him. If you don't want to go to bed, put your feet up and read a book or magazine. Don't worry about what else you should be doing. You will function far better if you take this time for yourself.

COPING WITH VISITORS
It is understandable that family and friends are eager to see the baby, and you, of course, are anxious to show him off to them. But whether they are there for an hour or a week, don't feel you have to entertain them – they can make their own coffee or meals,

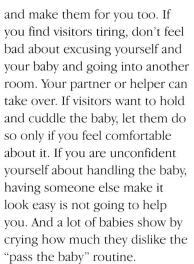

and make them for you too. If you find visitors tiring, don't feel bad about excusing yourself and your baby and going into another room. Your partner or helper can take over. If visitors want to hold and cuddle the baby, let them do so only if you feel comfortable about it. If you are unconfident yourself about handling the baby, having someone else make it look easy is not going to help you. And a lot of babies show by crying how much they dislike the "pass the baby" routine.

Similarly, while you and your baby are getting used to breast-feeding, you may be happier in another room. Mothers who have breast-fed, while happy to offer advice and encouragement, may make you feel a little inadequate (if it's so easy, why am I having trouble?). Those who did not breast-feed may ask why you are persevering when a bottle would be so much easier.

WHAT IS HAPPENING TO YOUR BODY
After the birth your stomach will look a little saggy and soft for a while, and you won't be able to get into your tighter clothes for at least a couple of months (probably longer). Although you have lost the weight of the baby, placenta and amniotic fluid, your muscles have stretched.

Breast-feeding and exercise will eventually restore your pre-pregnancy contours. You do not need to "diet" (dieting could, in fact, compromise your milk supply). Simply eat healthily and normally.

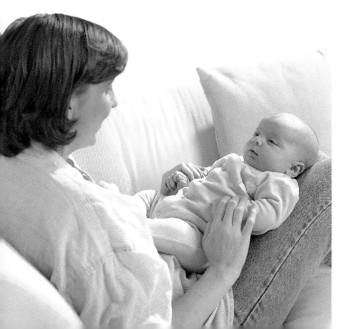

Your baby's waking hours are likely to be dominated by feeding at first, but while he is awake and not hungry, take time to sit with him. This time is important for you – you are resting – as well as for him. "Chatting" to him helps you to get to know each other.

Your uterus continues to contract in the days after birth as it returns to its pre-pregnancy size. The contractions are termed afterpains and may be more acute when you breast-feed. If you find that they are really uncomfortable, ask your doctor to recommend painkillers, but tell him or her if you are breast-feeding so those prescribed are safe for your baby.

Your breasts will get bigger when your milk comes in (see pp. 206–207) as a result of the increase in milk, blood and lymph in the breast tissue. Some women find they remain larger for several weeks, then start to get smaller. This does not mean you have stopped producing enough milk; it just means that the supply-and-demand mechanism of milk production has settled down, and you make more of the milk while your baby actually feeds.

Vaginal discharge after childbirth is called lochia and is a mix of blood and tissue from the inside of the uterus. At first it's bright red. It then changes to pinkish brown, then to greenish and finally cream. It's quite heavy at first, and you will need several changes of sanitary pads a day (don't use tampons because you risk introducing infection into the vagina). After the first week, the discharge will slow down, but you may find that it lasts several weeks before finally disappearing. Get medical advice if you start to lose a lot of fresh blood once the flow has slowed down, or if you pass any large clots after the first few days.

If you are sore from stitches, follow the advice on pages 186–87.

Postnatal exercise

It is never too early to start postnatal exercises, although they may be the last thing on your mind. The most important are pelvic-floor exercises (see pp. 44–45), and you should start as soon after the birth as you can. Not only will they pay dividends later, reducing the possibility of lasting stress incontinence while toning the vagina to make sexual intercourse more pleasurable, but they will also help alleviate pain in the perineum.

After a few more days (wait for your doctor's okay if you had a caesarean), add abdominal exercises to close the gap between the muscles of your abdomen.

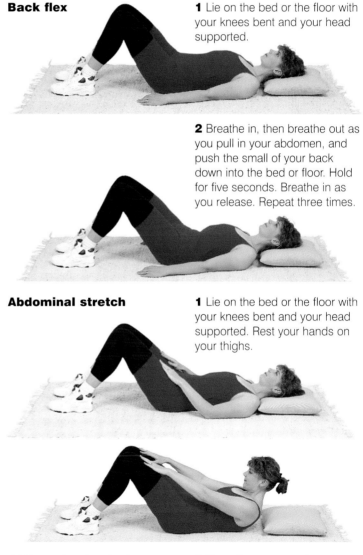

Back flex

1 Lie on the bed or the floor with your knees bent and your head supported.

2 Breathe in, then breathe out as you pull in your abdomen, and push the small of your back down into the bed or floor. Hold for five seconds. Breathe in as you release. Repeat three times.

Abdominal stretch

1 Lie on the bed or the floor with your knees bent and your head supported. Rest your hands on your thighs.

2 Lift your head and point your hands towards your knees. When you can feel the stretch in your abdomen, hold for five seconds, then relax.

3 From the same starting position, point your hands as close to the floor on your left as you can. Repeat, pointing to your right. Repeat the whole sequence three times.

AT HOME WITH YOUR BABY

The first few days at home with a newborn can be exhausting, but as you learn to care for your baby's needs, these days are also tremendously exciting.

Don't worry if your baby has a couple of days of restless crying when you first come home. This is very common – it may be a sign that he is aware in some way of the change in his environment. Do not try to get a new baby into a routine: what happens in the first few days or weeks will not set the pattern for the rest of his babyhood. Each day will be different when your baby is still new, in terms both of behaviour and of frequency and length of feeds. The best thing you can do is respond to his needs and be flexible.

SLEEPING AND WAKING
New babies sleep for at least some of the time between feeds, and they usually have their longest sleep at night. In total, a newborn normally sleeps between 12 and 18 hours of every 24. It's also normal for a newborn to wake up hungry a couple of times during the night (babies have small stomachs, and most simply can't take in enough to last for more than two or three hours at a time).

Your baby can sleep anywhere there's a firm, comfortable surface that is clean, out of draughts, and not too hot or cold. If you use a cot, put your baby's feet near the foot of the cot (so he can't wriggle under the bedclothes and overheat), and lay him on his back. Keep bedding lightweight, and don't

use duvets or pillows for a baby under a year old. He can sleep in a cot next to your bed for easy night feeding. Check that your baby is not too hot when he's sleeping by feeling his chest and neck. He should feel pleasantly warm, not hot or clammy.

If your baby does not want to sleep between feeds, he may not be tired, so play with him for a while, talk to him, or carry him in a front-pack sling while you do something else.

If he is crying or you sense that he is tired, you can soothe him in a variety of ways. Offer him the breast again – he could still be hungry. A bottle-

fed baby may also need more formula, or a drink of cooled, boiled water. Let him fall asleep in your arms first before putting him in his cot, but make sure he is fast asleep before you put him down (his body will be completely limp once he has relaxed into a deep sleep). You might rock him as you hold him against your shoulder, or pat his back rhythmically. This will release any wind that may be trapped in his stomach and make him more comfortable. You could also try whispering or singing

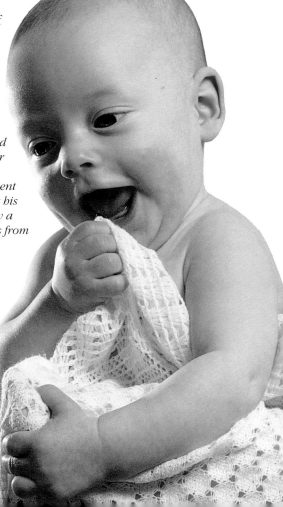

As your baby begins to spend more time awake, watch for his changing expressions. Although there is disagreement about when you can expect his first smile, most babies show a variety of facial expressions from the first few days onward.

My baby won't stop crying

Crying is the only way your baby can tell you that all is not right with his world. As he gets older, you will become more adept at working out what's causing his crying, and as he becomes more settled and "at home" in the world, he will probably cry less. But in the beginning, the best way to deal with his crying is simply to respond. Go to your baby, pick him up, and try to find the probable cause.

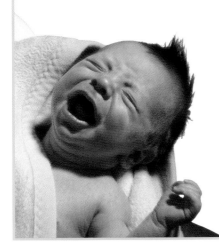

Hungry
This is the most obvious reason for crying. You may think you have only just fed your baby, but an hour or more could have elapsed, so offer the breast or bottle. He won't take what he doesn't want in the first few days.

Uncomfortable
He may be wet or soiled or both. Check his nappy and change him if necessary. Make sure the nappy is not too tight and that a pin is not sticking into him, or a tape is not stuck to his skin (mistakes that all parents of newborns make). Check that his clothes are not chafing his delicate skin. He may have trapped wind, so pat or rub his back.

Bored
He may simply need a change of scene or a change of arms. If he is lying in a cot without a view, put him in a baby chair; if he's restless in his chair, pick him up and take him for a walk around the room.

Sing a song to him (or get an older child to do this instead).

Overstimulated
When you have too many visitors passing the baby around among them, he can become upset. If the house is full, take him to a quiet corner while he calms down; if there is no quiet corner, take him outdoors for a while.

Tired
Follow the advice on getting your baby to sleep (see opposite page).

You are not spoiling your baby by responding to his cries. Babies cry for a reason, even if that reason is no more specific than just being slightly out of sorts. Make him confident that when he is hungry, he will be fed, and when he cries, he will be hugged and comforted.

You certainly can't teach your baby to be "good" by regularly letting him cry himself to sleep.

---

softly to him. If all else fails, movement may work: take him for a car ride (safely strapped into an infant car seat, as described on pages 136–37), or push him back and forth in a pram.

HOW TO DRESS YOUR BABY
A winter baby needs the same layers of clothing that you wear, plus one more layer (bedding or clothing) when you are outdoors. Just be careful not to overheat your baby, and when you bring him indoors, remember to take off the extra bedding and clothing.

For a baby born in the summer, keep bedding and clothing light. Cotton or cotton-blend fabrics are cooler than synthetics. On the warmest days, all your baby needs is a nappy and a cotton singlet. Never put your baby in direct sunlight. Use the sunshade on the stroller or pram to keep your baby shaded at all times.

If you didn't get everything ready in time, don't panic; a newborn's needs are basic. Send someone shopping for these supplies, which will last a couple of days, until you can make a more detailed list (see pp. 136–39).

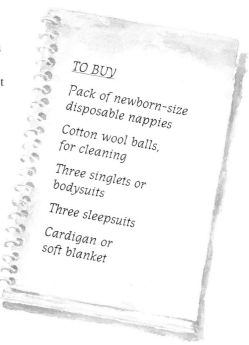

TO BUY

Pack of newborn-size disposable nappies

Cotton wool balls, for cleaning

Three singlets or bodysuits

Three sleepsuits

Cardigan or soft blanket

POSTNATAL DEPRESSION

After the overwhelming high of childbirth, most new mothers come back down to earth and their emotions normalize; a few have longer-lasting problems.

It is normal to suffer from "baby blues", to feel weepy, anxious or unhappy, or to veer precipitously between elation and depression in the first few days after the birth. Sleep deprivation and the drop in levels of oestrogen and progesterone that occurs after childbirth are usually responsible for these swings, and once your hormones stabilize, so does your mood. It is estimated, however, that 10 percent of new mothers experience more serious postnatal depression. Many more – perhaps half – go through spells of lacking confidence and feeling lonely, isolated and exhausted.

Postnatal depression is an illness, not a sign of inadequacy or self-indulgence. A mother who suffers from the disorder may be a good mother who cares for her baby's physical needs well. There may be nothing to indicate to outsiders her sadness and the turmoil going on inside her head. But they are there all the same.

SIGNS AND SYMPTOMS

Many of the signs of postnatal depression are common in new mothers, but if you have several of them, or if your ability to cope seems to be diminishing rather than improving as time goes on, seek help.

Sufferers often "lose" several hours of the day. You may look at the clock and wonder where the past two hours went. You may wake up in the morning feeling

A Case in Point
Beating Depression

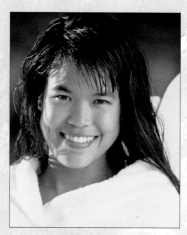

AMY, 30, WAS LONGING TO BE A MOTHER.

"We'd been married six years, while my partner David got his career together, before we started a family. Then he lost his job just before Victoria's birth. I breast-fed for only a month before I rushed back to work. David was a wonderful father, but I could see that he wasn't taking care of Victoria as I would have. It seemed so unfair that he was having it all, when I'd waited so long to be a mother. I felt shut out of their relationship, was working long hours to make ends meet, and didn't realize that my tiredness and disconnection from them both were part of an illness.

"The crunch came one weekend when my sister and her toddler were visiting. David was out, and my niece, Charlotte, fell off a rocking horse she was playing on. She wasn't hurt, but I went into hysterics, screaming that I'd nearly killed my niece, how could I possibly care for a baby, and I was a useless mother. My sister took the kids to another room, then called our doctor. I was still crying an hour later when David came home. The doctor and my sister took me to the hospital.

"I was a patient for six weeks and had Victoria with me for long visits for some of the time. I talked to a psychotherapist every day. He helped me to see what was obvious in retrospect: being the breadwinner did not make me less adequate as a mother. Like other parents, David and I had to do what was best in less than ideal circumstances; and Victoria wouldn't know that I wanted to do more, but she would love me for who I was. It didn't matter who took care of her, I would always be her mum.

"I slowed down when I returned to work, and, fortunately, David found a job a couple of months later. I was able to take up full-time motherhood again. Victoria seemed to suffer no ill effects from the shaky start to our relationship, but I sometimes wonder what would have happened if my sister hadn't been around."

that you have had no sleep at all. Tiredness is, of course, common, but exhaustion and listlessness – when even the simplest task, such as getting up to make a cup of coffee, seems daunting – may be a sign of depression.

You may realize that you don't smile or laugh much. New parenthood is full of amusing incidents (a nappy stuck on back to front, dinner at midnight), but you cannot see the humour in them. You may cry or feel tearful for no reason or for a trivial one.

Feelings that you don't deserve your baby or that you will never be able to care for her are common among sufferers of postnatal depression. So, too, is feeling numb, as if experiences don't touch you. The only person with whom you feel yourself may be your partner, and sometimes perhaps not even with him.

WHO IS AFFECTED?

Anyone can be affected by depression, but some women are more prone to it than others.

The illness is less common in societies in which there is a good support network of people who help a new mother with her baby. In Western societies, a new mother may feel friendless, as social contacts are hard to keep up and harder to make. Those who are alone or who have unsupportive partners are high on the list of sufferers. So, too, are those with a previous history of psychological problems.

Women who have unhappy memories of childhood, who were deprived or neglected, or whose relationship with their own parents is not a good one tend to suffer more, as do those

---

Postnatal psychosis

Postnatal psychosis, sometimes called puerperal psychosis, is a mental disorder that affects perhaps one or two women in every thousand. It usually starts just after the birth, and may worsen during the subsequent days and weeks. It is characterized by delusions, hallucinations, a personality change, and bizarre and perhaps compulsive or obsessive behaviour. You may wish you had never had the baby or wish she were gone. Some sufferers even contemplate suicide. All are obviously very ill to those around them.

Postnatal psychosis may require in-patient hospital treatment, and it can take a few months. Most women who suffer with depression make a full recovery. They are, however, at an increased risk of its happening again after a second birth.

---

who have had "disappointing" experiences with birth, which then become the focus of all the feelings of inadequacy ("if I hadn't had a caesarean, I would be able to deal with my baby's crying", for example).

Finally, problems that other women are able to handle – painful stitches, a demanding baby, sleepless nights, still not being able to get into regular clothes – tip some women over the edge.

GETTING HELP

If you think you are suffering from depression, get help. This is important for you, of course, but also for your baby. Mothers who suffer may not be able to respond to their babies' social cues, and the normal verbal and non-verbal playing and interaction between mother and baby is lessened. This may have longer-term effects on the way these babies develop and learn.

If you get nowhere with your doctor – even today, some only provide anti-depressants rather than tackle the cause of depression – persist, or get your partner to persist on your behalf.

Your partner's support is vital at this time. You may want to take him to the doctor with you, so that he can help you when you describe symptoms and give an account of any progress you make. He can remind you of advice the doctor gives you, too – sometimes depressed people don't take in everything that's said to them. Facing this illness together can speed your recovery.

Ask for help with the housework and with the baby. In order to sleep better when the baby allows, take a walk each day (take the baby in the stroller or pram). If you can, get some exercise. Some gyms have crèches, or you may be able to find a friend who can watch the baby for an hour or so. Make a bath or shower a priority. The better you look, the better you will feel. Contact a support group for women who have felt what you feel and have come through it.

Your doctor may check your thyroid if he or she thinks the cause of your depression is hormonal. Anti-depressants may be useful in the short term. Hospital admission is a last resort.

RECORDING THE FIRST FEW DAYS

When you bring your baby home, you may believe that every detail of his early weeks will be imprinted on your memory forever. But it is easy to forget.

Regardless of how busy they are caring for their baby and how exhausted they may feel as a result, almost all new parents find time to keep a record of the birth of their baby, perhaps the most momentous occasion in their life. Keeping memories of your baby's birth and early days can be fun.

You may also find that you want to write an account of your labour and the birth, as a way to make sense of what can be an overwhelming experience.

TAKING PHOTOGRAPHS

A photographic record of your baby helps you to retain memories of these early weeks and to keep track of the

fascinating ways in which the baby grows and changes.

Immediately after the birth, pictures are likely to be taken under fluorescent light, which will give a green cast to colour film. Use a filter to get a more natural result. Some automatic cameras focus on the first object the lens senses, so if your baby is in an incubator or you are shooting into the hospital nursery, take this into account. An image of mother, baby and the midwife who delivered the baby is a good memento.

Photographing your baby around the same time every day in the first week or so will record almost imperceptible changes. Try to take pictures of your child in similar poses with a similar

background to make an attractive sequence in an album or a frame.

You will probably be given photo albums, and it is worth arranging your photos in them as they are developed. Make sure you date each set of prints. (Some cameras record this information on the film.)

The risk exists of damaging your baby's eyes with flash photography, although the risk is small (babies, like adults, blink reflexively when a bright light shines in their eyes). Try to use natural light whenever possible; it will give a softer edge, and it avoids the possibility of eyestrain for your baby. If natural light is not available, and your camera allows, bounce the flash off a surface away from your baby's face. Remember, too, that a contented sleeping baby makes a beautiful study and eliminates any problems created by a flash.

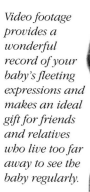

Video footage provides a wonderful record of your baby's fleeting expressions and makes an ideal gift for friends and relatives who live too far away to see the baby regularly.

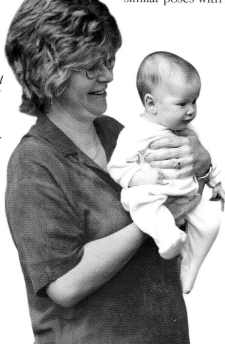

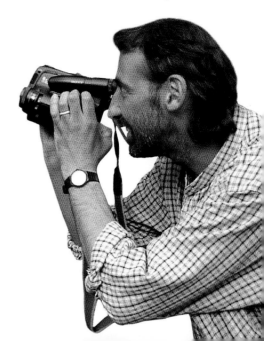

Photograph your baby doing everyday things – feeding, sleeping, showing interest in his hands – and bring out the camera on special occasions or for set-up poses, too. Photograph your baby with a soft toy such as a teddy bear or a rag doll throughout his first year and into toddlerhood. Looking back at the sequence, you will see the growth of your baby – he will appear tiny at first beside the teddy and then gradually outgrow it.

For more formal parent-and-baby portraits, consider using black and white film, which gives lovely, soft results. It is also a good way to look for family resemblances: ask your parents for shots they have of you as a baby. Keep such poses simple.

OTHER RECORDS

Fill-in baby books, which allow you to record "Baby's first smile", "Baby's first tooth" and other details throughout the first year or more, are popular gifts. If you receive one, take the time to complete it – your baby will love it when he is older. If you find this limiting – many parents do not want to be restricted to special happenings – buy a book and keep your own diary. Include such things as what the baby is wearing, how long he sleeps, how many feeds he has, what the weather is like, as well as milestones in his development.

Tape recordings of your baby are fascinating mementos, and good gifts for family and friends who live far away. Record your baby's first gurgles, his cry as he wakes from a sleep, his first babbles and – later – his laughter and attempts at words.

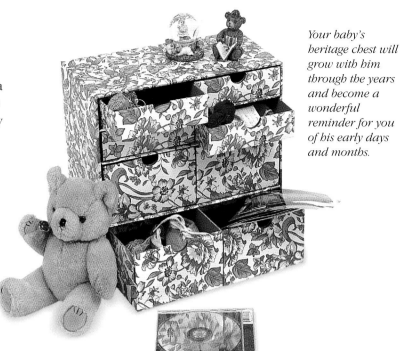

Your baby's heritage chest will grow with him through the years and become a wonderful reminder for you of his early days and months.

A HERITAGE CHEST

Serving as a collection of mementos of your baby's life, a heritage chest starts filling up as soon as you come home. An old shoebox is ideal for the first few items; later, a larger box may be necessary.

From the hospital, keep your baby's name tags and wrist and ankle identification bands, as well as the umbilical cord clamp and the cork from the bottle of champagne with which you toasted his arrival. Ask someone to buy a newspaper from the day of your baby's birth and keep it in pristine condition. If you like popular music, buy a copy of that week's number one single. Fashion magazines or other publications that show current life and times make fascinating memorabilia as well.

Take a foot print and a hand print of your baby (press his foot and hand against an ink pad and then against a piece of cardboard) and a snip of his hair, if he has any. Add a lock of hair when he has his first "real" haircut later.

Keep a day-by-day diary during the first week, complete it with photographs, and file it in the heritage chest. Your birth announcement published in the newspaper should be included, as should the cards you receive congratulating you on the birth. Pressed flowers from the bouquets you may have received make good additions, too.

As your baby grows, add his first shoes, any special clothes you thought made him look particularly appealing (or a photograph of him wearing them), and drawings and scribbles he made during his pre-school years. Once he starts school, certificates are worth keeping, as, of course, is his first lost baby tooth.

By the time a child is about six or seven years old and has some sense of "past", you can bring out the chest and continue building memories together.

USEFUL ADDRESSES

Acupuncture Association of Australia
5 Albion Street
Harris Park, NSW 2150
Tel: (02) 9633 9187

AGSA (Association of Genetic
  Support Australasia)
66 Albion Street
Surry Hills, NSW 2010
Tel: (02) 9211 1462
An umbrella organization providing
advice and information for
individuals and support groups
related to rare genetic disorders.

Al-Anon Family Groups
GPO Box 1002H
Melbourne, Vic 3001
Tel: (03) 9629 8327

Alexander Technique
PO Box 3020
Wellington, New Zealand
Tel: 473 5543

Alexander Technique International
11 Stanley Street
Darlinghurst, NSW 2010
Tel: (02) 9331 7563

Asthma Australia
Tel: 1800 645 130

Australian Association of Yoga in
  Daily Life
102 Booth Street
Annandale, NSW 2038
Tel: (02) 9518 7788

Australian College of Midwives Inc.
Suite 23, 431 St Kilda Road
Melbourne, Vic 3004
Tel: (03) 9804 5071

Australian Council for Rehabilitation
  of the Disabled
33 Thesiger Court
Deakin, ACT 2605
Tel: (02) 6281 2433
An umbrella organization which can
refer parents to appropriate
organizations dealing with child
disabilities or illnesses such as
deafness and blindness.

Australian Cystic Fibrosis Association
PO Box 254
North Ryde, NSW 2113
Tel: 1800 635 008

Australian Physiotherapy Association
Level 3, 201 Fitzroy Street
St Kilda, Vic 3182
Tel: (03) 9534 9400

Australian Society of Independent
  Midwives
77 Albert Drive
Killara, NSW 2071
Tel: (02) 9416 7289

Australian Society of Teachers of the
  Alexander Technique
PO Box 716
Darlinghurst, NSW 2010
Tel: 1800 339 571; Melbourne:
(03) 9853 1356

Australasian College of Natural
  Therapies
57–61 Foveaux Street
Surry Hills, NSW 2010
Tel: (02) 9211 7744

Australian Traditional Medicine
  Society
27 Bank Street
Meadowbank, NSW 2114
Tel: (02) 9809 6800
Provides a contact point for
alternative medical practitioners.

Centacare Pregnancy Counselling
  Service
PO Box 112
Curtin, ACT 2605
Tel: (02) 6281 1087;
fax: (02) 6281 1225
Refers callers to their nearest
counselling service.

Diabetes Australia
5–7 Phipps Place
Deakin, ACT 2600
Tel: (02) 6285 3277;
fax: (02) 6285 3703

Down Syndrome Association
31 O'Connell Street
Parramatta, NSW 2150
Tel: (02) 9683 4333

Drug & Alcohol Counselling Service
ACT tel: (02) 6205 4545
NSW tel: 1800 422 599
NT tel: 1800 629 683
Qld tel: 1800 177 833
SA tel: 13 13 40
Tas tel: 1800 811 994
Vic tel: 1800 136 385
WA tel: 1800 198 024

Endometriosis Association Victoria
37 Andrew Crescent
South Croydon, Vic 3136
Tel: (03) 9870 0536;
fax: (03) 9870 3007
Offers a national telephone
information and support service, as
well as operating a clinic in
Melbourne.

Family Planning Australia Inc.
9/114 Maitland Street
Hackett, ACT 2602
Tel: (02) 6230 5255;
fax: (02) 6230 5344

HIV Health Info Line
Tel: 1800 803 806

Homebirth Australia
PO Box 3198
Hamilton Delivery Centre, NSW 2303
Tel: (02) 4961 1626; (041) 929 4033

International Yoga Teachers'
  Association
34 Yaralla Crescent
Thornleigh, NSW 2120
Tel: (02) 9484 9848

Maternity Alliance
PO Box 789
Artarmon, NSW 2064
Tel: (02) 4961 1626; (041) 929 4033
An organization representing a wide
spectrum of groups dealing with
pregnancy and parenthood; provides
an information and referral service.

MBF Private Access
Tel: 13 1137
Provides a 24-hour national infant care helpline for members, staffed by midwives and nurses, with referrals to support groups and counsellors.

National Epilepsy Association of
Australia
Unit 2B, 44–46 Oxford Street
Epping, NSW 2121
Tel: (02) 9869 8444

NALAG (National Association of Loss
and Grief)
PO Box 79
Turramurra, NSW 2074
Tel: (02) 9988 3376
Support line: (02) 9489 6644

National SIDS Council of Australia
891 Burke Road
Camberwell, Vic 3124
Tel: (03) 9813 3099

Nursing Mothers Association of
Australia
1818/1822 Malvern Road
East Malvern, Vic 3145
Tel: (03) 9885 0855;
fax: (03) 9885 0866

Parentline
NSW/ACT tel: 13 2055
Qld tel: 1300 301 300
SA tel: 1300 364 100
Vic tel: 1800 134 883
WA tel: (08) 9272 1466
Provides a 24-hour telephone advice service for parents on any parenting issue.

Pen-Parents of Australia
PO Box 574
Belconnen, ACT 2616
A correspondence network of parents who have experienced pregnancy loss or the death of an infant.

Reducing the risk of SIDS Info Line
Tel: 190 229 1122

SANDS (Stillbirth And Neonatal
Death Support)
ACT: PO Box 450
Woden, ACT 2606
Tel: (02) 6244 2372
NSW: Block 4, RNS Hospital
St Leonards, NSW 2065
Tel: (02) 9906 7004
Qld: PO Box 49
Royal Brisbane Hospital, Qld 4029
Tel: (07) 3252 2865
SA: PO Box 308
Park Holme, SA 5043
Tel: (08) 8277 0304
Tas: PO Box 786
Rosny Park, Tas 7015
Tel: (03) 6344 6811
Vic: PO Box 302
Chelsea, Vic 3196
Tel: (03) 9773 0221
WA: Room G9, Agnes Walsh House
Bagot Road, Subiaco, WA 6008
Tel: (09) 382 2687
A parent-based organization which offers support to those who have experienced miscarriage, stillbirth, or neonatal or infant death.

Smokers Quitline
Tel: 13 1848

The Australian Multiple Birth
Association
PO Box 105
Coogee, NSW 2034
Tel: (02) 9875 2404

There are a number of other organizations which provide assistance and support but do not have a national referring body and operate separately in each state and territory. These can be contacted through your local telephone directory, and include Parents without Partners; Child Minding and Child-Care Centres; and Child Deaf and Blind organizations.

INDEX

ACKNOWLEDGMENTS

t=top; b=bottom; c=center; l=left; r=right

1 Laurence Monneret/Tony Stone Images; 2 Chris Harvey/Tony Stone Images; 3 Laurence Monneret/Tony Stone Images; 4t Matthew Ward, 4b Laura Wickenden, 5t Laura Wickenden; 5c Frans Rombout/Bubbles; 5b Laura Wickenden; 6 Andy Cox/Tony Stone Images; 7 Robert Harding Picture Library; 8 The Stock Market; 9 Susanna Price/Bubbles; 10–11 Laura Wickenden; 13 D. Oullette, Publiphoto Diffusion/Science Photo Library; 14 Jacqui Farrow/Bubbles; 15 Laura Wickenden; 16t Warren Morgan/Robert Harding Picture Library, 16b Matthew Ward; 17 Mattthew Ward; 18l CNRI/Science Photo Library; 18r Dr Tony Brain/Science Photo Library, 19l James Stevenson/Science Photo Library; 19c James Stevenson/Science Photo Library; 19r The Stock Market; 20t Marc Henrie; 20b The Stock Market; 21 Robert Kristofik/The Image Bank; 23t Sandra Lousada/Collections; 23b Laura Wickenden; 24–25 Jo Foord; 29 Stewart Cohen/Tony Stone Images; 31l John Greim/Science Photo Library; 31 Keith/Custom Medical Stock Photo/Science Photo Library; 32 Jennie Woodcock/Bubbles; 33 Hank Morgan/Science Photo Library; 34–35 Laura Wickenden; 36–37 Peter Myers; 38 Sterling K. Claren, Prof. of Pediatric Dept., University of Washington School of Medicine; 39 Loisjoy Thurston/Bubbles; 40-49 Laura Wickenden; 50 Anthea Sieveking/Collections; 52-53 Laura Wickenden; 50 Bubbles; 56–64 Laura Wickenden; 65 Emap Elan; 66 Matthew Ward; 67 The Image Bank; 68–70 Laura Wickenden; 72–75 F. Rombout/Bubbles; 76–79 Laura Wickenden; 80 Pauline Cutler/Bubbles; 81 Holy Name Hospital, New Jersey; 82 Laura Wickenden; 83 Petit Format/Nestle/Science Photo Library; 84–85 Laura Wickenden; 86 John P. Kelly/The Image Bank; 87t Laura Wickenden; 87 Loisjoy Thurston/Bubbles; 88–89 Gary Bistram/The Image Bank; 92 Laura Wickenden; 93 Jennie Woodcock/Bubbles; 94–95 Laura Wickenden; 96 Laura Wickenden; 97 Petit Format/Nestle/Science Photo Library; 98 Angela Hampton/Bubbles; 101 Howard Sochurek/The Stock Market; 102 Laura Wickenden; 103 Petit Format/Nestle/Science Photo Library; 104–106 Laura Wickenden; 108 Emap Elan; 109–111 Laura Wickenden; 113 Chris Harvey/Tony Stone Images; 114–116 Laura Wickenden; 117 Anthea Sieveking/Collections; 118 David de Lossy/The Image Bank; 119 Jennie Woodcock/Bubbles; 120t Nancy Durrell McKenna/Hutchison Library; 120tc Fiona Pragoff/Collections; 120bc Tony Stone Images; 120b Nick Oakes/Collections; 122 Anthea Sieveking/Collections; 123 Don Wood/Robert Harding Picture Library; 125t Sandra Lousada/Collections; 125b Laura Wickenden; 126 Lupe Cunha/Bubbles; 127 J. Croyle/Custom Medical Stock Photo/Science Photo Library; 128–130 Laura Wickenden; 132 Jennie Woodcock/Bubbles; 134 Laura Wickenden; 136t Andrew Sydenham; 136 Elizabeth Whiting Associates; 137–140 Laura Wickenden; 142 Jennie Woodcock/Bubbles; 144 Laurence Monneret/Tony Stone Images; 145t Laura Wickenden; 145b Jennie Woodcock/Bubbles; 146 Frans Rombout/Bubbles; 148–152 Laura Wickenden; 155 Robert Harding Picture Library; 156–158 Laura Wickenden; 159 Bruce Ayres/Tony Stone Images; 160–167 Laura Wickenden; 168 Laurence Monneret/Tony Stone Images; 170 Laura Wickenden; 173 Andy Cox/Tony Stone Images; 175 Jeremy Beckett/Bubbles; 176 Tim Brown/Tony Stone Images; 179 Ron Sutherland/Science Photo Library; 181 Jennie Woodcock/Bubbles; 184–185 Laura Wickenden; 192 Petit Format/Bubbles; 193 Michelle Edelmann/Bubbles; 196–197 Laura Wickenden; 198 Frans Rombout/Bubbles; 199 The Stock Market; 200 Laura Wickenden; 201 Robert Harding Picture Library; 203t Ian West/Bubbles; 203b Frans Rombout/Bubbles; 204 Laura Wickenden; 205 Jennie Woodcook/Bubbles; 206 Chris Harvey/Tony Stone Images; 208 Robert Harding Picture Library; 210–211 Laura Wickenden; 212 Susanna Price/Bubbles; 213 Frans Rombout/Bubbles; 214 Mark Lewis/Tony Stone Images; 216 Jennie Woodcock/Bubbles; 217 Laura Wickenden

All illustrations were produced by Mick Saunders